THE APHASIA THERAPY FILE

The Aphasia Therapy File

Volume 2

edited by

Sally Byng
Chief Executive, Connect—the Communication Disability Network

Judith Duchan
Emeritus Professor, State University of New York at Buffalo

Carole Pound
Director of Innovation, Connect—the Communication Disability Network

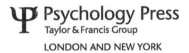

Psychology Press
Taylor & Francis Group

LONDON AND NEW YORK

First published 2007
by Psychology Press

Published 2014 by Psychology Press
27 Church Road, Hove, East Sussex BN3 2FA, UK

Simultaneously published in the USA and Canada
by Psychology Press
711 Third Avenue, New York, NY 10017

First issued in paperback 2014

Psychology Press is an imprint of the Taylor & Francis Group, an informa business

Copyright © 2007 Psychology Press

Typeset in Times by RefineCatch Limited, Bungay, Suffolk

British Library Cataloguing in Publication Data
A catalogue record for this book is available from the British Library

Library of Congress Control Number: 2000361735

ISBN 978-1-84169-270-8 (hbk)
ISBN 978-1-13800-605-8 (pbk)

Contents

List of Contributors

Wendy Best
Department of Human Communication Science
University College London
Gower Street
London WC1E 6BT

Sally Byng
Connect—the Communication Disability
Network
16–18 Marshalsea Road
London SE1 1HL

Deborah Cairns
Department of Language and Communication
Science
City University London
Northampton Square
London EC1V 0HB

Liz Clark
Speech and Language Therapy Department
Barts and the London NHS Trust
Royal London Hospital
2nd Floor
Outpatients Department
Stepney Way
London E1 1BB

Judy Duchan
130 Jewett Parkway
Buffalo
NY 14214
USA

Claire Gatehouse
Speech and Language Therapy Service
Plymouth Primary Care Trust
Building One
Brest Road
Plymouth
Devon PL6 5QZ

Debbie Graham
Department of Speech and Language Therapy
Burnley Pendle and Rossendale PCT
31–33 Kenyon Road
Lomeshaye Estate
Nelson
Burnley
Lancashire BB9 5SZ

Ruth Herbert
Department of Human Communication Sciences
University of Sheffield
Western Bank
Sheffield S10 2TN

Julie Hickin
Division of Speech and Language Therapy
De Montfort University
The Gateway
Leicester LE1 9BH

Fiona Hinshelwood
Speech and Language Therapist
Northumberland Care Trust
Merley Croft

Loansdean
Morpeth
Northumberland
NE16 2DL

Simon Horton
School of Allied Health Professions
University of East Anglia
Norwich NR4 7TJ

David Howard
Department of Speech
University of Newcastle
Newcastle upon Tyne NE1 7RU

Jayne Lindsay
19 Townley Road
London SE22 8SR

Jane Marshall
Department of Language and
Communication Science
City University London
Northampton Square
London EC1V 0HB

Sally McVicker
Connect—the Communication Disability
Network
16–18 Marshalsea Road
London SE1 1HL

Ann Montagu
Speech and Language Therapy Department
St Mary's NHS Trust
Praed Street
London W2 1NY

Felicity Osborne—deceased

Lisa Perkins
Department of Speech and Language Therapy
Jersey Health and Social Services
Overdale Hospital
William Knott Centre
Westmount Road
St Helier
Jersey JE1 3UH
Channel Islands

Carole Pound
Connect—the Communication Disability
Network
16–18 Marshalsea Road
London SE1 1HL

Jo Robson
c/o Jane Marshall
Department of Language and Communication
Science
City University London
Northampton Square
London EC1V 0HB

Carole Sacchett
Department of Human Communication
Science
University College London
Gower Street
London WC1E 6BT

Sam Simpson
14 Michelham Gardens
Strawberry Hill
Twickenham
Middlesex
TW1 4SB

Alex Stirling
Speech and Language Therapy Department
Aintree Hospitals Trust
Lower Lane
Liverpool L9 7AL

Janet Webster
Speech and Language Sciences
University of Newcastle
Newcastle upon Tyne NE1 7RU

Anne Whitworth
Speech and Language Sciences
University of Newcastle
Newcastle upon Tyne NE1 7RU

Leonie Winstanley
Occupational Therapist
North Herts & Stevenage NHS Primary
Care Trust
Solutions House
Dunhams Lane
Letchworth SG6 1BE

Acknowledgments

We thank our patient authors, who waited so long for their words to be published, Kate Swinburn and Jayne Lindsay for their work on a first draft of this manuscript, and the British Aphasiology Society for organising the therapy symposia at which the chapters in this book were first presented and which have provided such fertile ground for thinking about aphasia therapy in the UK.

ABOUT THE EDITORS

Sally Byng and Carole Pound are the co-founders of Connect and continue to work for Connect as Chief Executive and Director of Innovation respectively. Judy Duchan has been providing consultancy to Connect since it was founded in 2000. Connect is a national charity in the UK working collaboratively to promote effective services, new opportunities and a better quality of life for people living with aphasia.

the communication disability network

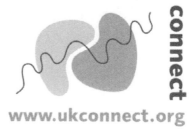

www.ukconnect.org

Introduction: Describing therapies for aphasia

Sally Byng and Judith Duchan

This book is about different ways of thinking about, describing, and carrying out aphasia therapy. The authors present one or more of their clinical practices in order to share their therapy experiences and reasoning with others. The book's aim is to provide aphasia therapy practitioners with new therapy resources and to challenge them to reflect on their own therapy decisions, processes, and successes.

This is the second volume to grow out of the aphasia therapy symposia organised by the British Aphasiology Society. This has been a biennial event at which speech and language therapists/pathologists, clinical linguists, and psychologists from across the UK and beyond come together to discuss in detail their experiences of doing therapy with people with aphasia. Feedback on the first volume of *The Aphasia Therapy File* (Byng, Swinburn, & Pound, 2001) was positive. Many felt it served to fill a gap in the therapy

literature, providing them with a forum for presentation of discussion to which both therapists and students could relate.

The papers here are slightly different from those published in the first volume. The first volume of *The Aphasia Therapy File* set out to provide a forum for the people who actually do the therapy, the therapists as opposed to the people who more generally get the opportunity to write, reflect, and talk about it, that is, academic researchers/therapists. This second volume has a slightly different authorship: More of the chapters represent collaborations between people in clinical practice and those working in academic practice. As a result some, but not all, of the chapters are closer to research papers than were those in the first volume. While different in format, this volume is like the first in that it is written with a spirit of exploration and with the intent of tackling difficult clinical issues. For these reasons the chapters vary considerably, reflecting to some extent the personal styles of the authors, as in the first volume.

ABOUT THE CHAPTERS IN THIS VOLUME

Below is a brief synopsis of each of the chapters in this volume. Together they offer readers a vivid sense of how aphasia therapies and their descriptions differ depending upon the clinician, the client, the framework that clinicians work in, and the chosen writing styles. The final chapter, Chapter 15, offers a way to examine the commonalities across the chapters, despite their differences, and a way to uncover some of the rationales the authors used to select their therapies. The synopses are presented in alphabetical order by the first author. This ordering is deliberate, even though it has the effect of separating chapters that address similar issues. We are keen not to categorise these therapies because we are concerned that the literature on aphasia therapy is littered with descriptions, and polarisations, of "approaches". Rather, we want the reader to take each therapy at face value for addressing the issues it seeks to address, rather than labelling it as being an example of a type of approach. We deal with this issue in further detail in Chapter 15.

The synopses provided in this chapter are intended to guide the reader to identify which chapters may address similar issues; these issues may be tackled using different methods of therapy. The commonalities and differences between the issues addressed are summarised at the end of this chapter.

Deborah Cairns' therapy with Tony (Chapter 2)
Deborah Cairns' story of her therapy encounter with Tony conveys how powerfully someone can communicate without language. So often therapists struggle to persuade people with aphasia to be prepared to use multimodal means of communication, and yet in Tony's case it seems that

the initiative came from him. Deborah describes how she and the students working with Tony had almost to run to keep up with Tony's clarity about what he was trying to get out of therapy. She conveys how Tony seemed to know just what he wanted—the job of the therapist was to figure that out and respond creatively to it.

The contribution of the therapy group comes across powerfully. Tony uses the group context effectively both to understand the impact of his communication on other people, and also to regain some of his identity by playing a leading role in the group—a role that was familiar to him prior to his stroke. How Tony's therapy would have developed without the opportunity to work in a group is hard to imagine.

Tony's story also conveys how communication strengths can turn out to cause barriers that have to be overcome. Tony's familiarity with communicating across language barriers seems to serve him well in being prepared to use all the means of communication at his disposal. And yet, the intrusion of one language upon another also causes both him and his interlocutors frustration as they try to pick out and follow Tony's meaning. His enthusiastic commitment to therapy could also prove to be overwhelming. His impatience to move on and yet his absorption in some aspects of the process sometimes made the therapists feel that he had lost sight of the practicalities and rationale of the therapy. However, through this process he also conveyed clearly his own rationale, which was different from that of the therapists.

The dynamic nature of goal setting with people with aphasia is revealed in this story. In the process of working towards one goal—in this case, developing a communication book—a different more subtle goal is revealed; that of creating a personal portfolio for Tony to convey who he is and his own story. This goal was set in a context in which (a) the therapist did not consider that a communication book could be used to help form an identity and (b) Tony had difficulty conveying what he really wanted out of therapy. The eventual outcome grew out of the ongoing interaction between the therapist and the person with aphasia.

Tony's experience of bilingualism offers opportunities to use his second language as an alternative means of communication, but creates its own difficulties. The "therapy" related to his bilingualism, which aimed to investigate the conditions under which one language intruded upon another, led to further communication breakdowns. Deborah Cairns described this therapy with inverted commas around the term "therapy". That is because there wasn't any therapy as we usually think of it. Rather it was "an opportunity to consider his own language in a more experimental spirit".

This spirit of experimentation corresponds well with the experience of many therapists, who report that people's aphasia changes during the process of assessment or exploration (hence the need for a category called "checks" in the framework described in Chapter 15, to account for the exploratory nature of some therapies). It seems that some people with aphasia can use that process for themselves as an opportunity to understand what is happening with their changed language—to see what happens when they try different tasks in different structured contexts. The therapist's role is to set up the appropriate range of structured contexts and then perhaps to provide explanations about *why* they have done *what* they have. It appears in Tony's case that this process in and of itself was sufficient to enable him to gain enough information about what he was doing linguistically to change aspects of his language behaviour.

Deborah Cairns' chapter offers a number of ways to consider a therapist's role, but a principal one might be as a developer of contexts in which people can do their own changing. That is, the therapist does not have to set up repeated practice exercises for the person to engage in. Rather she created the conditions to enable Tony to use those contexts to find what he wanted. She has done this by communicating in a group, enabling the group to develop its own topics, and through provision of models. Throughout, she has responded to his choices and reactions, through careful listening and attention to how Tony reacts and responds.

The therapy summarised in the framework (see Chapter 15) illustrates how some of the negotiation around the communication book was achieved, but more centrally, the summary shows how the whole therapy process really represents the creation of the conditions for therapy to take place, enabling Tony to make his own choices and to use the materials to develop the therapy as he wished to achieve his own ends.

Claire Gatehouse and Liz Clark's therapy with WL (Chapter 3)

The enormity of the impact of aphasia upon someone's life is underlined again in WL's story from Claire Gatehouse and Liz Clark. The list of positive factors and difficulties facing WL is daunting (see a summary in Table 15.3, Chapter 15). Yet this is the reality of aphasia for people who live with it. This story reveals the wide array of areas of work to be undertaken by the speech and language therapists trying to deal with that impact. The story chronicles the thinking of the two therapists principally concerned with providing therapy for WL's aphasia, and in so doing it also reveals the exclusion and isolation faced by people with aphasia.

Where do you begin when everything in someone's world has changed overnight? Gatehouse and Clark's chapter illustrates the pragmatic solution reached to deal with the small amount of time available to offer to WL. Therapy was carefully devised as language-focused tasks that could be done at home. However, this is not without its challenges—especially given the stigma of aphasia, which became apparent for LW as time went on. What must it feel like to work on language tasks at home, when the people around you do not understand what aphasia is and when the only other experience of doing this type of task is school-based?

The dilemma of managing it all—of trying to conduct well-controlled therapy, to monitor the effects of what you are doing, to see the impact of one aspect of language processing on another when you have one session available a week to see someone in an acute care setting and do not have the luxury of time to collect data, is well illustrated here. The therapist's frustrations are palpable. The difficulty of teasing out whether the effects are due to spontaneous recovery or therapy is enormous.

This is frustrating for a therapist wishing to understand the specific effects of the therapy or to illustrate the contribution of therapy to theoretical knowledge about language processing. This desire to know the impact of one's efforts is even greater in the professional atmosphere, where one is asked to provide evidence for the effectiveness of one's therapy. In situations where there is lack of service (presumably because of assumptions made by others about its relative effectiveness compared to other services), the pressure to prove the relevance and impact of your service feels all the more critical.

The story of WL's therapy includes how some of the social barriers that WL was facing were addressed through action by the therapist. The framework description (see Chapter 15, Table 15.3) reveals the different nature of the therapist's role in this type of therapy—involving negotiation, interpretation between people, explanation, preparation, and planning, to involve a much wider set of agencies. This role was carried out in a different setting, still involving just one session a week. However, the way that the session was used was very different—not necessarily involving face-to-face contact with the person with aphasia. This is very often the sticking point: Therapists are sometimes under pressure to monitor direct contact time with individual "cases". The results achieved by using therapy time flexibly, for interpreting, explaining, and negotiating, speak for themselves.

The long-term nature of the service WL required, the sense that issues revealed themselves over time, and that you cannot rush someone's coping process, are all important lessons from WL's therapy. One size doesn't fit all either: WL decided that counselling wasn't for him, and there is a clear sense that a lot more water has to go under the bridge with WL before he would be ready to develop a portfolio as Tony did in the previous chapter.

Debbie Graham's therapy with KB (Chapter 4)
Debbie Graham's chapter is written from the perspective of someone working in a busy rehabilitation setting, but who was able at that time to provide long-term and intensive rehabilitation—

something few clinicians are able to do these days. This short report from a clinician in practice reflects the real-life imperative of needing to get on with therapy, with the urgency that acute stroke and aphasia bring. Debbie conveys clearly how, in practice, therapists are often guided by their own implicit theory of the priorities to address through therapy. For most therapists the reality is that there is neither the time nor the appropriate resources and materials to do thorough, theoretically motivated and well-controlled assessment, let alone before and after evaluations, to demonstrate "scientific" evidence for change through therapy.

This chapter reflects KB's need to regain the use of, and control over, his language that he had before his aphasia struck, given its importance to his identity. This challenged Debbie Graham to keep up with his changing language and to continue, in turn, to challenge KB. The report captures the pressures and complexities of working with people whom professionals might see as having only relatively "mild" aphasia, in the same way that we often construe the complexities that people with more "severe" aphasia offer.

The therapist's familiar dilemma—whether to focus on repairing language, on developing strategies to circumvent difficulties, or on facilitating the gaining of confidence to use newly emerging language and communication skills in real-life contexts—is also clearly drawn. This author spells out the decisions she took, but also opens up the questions for others to consider.

Julie Hickin et al.'s therapy with HM and PH (Chapter 5)
The complex impact of changes to communication is again illustrated in Julie Hickin et al.'s work with HM and PH. This chapter describes a controlled experiment to compare and explore the effects of providing therapy in different ways. Opportunities to use specific words in a range of structured communication activities provided a context for two people with aphasia to see if they could regain ability to use the names of the learned words, and to see what the carryover effects were. Would they be able to use the words they learned in a highly structured task in conversation and

would they be able to find more words generally as a result of this therapy?

Both people showed positive changes in their ability to use the names learned after each of the therapies. Predictably, however, they showed different patterns of change following the two therapies, with one person appearing to make more gains after the first therapy than the other person, and only one of them making gains in finding names not learned in the therapy.

Interestingly, the person who made most gains from the two therapies was HM. The summary in the framework (see Chapter 15, Table 15.5) illustrates that, of the two of them, he is probably the person who has least opportunity in his day-to-day life to have conversations, and is possibly the more isolated of the two (although this is, of course, pure supposition). Could it be that having more opportunity to communicate purposefully in the therapy setting enables him to use latent communication skills, for which he has the potential but no opportunity to use?

The course of evaluating therapy never does run smooth, however. It is HM who has made the most measurable gains in naming and who perceives that words seem harder to find in conversation at the end of therapy than at the beginning. Is this because HM is attempting more conversation than he did previously, so could this perception of greater difficulty actually represent a positive outcome in some respects? This is an important issue for evaluators in an evidenced-based healthcare culture: From whose perspective are the outcomes that make up the evidence, and how do we interpret the potential meanings and complexities thrown up by those outcomes?

Sally McVicker and Leonie Winstanley's therapy with a group of people facing communication and cognitive difficulties following acquired brain injury (Chapter 6)

Sally McVicker and Leonie Winstanley describe a group for people coming to grips with living with cognitive and communication impairments, including in particular memory and attention difficulties. Negotiating different levels of awareness, self-perception, and retention of material proved challenging, but was supported by careful preparation of a programme with accompanying materials.

McVicker and Winstanley use a stringent gauge of the outcome of therapy, documenting not only whether goals have been attained but also whether group members have been able to apply the knowledge gained to make a difference in real life. For two of the group members this seems not to have been the case, representing a difference between knowing something about yourself and being able to act on that knowledge.

This further complicates the issues about assessing outcome that we referred to earlier. So much rehabilitation is now geared towards the attainment of goals. Unless the goals set also include application in real life then their relevance to real life cannot be assumed. The complexities of other life issues that affect the outcome of a specific therapy are also highlighted—sometimes the effects of therapies are compromised through circumstances well beyond the control of the therapist. Does this mean that the therapies are not effective, or rather that we should take a much broader and more subtle approach to appreciating evidence of outcome?

Ann Montagu and Jane Marshall's therapy with SH (Chapter 7)

Ann Montagu and Jane Marshall describe the therapy undertaken with SH, to enable her to say proper names. Although the therapy was essentially focusing on something SH could not do, it was designed in such a way as to allow her to carry it out without making any errors. This feature was built into the design in order to bolster what comes across as SH's fragile self-confidence and to reduce her frustration, a combination familiar to many people with aphasia. Much therapy in the literature seems to require people to focus on that which they can't do or is most difficult for them. This error-free approach seems to be an effective and constructive alternative.

SH was able to develop aspects of the therapy tasks for herself, and these authors incorporated her adaptations into the design. Much of their description of the therapy is about the preparation for the therapy—the careful assessment of SH's relative strengths and difficulties in naming, the design of the therapy tasks, the preparation of the materials for therapy, and the reassessment after the therapy. The implementation of the tasks with SH and her practising them at home on her own seem to represent a relatively small part of the whole process. Setting up the therapy appropriately is clearly a very important part of the whole therapy process.

The therapy was designed to capitalise on some of the language skills that SH had left, following her stroke. The therapy depends more on the design of the tasks themselves than on the therapist's interaction with the tasks. This is because the design was critical to making sure that SH could do the therapy both without error and by herself. Essentially, it seems that the tasks were designed and controlled in such a way that the therapy then took care of itself. The therapy in this case seems to have consisted of a process through which SH systematically learnt or recalled the orthographic and phonological form of the word. From it she seems to have developed for herself a way of recalling words that worked for words not practised in therapy. The therapist's primary effort seems to have been to set up the tasks, and then support SH in the process of going through those tasks, rather than giving precise feedback or information about the words: The tasks did that for themselves.

Montagu and Marshall track the impact of the specific learning of the words used in the learning part of the therapy on SH's language skills in other circumstances—other tasks and modalities using the same words, other words, and other activities such as conversation. They are also interested in discovering SH's perceptions of how her language skills have changed. SH is discerning about how she has changed, and can identify what she thinks has changed and what hasn't. Interestingly, she perceives herself to be more confident in talking to friends and strangers and on the phone, although she doesn't think she can talk more easily. She starts to attempt more language-based tasks on her own as the therapy progresses, like writing Christmas cards and writing using a computer. Perhaps the mechanism that mediates "generalisation", which much of the literature relates to cognitive or linguistic

origin, could, in addition, be related to self-perception, motivation, and confidence? This seems to be an area ripe for further research, although the research methodologies employed will need to be able to capture subtle issues.

This chapter demonstrates how, with careful planning, therapy can be made into a positive, successful experience, even when someone has considerable difficulty with the material. This enables a therapy, which has as its focus work on an aspect of impairment, to relate to wider issues such as emotional well-being, perceptions of competence, possibly self-esteem, and ability to engage with the world around them. Ann Montagu and Jane Marshall relate these issues implicitly to the WHO model of impairment, disability, and handicap, but they could as well be incorporated into the framework for therapy implemented by Simpson and Cairns in this volume. That is, perhaps the therapy, whilst focused on enhancing SH's communication, also addressed her identity and her psychological well-being. Arguably it could be said to have begun to open up more lifestyle choices, enabling her to feel able to attempt more computer-based activities.

The authors suggest that it might have been useful to explore more fully with SH the changes she felt she had made. A framework for life engagement, such as that used by other authors in this volume (e.g., Simpson, Cairns) can perhaps draw attention more explicitly to the interrelationships between the key areas in someone's life that are affected by aphasia. This might enable the implementation of therapy in such a way as to capitalise on the potential of those relationships. In this case this might mean more explicitly to extend the gains SH had made to bolster the lifestyle opportunities that might have been opening up, and the gains in confidence and perhaps self-esteem that she seemed to be beginning to make.

Lisa Perkins and Fiona Hinshelwood, therapy with FR (Chapter 8)

The difficulties experienced by FR, described by Lisa Perkins and Fiona Hinshelwood, in contributing to conversations in contrast to picture naming ability, sound familiar. FR has difficulty finding words, which they thought to be more marked in conversational speech than would be predicted on the basis of his picture naming ability. This observation motivated their quest to pinpoint why this might be the case, and led them to the now quite familiar finding that difficulties in producing language can be addressed through working on language without requiring any output. FR made gains in his conversational use of language through therapy that focused on raising his awareness and overt knowledge of verb argument structures. Interestingly, FR interpreted this therapy as akin to schoolwork, which he did not appreciate. This made him initially resistant to the therapy, but the success he could see for himself as he progressed through the structured stages of therapy encouraged him to persevere.

Interestingly, this therapy is contrasted with a therapy that was not based on a careful analysis of the origin of his word-finding difficulties. This earlier therapy (given during the period when conventional wisdom would suggest he was most likely to show change in his level of impairment) did not lead to any measurable change for FR, despite the consistent work he and his wife put into doing his exercises. The cost effectiveness of undertaking therapy that, although it required fewer resources, did not lead to any gains for FR, is called into question.

Carole Pound's therapy with Tony (Chapter 9)

The story of Tony's therapy, described by Carole Pound, has many echoes of the difficulties that LW was grappling with in Chapter 3. She describes two stages in Tony's therapy, the first stage when he was in active rehabilitation in a neurorehabilitation centre, and the second when he was a member of a centre providing long-term services to people with aphasia. The dilemmas that she and Tony faced are familiar: How to enable someone whose aphasia makes him profoundly anxious, lacking in confidence, and isolated to reconnect with the world around him in a way that is meaningful to him and with which he felt comfortable. The challenge of these dilemmas for the speech and language therapist/pathologist should not be underestimated. Indeed, Carole Pound ends her chapter by asking a difficult set of

questions, the first of which is whether connecting with others is an appropriate area of work for a speech and language therapist/pathologist. As Carole puts it, "issues surrounding language and life may seem inextricably linked, but how many of us feel equipped to respond to life issues in the way that we respond to requests to work on language processing and communication skills?"

This chapter presents some accessible and tangible ideas for beginning to address these issues. Carole Pound draws on materials and resources available for working with a range of non-communication disabled populations, and then adds the expertise that speech and language therapists/pathologists have in knowing how to interact with and support the communication of people with aphasia. She used a largely group therapy context to address these issues, since she considered this to be the most appropriate context to raise and air these issues.

She also describes having to deal with another dilemma familiar to many speech and language therapists. How can therapists and people with aphasia best negotiate goals of therapy where there may be a difference in perception of what is required? Tony's perception of what would be most useful to him was to work on verbs and prepositions: if he could speak better (normally?) then he would be better, feel more confident, and be able to pick up his old lifestyle. Carole Pound's view was that at about 4 years after his stroke his language was unlikely to return to its pre-stroke level. Therefore she had to devise a way to work with Tony to help him feel more confident and find an alternative, but still satisfying, lifestyle.

This is a big and significant difference of opinion between the therapist and the person with aphasia, representing a major ethical dilemma for the therapist. Should she concede to Tony's wishes, but implement therapy she feels to be inappropriate, or should she try to put her point of view across and negotiate a different solution? In the current climate of an emphasis on "client-centred" care and the importance of setting goals agreed by the client/patient, it would be all too easy to accede to the client's request (as students found it impossible to resist doing with Tony), and to continue doing what Tony wanted. But what therapist, hand on heart, could agree that, at 4 years after onset, an ability to use verbs and prepositions could overcome Tony's chronic lack of confidence and low self-esteem? Indeed, after the first therapy, which did focus on changing Tony's language skills, by his own admission it reinforced that "I'll never never gonna be normal".

What was required was discussion, negotiation, and reflection, with an active programme of alternative therapies, to see if the course of action that Carole Pound thought was most appropriate could indeed turn out to be helpful. The active discussion of alternative courses of therapy, of choosing from a menu of possibilities, and contributing expertise and experience from both parties in making that choice, is rarely described (or taught?) and yet requires considerable skill, confidence, and competence on the part of the therapist.

Perhaps there is always for the therapist a lingering desire to "fix" the breakdown, to "cure" the language problem, and to give the person what they very often want most of all—their former language and communication skills. If we can achieve this then there will be no need for alternative communication strategies and lifestyles, or renegotiated relationships. And what if we can't fix, cure, or restore—have we then failed? And how do we convey that to people with aphasia (and their families) in a way that they can take on board positively and constructively? What's for sure is that this process takes time, skill, and support, for all concerned.

Jo Robson and Simon Horton's therapies with people with jargon aphasia (Chapter 10)

The therapy described by Jo Robson and Simon Horton demonstrates the importance of finding residual skills that can be used as a springboard for therapy, (which the framework in Table 15.1 in Chapter 15 can reveal). The use of writing as a means of communication for people with jargon aphasia may not be immediately obvious, given that they apparently have as much difficulty with writing as with speech. However, Robson and Horton sought out aspects of preserved language

performance—an observation that some people with jargon aphasia can sort anagrams of words to match to pictures—and used this as evidence that the person with aphasia had some remaining representations of otherwise inaccessible words. They set out to find ways for people with jargon aphasia to access and use these representations.

The people with jargon aphasia who completed both the phases of therapy that these authors describe showed that they were able to use writing of single words, or parts of words, as a means of communicating even some novel information not explicitly worked on in therapy.

Jo Robson and Simon Horton use a definition of "improvement" that does not require the participants in their therapy to show that they have got the target words they are aiming for completely correct. They assume that if enough information is conveyed to make something comprehensible to the interlocutor then this is evidence of the utility of the strategy as a communicatively useful device. In these days of evidence-based healthcare, it seems important to hold on to this kind of outcome as useful evidence. We should not fall into the trap of assuming that all therapy has to lead to errorless performance: We are in the business of supporting people to communicate effectively, and if the means by which that is achieved are unconventional or incomplete, so be it, and so be our robustness in accepting this.

Carol Sacchett and Jayne Lindsay, therapy with FM (Chapter 11)

Carol Sacchett and Jayne Lindsay report two distinct but related phases of therapy with FM, with whom they both worked at different times. FM had no reliable means of communication prior to therapy, and the extent of his aphasia suggested that the most effective place to start in therapy was to focus on non-verbal means of communication. The first phase of the therapy described here was to develop drawing as a more reliable means for FM to get his message out. The second phase focused on developing a communication book as a means for FM to interact and share personal information and knowledge with other people. The non-verbal means of communication that he had developed in the first phases of therapy proved useful for negotiating the content and layout of the communication book.

The therapy shows that, even though FM's non-verbal skills still required interpretation, they had developed well enough to give him an additional means of communication. This change is important. FM is a good example of finding a way forward with someone who was facing profound difficulties in communication. After the therapy he remained profoundly disabled, but had gained a route for at least making external some of his internal thoughts, and of revealing his retained competence as a person.

The therapy demonstrates the importance of not only the tasks and content of therapy but also the dynamics between FM, his wife, and the therapy team (including students). The need for FM to feel ownership of the process of developing the book was perceived to be as important as establishing the content. The importance of including his wife in the establishment of drawing as a medium for communication is also evident. She needed to focus on developing new interpretation skills as well as FM because, even though his generative drawing skills developed, his drawing was often hard to interpret. This chapter, like the ones preceding it, shows the importance of working with a broad context for therapy, and paying attention to the impact of the dynamics of therapy on the lives of those receiving it.

Sam Simpson's therapy with Carlos (Chapter 12)

Sam Simpson tells the story of a young man, Carlos, with whom she worked over a period of 2 years. But as we will see with a number of the studies in this book, the story is not just about Carlos but also to some extent about Sam Simpson's own thinking about therapy, how her perspective and judgement interacted with Carlos, and what she learned about therapy through working with him. Carlos was very young to have a stroke—he was 20. Simpson describes the impact of Carlos's age on how the therapy proceeded, the kinds of decisions and discussions that took place, and the issues and expectations with which Carlos was dealing.

The therapies undertaken are described chronologically. First, Simpson focuses on therapy designed to enable Carlos to confront his aphasia directly, to understand it, and to try to live more overtly with it. Her second main focus is on therapy to support Carlos to make realistic decisions about his own life and to take a direction that was both satisfying and sustainable for him. She portrays vividly the complexities inherent in supporting people who are going through difficult times in their lives. She also unpacks a number of the subtle and profound components required of rehabilitation and the range of skills that a multi-disciplinary team can offer. Rehabilitation is clearly conceptualised here as requiring that the person with aphasia both acquires knowledge and skills and also goes through a process of personal growth and development. This growth and development needs to involve families and friends, who are integral to the whole process. The range of people and contexts that have an impact on Carlos and his journey of recovery are lucidly illustrated in the story that Sam Simpson tells.

Alex Stirling's therapy with B (Chapter 13)

The challenge to the therapist's perception of his or her role is also apparent in this therapy study. The impact of even a very "mild" aphasia on language functioning and self-perception is brought out yet again, in the story told by Alex Stirling. She worked with a young man who had elective neurosurgery for epilepsy. Although she describes B as having excellent communication skills, even the very mild (in professional terms) difficulties that B experienced were sufficient to make return to work hard for B and had an impact on his self-perception.

Stirling devised a therapy programme to address both of these issues. She suggests that speech and language therapists/pathologists cannot avoid addressing psychological issues since the person's communication is "part of them and influenced by how they feel". "If we address the language difficulty but not how the person feels about it, our goals of communicative effectiveness and confidence surely are not met." However, she also says that it is important for the speech and language therapist to recognise the issues that they do not feel capable of addressing and to ensure that the person has opportunities to address these elsewhere. A problem arises when speech and language therapists have nowhere else to suggest that someone might go.

Several of the people discussed in the chapters to follow experienced a considerable loss of confidence as a result of their aphasia, which seemed to have been improved as a result of the therapies that they received. The inter-relationship between confidence and communication is clearly highly significant, and seems to be present as a factor in therapies of very different kinds.

Janet Webster and Anne Whitworth's therapy with AL (Chapter 14)

This chapter describes the implementation of the same programme as that used by Lisa Perkins and Fiona Hinshelwood, with broadly the same aims and with similar outcomes, namely that those aspects of sentence production that had been the focus of the therapy showed change in the intended direction. AL's wife began to use the "wh" question prompts during conversation for obligatory information that had been omitted, and AL began to show evidence of self-monitoring, and reported that he thought this helped him in conversation. In a narrative task after therapy, although he was able to use more lexical verbs, the analysis of his performance showed that he was still "outside normal limits".

This begs the question of what AL means by improvement in conversation—does he feel more able to have conversations in the social situations that he felt inadequate in previously, or that the content of his conversation is better? Are people gaining insight into, and control over, their language through this kind of task?

Sally Byng and Judy Duchan, viewing the previous chapters within a uniform framework (Chapter 15)

In this final chapter, Sally Byng and Judy Duchan offer a way to view the therapies in the earlier chapters within a uniform framework. The need for the framework became apparent when trying to make comparison across the disparate chapters.

The differences among the chapters were not only due to the different people with aphasia and therapies; they also differ in style, ranging from free-flowing discussion to a structured, prespecified set of routines. The chapters also range from a more traditional academic form of writing to descriptive personal reflection—with others falling somewhere in between. Some of the chapters describe one specific period of therapy, while others describe therapies with the same person carried out at different lengths of time after the start of life with aphasia. Finally, the frames of reference underpinning these authors' thinking about therapy lead to their writing in different ways, choosing to highlight or bring to the foreground different issues about both the individual with aphasia and the therapy.

These differences can make it hard to see what is shared between the studies, except that all the authors are trying to do something about the impact of aphasia on an individual or a group of individuals. How might readers who are trying to compare the information across studies be able to see the overall forest when immersed in the details of the trees?

In Chapter 15, we offer a common framework for describing the different therapies, *regardless* of the frame of reference adopted by the authors writing about them. The framework offers a common format for outlining the impact of the aphasia and what the therapists did in the therapy. We then use this framework to pull out the key features about each of the therapies, examining what was done and possible reasons why.

We see this framework as potentially useful not only for comparing therapies described in this book, but also for speech and language therapists/pathologists to apply to their own therapies, so that they can reflect on them and talk more explicitly about them with their peers.

SUMMARY

We will end this introductory chapter with a brief summary of some of the overarching themes for aphasia therapy raised across the studies.

- *Therapies that create the conditions for language change to take place*
The chapters by Deborah Cairns, Claire Gatehouse and Liz Clark, Debbie Graham, Ann Montagu and Jane Marshall, Lisa Perkins and Fiona Hinshelwood, and Janet Webster and Anne Whitworth, all describe therapies in which the role of the therapist was to set the therapy up so that the materials used enabled the people with aphasia to learn about their language, and make changes to it. These therapies contrast with those where the therapy seems to take place in the interaction between therapist and person with aphasia (Sally McVicker and Leonie Winstanley, Carole Pound, Sam Simpson), and where the materials used are less critical to the design of the therapy.

- *The complexity of getting the goals right*
Negotiating goals and arriving at a mutual understanding and agreement about appropriate goals is clearly a complex process (e.g., Deborah Cairns, Sally McVicker and Leonie Winstanley, Carole Pound, Sam Simpson). Yet it is clearly critical to both the outcome of therapy and the whole relationship between the therapist and the person with aphasia. The processes required for this negotiation deserve more attention than they perhaps receive, especially in training for speech and language therapists/pathologists.

- *Involvement of families and others in therapy*
A number of the studies reported here included working with people other than the person with the aphasia as integral to the therapy (e.g., Claire Gatehouse and Liz Clark, Carole Sacchett and Jayne Lindsay, Sam Simpson). Their involvement was necessary (a) to ensure that the communication skills being learned in therapy were useable in everyday life, (b) to facilitate the re-engagement of the person with their day-to-day life, or (c) to enable family members to learn to live with the impact of aphasia as much as the person with the aphasia.

- *Basing therapy on preserved language and communication skills*
A number of authors specifically base their therapies on aspects of language skill that are preserved, with these forming the starting point for the design of a therapy activity (e.g., Deborah Cairns, Ann Montagu and Jane Marshall, Jo Robson and Simon Horton, Carole Sacchett and Jayne Lindsay). This seems to be a very effective technique for designing therapies, especially where it is hard to see where to start given the density and complexity of someone's impairment.

- *Complexities raised by evaluating outcomes from the perspective of people with aphasia*
A number of the studies describe evaluating the therapy on both measures of communication and language skills as well as seeking the perspectives of the people with aphasia about how they had changed. Interestingly, in quite a number of studies, there were differences between how people "performed" and their perceptions of what had changed for them. This raises interesting questions for efficacy studies: What should be regarded as a mark of efficacy—how someone feels or how they perform? The studies also reveal the many factors that impinge on measuring or establishing outcomes, which reveal why outcome data often feel as if they do not reflect the reality of a situation.

- *Confidence-building as a critical component in or an outcome of therapy?*
Many of the studies describe how one of the outcomes of therapy was enhanced confidence. It is not possible to tell whether language and communication skills improve because of having greater confidence or whether having better language and communication skills leads to enhanced confidence. What it does suggest, however, is that perhaps more attention should be paid explicitly to confidence-building processes in therapies. Who knows, these might turn out to be the critical ingredients in making therapies effective and their effects generalised.

- *Whose role is it to provide therapies to promote reconnection with life and addressing the psychological impacts of aphasia?*

  Carole Pound and Alex Stirling, whose therapy studies describe the need to address issues to do with learning to adapt to living with aphasia, raise the question of whose role it is to carry out this kind of therapeutic work. Whilst neither of them answer the question unequivocally, there is a worry that if it is not the role of the speech and language therapist, then whose role is it? Who else has the communication and interaction skills to know how to negotiate or frame the discussions needed with people with aphasia?

- *The length of time of the process of learning to live with aphasia*

  There are few quick wins in therapy for aphasia. Therapists of course know this, but all of these studies demonstrate just how much has to go into a service for people with aphasia, if it is going to be able to meet the multiple and complex needs of someone embarking on the long and often arduous journey of learning to live with their condition.

- *Managing roles and resources*

  Given these timescales and the pressures felt by therapists to produce sound results with limited resources, it is unsurprising that many question explicitly how best to use precious therapy time (e.g., Sally McVicker and Leonie Winstanley, Lisa Perkins and Fiona Hinshelwood, Carole Pound). In addition to questioning best use of resources, the studies demonstrate methods of extending therapeutic capacity by working with students, enlisting the support of others around the person with aphasia, and working with groups in addition to one-to-one interactions with the therapist.

- *Developing new identities*

  Many of the authors reflect on the complex relationship of language and communication with identity. Within some studies this represents the primary focus of an intervention (e.g., Claire Gatehouse and Liz Clark, Carole Pound, Sam Simpson, Alex Stirling). In others (e.g., Deborah Cairns, Julie Hickin and colleagues, Ann Montagu and Jayne Marshall, Jo Robson and Simon Horton, Janet Webster and Anne Whitworth) there is an implicit or explicit question over the way control over language through careful language assessment, exploration, and explanation relates to control over life. As different authors grapple with their role and skills in supporting people with aphasia to live more comfortably with who they are once aphasia has changed their life irrevocably, the studies tell another set of stories, those of therapists exploring their own narratives about who they are and what they do.

USING THIS BOOK

We hope that the ideas from the therapy studies described herein, our above analysis of some of the issues they raise, and the framework we provide for describing therapies in the final chapter, will give speech and language therapists/pathologists some additional tools in their therapy toolbox to assist them to discover the implicit frames they are working from to carry out their everyday practices. This is crucial for all areas of professional practices for a variety of reasons. It allows professionals to examine their taken-for-granted ways of doing things so that they can improve upon them. It allows those who see and do things differently to examine their differences, and, when working together, to combine or alter their thinking so that they can all be on the same page. It opens new avenues of practice, ones that derive from thinking outside the box.

REFERENCES

Byng, S., Swinburn, K., & Pound, C. (2001). *The aphasia therapy file, Vol 1*. Hove, UK: Psychology Press.

Duchan, J. (2001). Impairment and social views of

speech-language pathology: Clinical practices re-examined. *Advances in Speech-Language Pathology*, *3*, 37–45.

Duchan, J. (2004). *Framework in language and literacy: How theory informs practice*. New York: Guilford Press.

Petheram, B., & Parr, S. (1998). Diversity in aphasi-ology: Crisis or increasing competence. *Aphasiology*, *12*, 468–473.

Weniger, D., & Taylor Sarno, M. (1990). The future of aphasia therapy: More than just new wine in old bottles? *Aphasiology*, *4*, 301–306.

2

Controlling language and life: Therapy for communication and identity in a bilingual speaker

Deborah Cairns

Tony is a bilingual Portuguese/English-speaking man with aphasia. This study presents some of the projects in which Tony was involved at the City Dysphasic Group (now Connect—the Communication Disability Network). This is a therapy and support centre in London for people with aphasia. The therapies are discussed within the framework for interventions described by Byng, Pound, and Parr (2000). This sets Speech and Language Therapy within the context of a person's whole life, taking into account not only their language and communication impairment but also their psychological state, sense of autonomy, and social identity.

Two projects carried out with Tony are described in detail. The first is an investigation of his bilingualism. This project explored Tony's tendency to code-switch between Portuguese and English, which could lead to communication breakdown. Tasks were devised to consider the linguistic and pragmatic contexts in which he was more likely to code-switch. The clinical implications of the results are discussed, especially in relation to Tony's communication and sense of identity.

The second project was the construction of a personal communication book or portfolio. Aspects of the book's development are described, as well as some of the clinical challenges that arose. These involved the roles of therapist and client in decision-making, and the influence of the therapist's constructs in determining therapy.

The project illustrated the difficulty of listening and responding to what a client wants. It also highlighted the distinction between a communication book and a portfolio, and some of the clinical implications of this difference are suggested.

The outcomes of these projects are discussed in the context of the Byng et al. framework. Drawing on evidence from Tony and his wife Nanda (both asked that their real names be used) and from external observers, a number of possible changes are suggested in Tony's communication skills and sense of identity. Finally some remaining challenges are outlined.

INTRODUCTION

Tony is a 74-year old man who had a left fronto-parietal haemorrhage in 1997. He now has severe non-fluent expressive aphasia as well as some comprehension impairment. He expresses himself through a skilful combination of writing, intonation, facial expression, gesture, and occasional drawings, and the use of a personalised communication book. This case study presents work done with Tony over a 15-month period through a variety of group and individual projects. An overall theme is Tony's sense of confidence as a person with aphasia, and the way in which some of the projects, whether directly identity-related or not, may have contributed.

The work presented is based on a framework of aphasia therapy that relates interventions to a person's need to live with aphasia (Byng et al., 2000—see Appendix 2.1). This is also related to the Life Participation Approach in Aphasia (LPAA Project Group, 2001). Byng et al.'s framework includes the person with aphasia, their immediate social context (e.g., relatives and friends), wider community (work, education, leisure, or religious context), and society in general. Interventions are divided into six broad and sometimes overlapping categories:

- enhancing communication
- adaptation of identity
- access to autonomy and choice of lifestyle
- identifying barriers to social participation
- health promotion/illness prevention
- healthy psychological state.

The framework is sensitive to the need for work on a person's communication skills in themselves: "Therapy needs not just to enable the aphasic person to transmit information but also to engage in the exchange of ideas, thoughts and opinions which represent a reflection of who they are" (Byng et al., 2000). It is suggested that the aim of all intervention in aphasia is to promote, either directly or indirectly, "healthy living with aphasia", where "health" encompasses both mental and physical aspects.

The concept of identity, in relation to the individual and to society and culture, is increasingly discussed within the general disability literature (e.g., Corker & French, 1999). The importance of developing a strong sense of identity after the onset of aphasia has also been highlighted (e.g., Brumfitt, 1993; Harding & Pound, 1999; Simpson, 2000), but few therapy studies have reflected on the process in detail. As Byng et al. (2000) point out, the concept of "functional therapy" is a familiar one, but has rarely been put into the context of the expression of identity. One of the difficulties in addressing such concepts is, of course, that of measuring and attributing change. This is particularly acute when, as here, the theme of identity was not explicitly stated early on, and was often an unconscious or subsidiary goal. Feelings about oneself are so intangible that it is very difficult to make therapy aims explicit, particularly in the context of considerable communication impairment. And yet both Tony and his wife felt strongly that their contact with the centre had played an important role in the way Tony saw himself.

It is not surprising that it was difficult to discuss therapy and to attribute its effects, given how hard I found it to articulate ideas in an aphasia-friendly fashion. It remains an ongoing challenge to find ways of talking clearly about such themes, both with colleagues and with clients. Without doing so, however, it is difficult to gain clients' real consent and collaboration in therapy that aims to affect language in "real" life.

TONY—BACKGROUND INFORMATION

Tony was born in Switzerland, of Swiss-Portuguese parents, but spent most of his child-hood in Portugal. He also lived in Brazil and France, moving to the UK in 1959. After arriving in Britain he worked as a hospital theatre porter, later training as an operating theatre technician. He worked in the theatre at a major London hos-pital until his retirement in 1991. Tony married his Portuguese wife, Fernanda (known as Nanda), 50 years ago. They have no children, but maintain close contact with their families in Lisbon.

Nanda reports that their marriage has always been particularly close. She describes them as "always talking" and as having done everything together. They are deeply protective of one another. Nanda expresses a great sense of upset and shock at his uncharacteristic irritability and frustration in the period after his stroke. Tony similarly mimes a sense of bewilderment at his own reaction. Nanda is quick to talk with pride about Tony's professional background and com-mitment to his other interests. Conversely, it is clear from Tony's behaviour whenever anything is wrong with Nanda, particularly when he is wor-ried about her health. Normally exceptionally friendly and cheerful, Tony then becomes with-drawn and obviously unhappy. This is noticed by other group members at the centre. One woman described him in the following terms:

> Slow, slow, down and nothing, nothing . . .
> very quiet and miserable . . . other times, ah,
> beautiful day! (mimes someone beaming
> and patting others on the back).

Before Tony's stroke, both he and Nanda spoke Portuguese and English fluently. They used mostly English at work and Portuguese at home and in their social life. Both used to play an active part in the local Portuguese community, Tony acting as chairman of the Portuguese club. As well as his two main languages, he spoke French, Spanish, and a little German, a matter of great pride. Nanda describes his competence in languages as one of the skills drawn on in Tony's work, where he was often required to translate for foreign patients and staff members. Tony's bilingualism proved to be one of the main themes of our work. This is linked with the wider aim of enhancing his communication and improving his success in transaction and interaction, and also with his consolidation of identity as a skilled controller of more than one language.

When asked what three areas of life were the most important to him before his stroke, Tony was quick to answer "politics, sport, work". He was a member of the World Championship-winning Portuguese roller-hockey team in the 1940s. He is also keen on rugby and athletics, and until his stroke belonged to his local sports club. His political commitment led to imprisonment in Portugal, and was the cause of his and Nanda's leaving as refugees from Salazar's regime. They both portray Tony as a passionate discussant, who loved to debate politics whenever the opportunity arose. When asked to describe his political role, Tony clearly mimed a confident chairman of meetings, expressing his own views fluently but also inviting contributions from others. A chance occurrence provided an insight into his continu-ing commitment to politics. During an activity in which group members were describing the person with whom they would most like to have a one-to-one conversation, Tony immediately indicated that he would like to ask the president of China about his involvement in East Timor.

Medical background and previous speech and language therapy

Tony had his stroke in July 1997. According to reports, this resulted in severe aphasia and dys-praxia and a mild right-sided weakness, although Tony remained fully mobile. He had a number of other health problems including diabetes and mild heart failure at this time. He is also reported to have had repeated ear infections, which resulted in serious bilateral hearing loss. This greatly affected his Speech and Language Therapy. Tony was seen by his local Community Rehabilitation Team for a number of months; however, direct work on his dyspraxia and aphasia was impossible. Speech and Language Therapy at this stage instead aimed to offer support and information to him and Nanda.

Tony's comprehension was described as being greatly affected by his hearing loss. However, when hearing better, he was reported to be able to follow conversations. He could read single words and some simple phrases. His spoken expression was severely limited by verbal dyspraxia; he was not able to produce any intelligible sounds other than indicating "yes" and "no". His access to written words was better in Portuguese than in English, and he was able to spell or part-spell some Portuguese words. This was a source of frustration as he wanted to be communicating in English. Tony is also reported to have quickly learned to convey a wide range of messages through gesture and pointing, particularly in more natural settings. In addition he worked to produce a picture/word communication book, which he used to convey basic needs.

Tony's emotional status at this time seems to have been very fragile. He is said to have become very depressed soon after his stroke, and this appeared to worsen as his health deteriorated. Nanda too was reported to feel very low and both were experiencing a great deal of frustration and anxiety.

Tony was initially referred to the centre 1 year after his stroke, with the aim of "practising using his current skills, gaining confidence and self-esteem and offering and receiving support". His family doctor also raised the possibility of counselling. Tony and Nanda initially started attending counselling sessions together. A major issue for both of them at this time was his tendency to angry emotional outbursts when not understood. Tony also continued to see his local Speech and Language Therapist, compiling a communication book containing useful written words, and developing strategies to help him access words from his Portuguese/English dictionary. Some improvement was also reported in his ability to spell a small set of English and Portuguese words.

Initial contact at the centre

I first met Tony and Nanda in February 1999. At this point they were reporting that the intensity of Tony's outbursts had lessened, and that they were both feeling calmer. Nanda described him, with great relief, as being much more "back to his own self". They were keen for him to join a therapy group so that he could build on his communication skills in a supportive and social environment. They wanted him to develop skills in a range of communication modalities, as they recognised that speech was still extremely difficult. In fact, in the time I have known him, Tony has never asked us to work directly on his speech, although he regularly expresses a powerful desire to speak again. At this stage Tony particularly wanted to develop his existing communication book and to work further on his use of the Portuguese/English dictionary.

Nanda was under a great deal of strain. Her health was not good and regular attendance at the centre was (and remains) difficult. We discussed the possibility of doing some joint work with them both at a later stage. For the moment it seemed that Nanda needed above all to be reassured that she was doing well as Tony's main communication partner. She regularly expressed anxiety about this, and a great sense of responsibility for conversation breakdowns. I was relieved, therefore, since we were not to address interaction with them more directly, that she was able to attend occasional relatives' information and support days.

Tony's goals for himself at this stage ranged very broadly. So, for example, while he wanted to improve his writing, he was keener to develop use of his communication book in interaction with others. He wanted to be able to lessen the confusion in his head between his two main languages by learning to translate more reliably. He also felt strongly about working on areas of activity such as using the telephone, which was impossible for him, and accessing the computer, a skill he associated with his working life. Perhaps less tangibly, he seemed to have a real hunger for discussion with others. He was extremely enthusiastic about talking about what aphasia is and means, how to raise awareness of it, and how to make information more accessible to those who have it. He expressed a polite dissatisfaction with group work focusing on worksheets—he wanted more structure, and more opportunities to discuss and to share experiences. Though we did not think of it in such terms at the time, this might be seen as the beginning of Tony's work to address his identity as a person with aphasia.

Unfortunately, I did not have the vocabulary to discuss these issues properly with Tony or Nanda at the time. However, their responses to questions about Tony's communication and feelings give some idea of their views (see Table 2.1). Although the simple Likert scale used was very crude, it does suggest some differences between them. For example, Tony responded to the question, "How confident do you feel about communicating with Nanda?" with a rating of 5/7, while he rated communication with others as more problematic (2/7). Nanda, on the other hand, rated Tony's confidence in communicating with others much more highly, and indeed more highly than his feelings about communicating with her. While Tony gave his speech a rating of 0, he felt somewhat better about his writing and reading, and fairly confident about his ability to understand others. However, he immediately indicated that his feelings about himself were at a very low ebb (0/7).

It was agreed that Tony would initially join a group of people who have more severe difficulties with communication. We hoped that this would allow him to focus on his skills in Total Communication, which was a constant theme in this group's work.

Language and communication profile

We knew from our first meeting that Tony was an eager and resourceful communicator, and that he would spontaneously use a wide range of means to get messages across. Over time we began to build a clearer picture of Tony's language and communication profile. A transcript of a sample from a recorded conversation between Tony and Nanda is included in Appendix 2.2. This illustrates some of the observations made below.

Understanding conversation

Tony gave the impression of being able to follow most conversational speech at a fairly steady pace, although he benefited from having topic changes marked with written supports. It later became clear that Tony was making considerable

TABLE 2.1

Rating scale: Before therapy

Topic	Tony's rating of himself (0 = very poor, 7 = very good)	Nanda's rating of Tony (0 = very poor, 7 = very good)
Confidence in communicating with Nanda	5	4
Confidence in communicating with others	2	6
Feelings about speech	0	0
Feelings about writing	3	0
Feelings about understanding others	6	6
Feelings about reading	3	3
Feelings about himself (his identity)	0	0

use of contextual supports to aid his understanding, which led at times to misunderstandings. He would often also "go with his hunch" if he was not certain that he had fully understood, which could lead the conversation on to an unexpected tack. Tony would, however, indicate when he felt sure he had not understood what had been said, and would ask for repetition. He appeared to be greatly helped by the writing of key words or concurrent "minutes" of discussions, and he made effective use of these to indicate choices, to clarify points, or to refer back to a previous conversation.

Formal assessments supported these observations. Results from key sections of the PALPA (Kay, Lesser, & Coltheart, 1992) are summarised in Table 2.2. Tony scored 38/40 and 39/40 respectively on the tests of single spoken and written word comprehension. His scores for

TABLE 2.2

Details of language assessments

Assessment	Score	Error types
PALPA 47 (spoken word-to-picture matching)	38/40	1 close semantic 1 distant semantic
PALPA 48 (written word-to-picture matching)	39/40	1 close semantic
PALPA 55 (spoken sentence-to-picture matching)	46/60	Reversible directional verbs Converse relations
(written sentence-to-picture matching)	36/60	Reversible sentences Gapped sentences Converse relations

sentence comprehension indicate greater difficulty, at least when out of context. On the spoken version he scored 46/60, having trouble with reversible directional verbs (e.g., follow, chase, pull) in particular. Converse relations (buy, sell, take) were also troublesome. A similar pattern emerged with the written version, where Tony's score overall was lower (36/60); here reversible sentences in general proved problematic.

Spoken output

Tony's speech was still severely limited; he could produce "no", "si", and an approximation to "yes", but not always consistently with his nonverbal communication. He tried also to say a small number of other words, especially Nanda's name, but these were almost always unintelligible except to very familiar listeners. The only close relation to the target was usually an approximation to the vowel. Attempting spoken production of any words was extremely effortful, and he was very aware of his unintelligibility. At other times Tony would produce a range of non-specific vowel sounds or other non-verbal vocalisations, which were often extremely expressive. By combining these with facial expressions, intonation, and a small range of gestures he would convey, for example, disagreement, surprise, frustration,

delight, bewilderment, unhappiness, or uncertainty. No attempt was made to assess Tony's spoken output formally, as to do so seemed futile and likely to be distressing.

Writing

Tony's main mode of communication was, and remains, writing. He spontaneously writes mostly single words in English, and occasionally some longer phrases in Portuguese. His writing is often intelligible in context, but contains frequent letter inversions and omissions and occasional additions. Tony often writes the beginning of a word only. In addition to single words or phrases, he makes resourceful use of written place names and numbers, and will underline words or draw arrows between them to indicate links or emphasis. As shown in the conversation sample, he is able to access some nouns and verbs in both languages. He has some access to morphology, too; for instance, earlier in the same conversation he had written "FALO EU" ("I am speaking now") to indicate that he wanted a turn. However, in general he relies more on nouns and numerals than verbs. Tony's performance on tests of written naming will be discussed below in the context of the bilingualism project.

Gesture and mime

Tony used a small number of specific gestures such as holding his lips together and indicating "no" with his other hand to convey that he was unable to speak. More often, his gestures were used pragmatically to control the flow of communication, as when he would indicate the need for people to slow down. An example of his controlling conversation in this way can be seen at the start of the conversation sample, where Tony indicates very clearly that he wants Nanda to wait while he writes.

At times Tony's gestures were very non-specific and could prove confusing for his communication partner, as when he used his hands to indicate strong feeling but in a way that was difficult to interpret as "yes" or "no". This kind of misunderstanding often proved difficult to disentangle. Repeated questioning using different wording or written supports frequently seemed more confusing than helpful. It was often necessary to take the lead by going right back to the beginning of a conversation and re-checking every step, a process of which Tony was extremely tolerant but which he clearly found extraordinary and frustrating. A similar feeling of frustration is evident in the conversation sample where Nanda misunderstands Tony's written message ("AMIGOS RECOMEND CITY"), thinking he means that a friend recommended the therapy group to him. Both his frustration with himself and her, and her anxiety at having misunderstood him, are clear.

Using conversation partners

For some people Tony in fact proved one of the most challenging communication partners in the group, despite his eagerness to engage in conversation, his wealth of ideas, and his determination to make himself understood. His very eagerness could prove intimidating, and his lack of inhibition about expressing frustration or insisting that people slow down, could be nervewracking. On the other hand, one student commented that Tony's determination, coupled with his good humour, made interactions in the group easier for her: "It was good to have someone who gets involved, even if on slightly the wrong track". Tony very quickly saw students and therapists as a resource to be used in getting messages across. In particular he would write messages and indicate to students that he wanted them to act as his "mouthpiece" by reading aloud his words. A similar process is evident in the conversation sample, where Tony wishes Nanda to read or interpret what he has written.

Modelling communication

Interestingly, a number of students felt uncomfortable about reading aloud Tony's messages, as they were aware of the possibility of "taking words from him" or of misinterpreting his intention. We discussed whether this collaboration would have an undesirable effect on the group as a whole. They worried that other group members might feel inhibited about producing "imperfect" communication if they saw Tony modelling the use of a spokesperson in this way, or might feel more inhibited about using non-speech methods. In fact, both Tony's collaboration with students and his use of non-speech modalities seemed to have a positive effect. Whilst other group members were quick to acknowledge his difficulty in speaking, they rated him consistently highly on his writing whenever comparisons came up. They also seemed to regard him as a "model" for the use of non-verbal methods, something that the students also used with relief in sessions. This was a role Tony took on, apparently, very easily. He was quick to rate himself and others, and was passionate in encouraging them to try other methods of communicating. We began to make a habit of incorporating discussion about people's strengths within conversations about aphasia.

THERAPY INTERVENTIONS

When Tony joined the centre, people typically attended for 2 days per week. The majority of the time was spent in group programmes, with one individual session (45–60 minutes) of individual therapy per week. Therapy sessions and key-working activities were carried out by a team of students supervised by a Speech and Language

TABLE 2.3

Examples of projects within a framework for therapy interventions (Byng et al., 2000)

	Enhancing communication	Identifying barriers to social participation	Access to autonomy & choice of lifestyle	Healthy psychological state	Health promotionlillness prevention	Adaptation of identity
Project	Total communication	Access to information	Access to information	Counselling	Relaxation	Video
	Computer work	Conversation	Transport	Conversation		Portfolios
	Interaction work	Outings				Aphasia awareness

Therapist. Clients also had the opportunity to take part in a range of education, research, and consultation initiatives. Table 2.3 relates elements of the therapy programme to the Byng et al. framework presented above.

As the table suggests, there were aspects of Tony's therapy that addressed a number of different areas within the framework. For example, an important theme at this time was the group members' need to express their experience of having aphasia. It seemed important to build in as many opportunities for this as possible within the projects we undertook. These included projects aiming to educate others about aphasia, such as drawing up guidelines for a publicity leaflet about the new centre, or making a video film about aphasia for families and friends. At other times reflection about the experience of aphasia took place during more explicit discussion of language impairment, as in the Cognitive Neuropsychology project. Here the group members used a processing model (Patterson & Shewell, 1987) as the basis for discussion of their strengths, difficulties, and strategies.

Negotiating themes of therapy

It was certainly not always the case that each component of Tony's therapy was carefully planned in sequence. The content was decided on a termly basis through consultation among the group members, therapist, and student key workers. A range of supports was used to assist in this process, including:

- listening to clients in group and individual sessions, in conversations with family members and in informal social contacts
- pulling together common themes in people's experience and discussing exceptions
- exposing group members to other sources of information on disability and aphasia, e.g., videos from other organisations
- discussing models of practice in Speech and Language Therapy, e.g., the social model of disability
- reviewing and evaluating past programmes, which involved use of:
  — pictographic icons and artefacts as reminders of content
  — icons representing a range of positive or negative feelings
  — accessible rating scales
- checking, verifying, and modifying in response to feedback
- using ground rules to guide discussion
- agreeing a process for reaching consensus, e.g., by voting
- agreeing an explicit set of goals and means of measurement.

Tony worked individually on two therapy projects. The first was an investigation of his bilingualism and its effects on his current communication, the second the development of a personal communication book or portfolio.

THE BILINGUALISM PROJECT

Background to the Bilingualism Project

One of the issues that most affected Tony's communication, at least in English-speaking contexts, was his tendency to move into Portuguese or to mix English with Portuguese, without being aware that he had done so. There are examples of both of these processes in the conversation sample. Tony combines the two languages when he writes "AMIGOS RECOMEND CITY". In the same conversation, he also wrote complete utterances in English and in Portuguese ("FRIDAY NEXT WEEK"/"POR ISSO NO ESPERAR NOSSOS"). Sometimes it seemed that the influence of Tony's other languages and his personal history was also evident; for instance he consistently wrote "SUISSE" for Switzerland and "ITALIANO" for Italy. This mixing of languages was a source of frustration and distress, and was observed to lead to a number of communication breakdowns, both in therapy groups and in conversation with monolingual students and therapists.

When Tony switched languages in conversation with an English speaker, he seemed almost always to be unaware that he had done so. He would react with surprise and immediate recognition when it was pointed out, or when asked to translate. This was something he found very difficult, however. He would sometimes attempt to use his Portuguese/English dictionary but this almost invariably proved a painfully slow process during which he risked losing the interest of the other group members. However, Tony was insistent that he wanted to be writing in English rather than Portuguese, and he displayed frustration when he found himself writing Portuguese words. He was very aware that English was the language of group discussions and that by which the centre functioned. He indicated that he felt it would be confusing for him to consider both languages, and that he wanted to be able to fit into his

English environment by communicating in English, even at home.

There seemed to be a mis-match between our view of Tony's bilingualism and his own. While students often commented that they felt inadequate as non-Portuguese speakers, Tony clearly felt that the responsibility for breakdowns was his, and that the solution was for him to write better in English. This was the spur behind an investigation carried out by Anna Heino, a student Speech and Language Therapist (Heino, 2000). Therapy in this project related to Tony's control of his two languages and to his feelings of communicative competence as a bilingual speaker. We wanted to investigate what factors within conversations, if any, made Tony more likely to code-switch from English into Portuguese. Our hope was that, if Tony could become more aware of his code-switching and of the factors that were likely to produce it, he might gain increased control. This might translate into a lower rate of code-switching, or Tony might be able to indicate more effectively when he was switching languages.

The "therapy" involved did not try to change Tony's language processing, but rather aimed to give him the opportunity to consider his own language use. This sense of jointly discovering aspects of his language, in the context of his expertise as a bilingual speaker, was very important. Although one of the aims was for Tony to experience increased success in communication as a result of achieving greater control over his languages, it was equally important for him to feel that he was contributing his expertise to a joint undertaking.

Three possible explanations for Tony's code-switching were hypothesised, and tasks devised to investigate them. The first was that his code-switching was a strategic response to compensate for word-finding difficulties in English (as suggested by Muñoz, Marquardt, & Copeland, 1999). The second possibility was that Tony's code-switching was "pathological": the result of a deficit in his language-production system (Perecman, 1984). Alternatively it may have had a pragmatic origin, for example, if Tony was having trouble working out which of his languages to use in a given situation.

TABLE 2.4

Responses to PALPA 54 (picture naming × frequency): English version

	High frequency (N=20)	Medium frequency (N=20)	Low frequency (N=20)
Correct without self-cue	10	5	1
Correct with Portuguese self-cue	14	5	1
Total Portuguese words produced	7	6	7
With awareness	5	3	6
Without awareness	2	3	1

Assessment of code-switching in naming, letter selection, and conversation

Written naming

A series of written picture-naming tasks probed for linguistic effects on Tony's naming. If Tony's code-switching was a response to word-finding difficulties, he should be more likely to code-switch on items that he found harder to name in English. This might include lower-frequency words or (perhaps) verbs.

Frequency effects on written naming

Tony completed PALPA test 54 (Picture naming/ Frequency) in each of his languages, in order to test for effects of word frequency, and also to see whether, as seemed likely, he had more ready access to Portuguese words than English words. (We assumed for the purposes of the test that the frequency of the targets in Portuguese would more or less match their frequency in English, although this assumption may not always have been valid.) Both the results and the way in which Tony went about this test were interesting.

On the English version, he divided his responses into two columns, one for English words and one for Portuguese. He then used this system to cue his naming. For a number of items, where he could not immediately find the English target, he wrote either the complete Portuguese word or the initial letter in the Portuguese column and consciously attempted to use this to cue the English name. As shown in Table 2.4, this cueing strategy was only helpful in four cases. There was also a

frequency effect in Tony's English naming ($\chi^2 = 10.45$, $p < .01$), but frequency did not affect the number of words he initially wrote in Portuguese.

On the Portuguese version of the test, Tony's naming was much more successful, and here there was no obvious frequency effect. Tony again cued himself, sometimes by initially producing an English word (e.g., TREN for the Portuguese "COMBOIO" [train]), sometimes with a mixture of semantically related Portuguese and English words. For example, for the target "CASACO" [jacket], he wrote "CAMISA" [shirt], "SUETER", then "CASACO". He achieved 42/60 names correctly without the use of this strategy; when self-cued words were additionally credited this rose to 52/60.

Word class effects on written naming

Tony was also asked to name a series of noun and verb pictures in English. Each pair was matched for word length and frequency. Results are presented in Table 2.5.

Tony was slightly more successful overall at naming nouns than verbs. The amount of code-switching was not affected by word class, but the degree of success was. Of the 10 nouns on which Tony switched into Portuguese, 9 were correct, whereas only 2 of his 7 Portuguese verbs were correct. In other words, Tony's code-switching was more successful on nouns than on verbs.

Letter selection task

A final linguistic task aimed to probe which word most readily presented itself to Tony, without

TABLE 2.5

Responses to word class naming task (N=23)

	Nouns	Verbs
Correct in English	7	3
Code-switches:	10	7
With awareness	7	4
Without awareness	3	3
Correct in Portuguese	9	2

TABLE 2.6

Responses to letter judgement task

English initial letters	23
Portuguese initial letters	34
Random letters	0
No response	12
Total	69

requiring him to produce the whole word. Tony was asked to choose the first letter of an item's English name from a choice of three: the English initial, the Portuguese initial, and an unrelated distracter. It was hypothesised that the letter he chose would correspond to the language for which he had the highest "activation level" for that word. Sure enough, as illustrated in Table 2.6, Tony demonstrated that he was more likely to think of the Portuguese than the English initial or a random letter. This was not influenced by word frequency or class. Tony would then use the Portuguese letter to cue the English word. It seemed that giving him the initial letter helped him access items in his lexicon, and in many cases this enabled him to produce a whole word.

Code switching in conversation

We were aware that the test situation was very different from everyday conversation, and suspected that this was making a significant difference to Tony's control of his languages. In particular, he was very aware of which language was being targeted, and was making conscious use of columns to separate them. The tasks were also highly constrained, with clear targets and plenty of time to respond. It seemed possible that the conversational situation, especially that within the group, was much more linguistically and pragmatically demanding for Tony, leaving him less able to sort out his languages.

A final investigation looked at the influence of pragmatic variables on Tony's code-switching. We recorded conversations held in English between Tony and two different conversation partners, a monolingual student and a Portuguese-speaking student, in order to investigate the effect of his conversation partner's linguistic background. We also wanted to look at the effect of topic, so each partner talked to him about a range of topics that we judged to be more associated with either Portugal or England. Examples were Tony's childhood in Portugal and his Speech and Language Therapy in England. Results for this task are summarised in Table 2.7.

Overall, Tony used Portuguese significantly more often with the bilingual partner than with the monolingual ($\chi^2 = 4.69$, $p < .05$). The effect of topic also differed between the two partners. With the monolingual speaker, the proportion of Portuguese and English words produced did not change with topic. With the bilingual partner, however, Tony switched into Portuguese significantly more often on Portuguese topics than on English ($\chi^2 = 15.35$, $p < .001$). Interestingly, a recorded conversation between Tony and Nanda indicated that he was more likely to code-switch with her than with either of the conversation partners involved in this task.

Summary of assessments and implications for the Bilingualism Project

These investigations as a whole suggested that, although Tony seemed to have better access to Portuguese words than to English, he was not using his Portuguese strategically when he experienced word-finding difficulties in English. There were many words that he could access in Portuguese, but he was rarely able to use them as self-cues. It seemed likely that his code-switches were the result of reduced linguistic control rather than

TABLE 2.7

Responses to conversation task

	English topics	Portuguese topics	Total
With monolingual partner			
Total words produced	54	96	150
English	25	44	69
Portuguese	5	10	15
Other—numbers, proper names & unknown targets	24	42	66
With bilingual partner			
Total words produced	33	47	80
English	20	10	30
Portuguese	1	15	16
Other—numbers, proper names & unknown targets	12	22	34

a conscious strategy in most cases. On the other hand, his awareness of which language he was using in the naming tasks, and his response to the conversational task, suggested that he had very good pragmatic skills that enabled him generally to be aware of code-switching when it occurred. Pragmatically speaking, he seemed to be following a more or less normal pattern, in that he switched languages more with someone whom he knew spoke both, and more still with Nanda. With her, he seemed to be perhaps using the strategy of "most available word" (Grosjean, 1982). That is, because he knew that she would understand him in either language, he used his linguistic resources to access as many words as possible, rather than to control his language. In the group setting, where he was experiencing more linguistic and pragmatic processing load, he code-switched more, and with

less awareness, because he had fewer resources to spend on controlling his language.

Outcomes of the Bilingualism Project and clinical implications

This process of investigation had a number of useful outcomes for Tony. One was that he became more aware of code-switching as a phenomenon within his language, and in particular developed an awareness that it was more likely to occur in less structured situations. This meant that, even if he was not able to translate Portuguese words into English, he was more likely to notice when he had produced them, and to indicate this to his conversation partner.

This realisation or "taking control" of his code switches had an interesting effect on the group dynamics as well as on Tony. By chance there were a number of other bilingual people in the group at the time. Tony's greater readiness to discuss his code-switching, which we tried to facilitate, seemed to allow the other members to discuss their experience as speakers of more than one language. Bilingualism, and the particular issues of being bilingual and aphasic, became part of the currency of the group. This provided a means of acknowledging the bilingual group members' expertise, and provided opportunities for discussion of their often international histories. For Tony, talking about his unique language difficulties, even when he could not deal with them any more strategically than before, seemed to provide a way into discussion about himself and his aphasia. Relating this back to the Byng et al. framework, we seemed at least to have opened up discussion on his pre- and post-stroke identity.

A second outcome of the project, which related to enhancing communication within the framework, was that we were able to discuss Tony's readier access to Portuguese than to English words. This allowed us to re-evaluate his options as to choice of language for communication in different settings. We focused in particular on his use of English rather than Portuguese with Nanda, and talked about his perhaps using the "most available word" strategy in situations where he knew that either language would be acceptable. The outcome of this is still uncertain. Tony now recognises that Portuguese might be a more economical option in some contexts, and he certainly continues to use Portuguese words with Nanda. It is hoped that this may increase.

I hoped that Tony might use his greater awareness of his language, together with his ability to specify which language he was using in structured contexts and his easier access to Portuguese, to develop some means of translating into English. We therefore worked to help him develop the use of his Portuguese/English dictionary. A number of strategies were devised:

1. Tony labelled the section of his dictionary corresponding to each letter with a different colour to promote speed of access.
2. If possible he wrote down the whole Portuguese word as a reference.
3. He was given a grid with three spaces, into which he copied the first three letters of the Portuguese word.
4. He was also encouraged to use an alphabet chart to help him locate each letter.
5. He would then look up each letter of the word in turn in the dictionary. He found it very difficult to use the "headline" words at the top of each column as guides; instead he had to scan down the whole of each column until he found the target.
6. As he found each letter, he checked it back against the letters in his grid, which he could then tick off.
7. When he accessed the correct English word, he copied it alongside the Portuguese one.

Tony's progress with this system was slow and laborious, and his use of the dictionary when he code-switched in the group could be extremely time-consuming. However, he became adept at indicating when he wished the conversation to carry on without him, and would reclaim his turn once he had found his target. Although this resulted at times in disjointed conversations, and still risked Tony's contributions being misunderstood, his use of the dictionary was a source of great interest to the other group members and students. It was later combined with a portable electronic translation device, which Tony found more acceptable. Like his work on code-switching itself, these tools served to mark Tony out as a bilingual speaker, someone whose language, and therefore his aphasia, was interesting. It was almost as if his skill with them was a marker of his skill with both languages. What had been seen as a barrier to effective communication and a source of difficulty was still at times a cause of misunderstanding, but had also become a symbol of Tony's particular expertise.

Summary of the Bilingualism Project

We hoped that by discussing what might be seen as a deficit in terms of linguistic expertise, we might contribute to Tony's sense of himself in relation to his pre-stroke identity. The therapy involved was the process of drawing attention to Tony's language and communication, without any direct attempt to change his skills at this stage. Any changes that occurred happened not so much because of the investigations themselves, as in the process of discussing and feeding back their results. In order for this to happen effectively, information sheets summarising the assessments were adapted to suit Tony's language skills. These then served as the basis for discussion, and provided a spur to elicit Tony's feedback on the findings.

THE COMMUNICATION BOOK / PORTFOLIO PROJECT

Aims of the project

One of Tony's aims when he started individual sessions was to develop his personal communication book. This was a small book with words grouped under headings, which he used to convey basic information and needs. Over the course of a term we worked with him to develop and extend this book, including more information about Tony and his past. This process raised some interesting and challenging questions, which in retrospect have affected my thinking about communication books and portfolios in general. This work was much influenced by the discussion in Pound, Parr, Lindsay, and Woolf (2000).

Process of constructing the portfolio

The initial sessions were spent discussing Tony's ideas about his new book and what he wanted it to contain. He spent some time looking at other group members' communication books to get an idea of what was possible. We also used icons and pictures from the Pictographic Communication Resource (Kagan, 1995a) to facilitate discussion of possible topics. However, Tony very quickly indicated the sections he wanted to include, with photographs and information on:

- family and friends
- medical staff, therapists, and students at the centre
- his job and work colleagues
- his birth history and nationality
- a set of maps to illustrate the countries he had lived in
- his hobbies and interests
- places he visits, including local shops and restaurants
- a weekly diary to indicate his current timetable
- his medical background and current medication
- his stroke and aphasia
- his current communication skills.

Further discussion centred on questions of style and layout. Again using a range of non-verbal resources and pictographic icons, we considered whether he wanted words, pictures, photographs, or all three, and how many of each per page. Again Tony had very strong ideas. He quickly decided on size and style, and the following week produced a notebook that he liked. While he wanted most of the book to be handwritten, and chose to write it himself, he also indicated that he would like to use its construction as a means of re-accessing the computer. He had been a proficient typist, and wanted to try typing again. He also wanted to use photographs of people around the centre, which we arranged for him to take. We spent some time discussing how he would represent the ways in which he communicates and his relative strengths in the different modalities. Tony decided to use a pictographic representation of Total Communica-tion that had been put together by one of the groups, adapted to convey his own skills.

We set a series of goals and deadlines for completion of the various tasks, clearly delineating who was to take responsibility for each. This was in response to Tony's desire to finish the book as quickly as possible. I also hoped that by explicitly breaking down the process into smaller steps, we might achieve a clearer focus on the rationale for each section and on the best way to achieve the desired outcome. Tony produced a mass of photographs and other materials for each part, which made the process of selection and discussion very time-consuming. He responded very positively to the idea of drawing up a schedule, particularly as this would allow him to have the book completed by the start of the following term. While speed in producing a finished product was clearly important for both Tony and myself, on reflection we may have missed the therapeutic potential of this process by limiting discussion of the materials he brought in.

We discussed in some detail where and with whom Tony was going to use his book, in order to tailor its design to be most useful. However, I gradually came to realise that my thinking was being heavily determined by my construct of a communication book. So my notion that Tony would use his book when he experienced a communication breakdown, or in situations where he regularly had trouble conveying particular messages, coloured the way in which I negotiated its construction. My repeated insistence on where the book was to be used, or with whom, was missing the point. For Tony, the lists of vocabulary, however well supported with accessible photographs or icons, were never going to be useful in the transaction of messages. It was the unexpected person or the unknown quantity with whom Tony needed help. And it was not in *transaction*, or message-exchange, that he needed the book, but rather in *interaction* and facilitating social connection. This recalls Simmons-Mackie and Damico's (1997) study of the use of compensatory strategies, in which social interaction and the organisation of discourse were found to be more important factors than transmission of messages.

It became clear later on, from the way in which he used the finished item, that Tony wanted help in introducing himself to people in a more satisfying way. He was forced to rely on his own writing and on his conversation partner's questions to lead and structure introductory conversations. Perhaps with a more subtle or sensitive process of goal-setting, we might have been able to discover this. I have the feeling, though, that it was only in the process of constructing the book that its ultimate use became clear even to Tony, and that, had we not gone through such highly structured routes, he may not have been able to adapt it to suit his real need.

Portfolio Project—questions and challenges

One of the issues arising from the construction of Tony's book centres on the way in which our constructs as therapists affect the process of decision-making. How do we relate what we do to what people ask for? How, in this case, did my expectations of communication book construction and use relate to Tony's? We started off with something of a mismatch of expectations, both in terms of the therapy process and in terms of his use of the finished item, perhaps by not delving deep enough into Tony's aims to facilitate a full discussion.

When a misunderstanding arose involving Tony's use of the book to convey a message, I saw it as a fault in our design or in the limited specific therapy we had dedicated to its use. I thought he was asking for a tool to help him through communication breakdowns related, essentially, to his difficulty in word-finding. The greater issue for him was not being able to convey who he was in a satisfying way. For him, the book was not essentially a tool to circumvent word-finding difficulties. So when he was asked, for example, the name of a particular family member or a fact about his past, he was frequently unable to find it, even though the book contained a great deal of information on these topics. It sometimes seemed difficult for Tony to find his way around the book in time to repair a conversation breakdown. If the topic of family arose, he would show the whole section on his large extended family, and more or less leave his partner to work out who was who,

confirming or correcting as they read. It seems that Tony was expressing a clear desire to construct a personal portfolio, rich with illustration of his identity, rather than a communication book with a focus on transacting information.

The students who worked with Tony on the book found the process very challenging, reporting frequently that he was jumping ahead of them in decision-making, and not allowing the necessary time for discussion or practice in real communicative situations. They worried that their discussions about the book's layout and Tony's ability to access information were not sufficiently focused, and that because of his hurry to finish the book they were not being able to equip him to use it successfully. While their concern for the book's functional practicality was entirely appropriate, this sense of unease at relinquishing responsibility for its success now seems more related to our misunderstanding of what Tony wanted. Some quotations from the students' notes illustrate the re-negotiation of aims:

> Tony is very keen to develop a communication book. This will provide him with the means to a useful communication strategy beyond [the centre] and his home environment. It is hoped that it will add to his independence, promoting his confidence in social situations and reducing his social isolation. (Week 1)

> It was decided to include a section with useful vocabulary for when Tony goes shopping, or to the gym, park, café or hospital. His week is organised in such a way that these are regular places he goes, where a communication book would enable him to communicate with staff. (Week 2)

> Tony expressed that shopping is not a problem for him as he goes to the supermarket and picks things off the shelves, i.e., there is no real communicative need. Similarly at the gym, the manager and staff know him and he does not encounter any real communication difficulties ... In view of Tony's ability to function adequately in these situations, it

may be more useful for him to use his book for social reasons. Therefore we should consider taking more of a personal portfolio approach with personal information about himself and what he does, and less emphasis on functional needs and vocabulary. (Week 3)

Outcomes of the Portfolio Project

The continuing importance of the Portfolio as a way for Tony to represent himself to others is perhaps most tangibly demonstrated by the fact that he rarely travels anywhere without it, and by the frequency with which he takes it from his briefcase at the centre. This may be to smooth the introduction process with a new person or it may be to extend a conversation with someone he already knows. Interestingly, Tony has also begun to extend the use of his book as more of a problem-solving tool. In group sessions he has been observed to reach for it spontaneously when communication breakdowns have arisen, not necessarily those involving himself. He has used his set of world maps to provide information about place names when another group member had difficulty in discussing his holidays. He also offered his map of the London Underground when a student came under-prepared to a discussion on transport. This blending of uses is not something that has been objectified or measured. However, I have the feeling that it may be at least partly because of the earlier work using the book to express his identity, that Tony is now able to begin using it to solve communication problems in this way.

In summary, some of the outcomes of this project for Tony were:

1. the opportunity to:
   - review materials from different areas of his life, and to select those he felt best expressed his identity
   - present himself in his own terms to other group members, therapists, and students
   - tell his experience of stroke and aphasia, leading to useful group discussions of aphasia and its implications
   - demonstrate his expertise, e.g., in terms of his professional life, bilingualism or politics

2. development of:
   - a means of introducing himself more autonomously to new people
   - a tool to help in explaining aphasia to others
   - a tool to assist in communication breakdowns
   - a spur to gaining support in re-accessing the computer.

REVIEWING THE BENEFITS OF THERAPY

Returning to the Byng et al. framework once more, the Bilingualism and Communication Book/Portfolio Projects could be said to have touched on a number of different areas. Both included a focus on enhancing Tony's communication. Both, however, also worked at the level of his identity—in relation to himself, his wife, and his immediate social context.

It remains very difficult to assess the contribution of any single piece of work to the way in which Tony feels about himself. However, the repeated rating scale (Table 2.8) suggests that something had changed in Tony's sense of personal identity. Only small changes were reported in other areas, such as his confidence in communicating with other people (which he related to his experience in the group) and, interestingly, his feelings about his speech. Nanda felt that this would not have changed. Tony, however, indicated that, although the improvement was very small, he was pleased with what he saw as some progress and more relaxed about his difficulties. His dream, though, is still to be able to speak again, and this was his resolution for the millennium.

I attempted to elicit Tony and Nanda's feelings on the role that coming to the centre had played. Asked first about the past, Tony wrote "UTIL" and made a negative gesture to describe his feeling of uselessness. Nanda added, "Was not a life for him. He don't feel he can be 'util' to anything, do anything or achieve anything." When asked about the effect, if any, of the group, Tony pointed to the counsellor's name and indicated a

TABLE 2.8

Rating scale: After therapy

Topic	Tony's rating of himself (0 = very poor, 7 = very good)	Nanda's rating of Tony (0 = very poor, 7 = very good)
Confidence in communicating with Nanda	6	3
Confidence in communicating with others	4	6
Feelings about speech	4	0
Feelings about writing	4	0
Feelings about understanding others	6	6
Feelings about reading	4	5
Feelings about himself (his identity)	4	0

forceful "thumbs up". He then indicated the names of the therapy groups, gesturing that he valued the contact with others. He wrote "STU-DENTAS" and gestured working with therapists. He felt he had developed a role within the centre as a teacher or trainer. For instance, he indicated that he feels confident about training students to slow down, and enjoys teaching them about stroke, although he feels he has more ideas than he is able to express.

When asked to reflect on himself now, Tony wrote:

PATIENCIA NOW
UTIL LIFE
CALM—TRAVEL—NACTING   (i.e.,
nothing)

Describing the role of the centre, he used his hands and face to gesture a growing feeling of confidence and happiness. Nanda interpreted: "The way he explain to me, he feels he achieve something, some goals".

Tony represented his feeling of loss with a drawing, showing a long column with the bottom section chopped off, and indicated that this represented his speech. Nanda commented:

> His feelings, his nature . . . is the same person. He was a person always looked at the other first—he still do it. For him, because he don't speak, he believes he changed so completely. He didn't, it's not true. He changed of course, he can't communicate or anything, and for him, one part of him gone. And for us of course, but not so big as he think.

Some observations from a project advisory committee on which Tony sits are interesting. In the course of a discussion on what constitutes severe aphasia, Tony was very clear that for him being able to speak (whilst being a dream he was unwilling to abandon) was not the most significant factor. More important was his sense of confidence in what he does, and the recognition that aphasia is a long-term, incurable condition. There was a strong sense around the table that Tony was a confident, able man, and that the fact that people treat him as such was as important as his language ability in his view of himself. One of the research team commented:

> Tony is not playing the role of chair on the advisory group but is a keen contributor and is not abashed either at volunteering a response or about taking a long time, stopping the meeting for a while to make a point . . . If he doesn't feel his point is understood he pursues it and won't accept a half-way house. He comes into the room carrying his papers in what looks like a very familiar way, in a file tucked under his arm—the pro. He pulls out his chair with assurance, no timidity. He doesn't feel he's there apologetically. I

think he feels this is not a therapy setting—this is work and he is working, not having therapy.

FUTURE CHALLENGES

I am very aware that most of our work so far has been with Tony, and has not directly addressed the issues that continue to affect Nanda. She still expresses a great deal of anxiety about her own competence as a communication partner for Tony, and is concerned that he seems less willing to use writing with her at home than at the centre. She also continues to express anxiety that he might find others easier to communicate with than herself. We have recently negotiated that some sessions would be held at Tony's home, and would look more directly at interaction between him and Nanda. It seems particularly important to highlight their communication skills; therapy may therefore focus on acknowledging and revealing both Tony's and Nanda's competence (Kagan, 1995b; Kagan & Gailey, 1993).

The issue of whether further work on Tony's language would be useful is still current. He is certainly very keen to build on his use of the computer, and some preliminary work in this area has focused on using the spell checker. We hope that this may help Tony to recognise potentially misleading errors or code-switches and, perhaps in combination with the dictionary, assist him in selecting targets. Another issue that remains a real challenge is that of Tony's leaving therapy. Whilst he is already making the transition from direct therapy to teaching and advisory roles, this process will inevitably call for a gentle and ongoing renegotiation. It will entail exploration of how therapy and Tony's other centre activities contribute to his quality of life. It may also entail unpicking the delicate interplay of communication, lifestyle, and identity as they affect him in all contexts. My hope is that we will be able to use what Tony has taught us about therapy to help him plan a satisfying future.

ACKNOWLEDGMENTS

I am extremely grateful to Tony and Nanda for their time, energy, and generosity. Many students have worked with Tony; my thanks to all of them, and to the staff at Connect, especially Carole Pound. I am particularly indebted to Anna Heino, who worked on the Bilingualism Project, and to Jane Marshall, who co-supervised it.

REFERENCES

Byng, S., Pound, C., & Parr, S. (2000). Living with aphasia: A framework for therapy interventions. In I. Papathanasiou (Ed.), *Acquired neurological communication disorders: A clinical perspective*. London: Whurr Publishers.

Brumfitt, S. (1993). Losing your sense of self: What aphasia can do. *Aphasiology, 7*, 569–575.

Corker, M., & French, S. (1999). *Disability discourse: Disability, human rights and society*. Buckingham, UK: Open University Press.

Grosjean, F. (1982). *Life with two languages: An introduction to bilingualism*. Cambridge, MA: Harvard University Press.

Harding, D., & Pound, C. (1999). Needs, function and measurement: Juggling with multiple language impairment. In S. Byng, K. Swinburn, & C. Pound (Eds.), *The aphasia therapy file*. Hove, UK: Psychology Press.

Heino, A. (2000). *Pathological code-switching: A deficit or a strategy?* Unpublished BSc dissertation, City University, London.

Kagan, A. (1995a). *Pictographic communication resources binder*. Toronto, Canada: The Aphasia Institute.

Kagan, A. (1995b). Revealing the competence of aphasic adults through conversation: A challenge to health professionals. *Topics in Stroke Rehabilitation, 2*, 15–28.

Kagan, A., & Gailey, G.F. (1993). Functional is not enough: Training conversation partners for aphasic adults. In A.L. Holland & M.M. Forbes (Eds.), *Aphasia treatment: World perspectives*. San Diego, CA: Singular.

Kay, J., Lesser, R., & Coltheart, M. (1992). *Psycholinguistic assessments of language processing in aphasia*. Hove, UK: Lawrence Erlbaum Associates Ltd.

LPAA Project Group: R. Chapey, J. Duchan, R. Elman, L. Garcia, A. Kagan, J. Lyon, & N. Simmons-Mackie (2001). Life participation approaches to aphasia: A statement of values for the future. In R. Chapey (Ed.), *Language intervention strategies in aphasia and related neurogenic communication disorders* (4th ed.). Philadelphia, PA: Lippincott, Williams & Wilkins.

Muñoz, M.L., Marquardt, T.P., & Copeland, G. (1999). A comparison of the code-switching patterns of aphasic and neurologically normal bilingual speakers of English and Spanish. *Brain and Language, 66*, 249–274.

Patterson, K., & Shewell, C. (1987). Speak and spell: Dissociation and word-class effects. In M. Coltheart, R. Job, & G. Sartori (Eds.), *The cognitive neuro-psychology of language*. Hove, UK: Lawrence Erlbaum Associates Ltd.

Perecman, E. (1984). Spontaneous translation and language mixing in a polyglot aphasic. *Brain and Language, 23*, 43–63.

Pound, C., Parr, S., Lindsay, J., & Woolf, C. (2000). *Beyond aphasia*. Bicester, UK: Winslow Press.

Simmons-Mackie, N., & Damico, J. (1997). Reformulating the definition of compensatory strategies in aphasia. *Aphasiology, 11*, 761–781.

Simpson, S. (2000). *Making sense of aphasia and disability: The impact of aphasia on sense of self and identity and factors influencing the reconstruction process*. Unpublished MSc thesis, City University, London.

World Health Organisation. (1999) ICIDH-2. *International classification of functioning, disability and health*. [http:/www.who.int/icidh]

APPENDICES

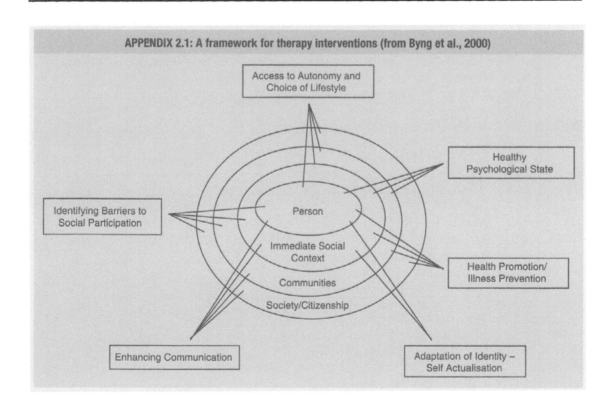

APPENDIX 2.1: A framework for therapy interventions (from Byng et al., 2000)

APPENDIX 2.2 Sample of conversation between Tony and Nanda

At home, January 1999
Tony and Nanda are talking about the new therapy centre building

T: (writes) POR ISSO NO ESPERAR
      NOSSOS
{N: And also—
{T: (gestures "Wait")
N: Ah, all right, I wait
T: (writes) AMIGOS RECOMEND CITY
N: Yes, was a friend recommend. Was, um. . .
      Monica
T: No, no, no, no
N: No?
T: Ooo
      (gestures that what he has written is wrong,
      and tries to correct it)
N: You want to say when you start there—
T: No
      (bangs table with fist; looks fed up)

N: Calm, calm down, calm down darling
T: (drops pen on table)
      (points at word "AMIGOS")
N: Friends recommend City?
T: (nodding) Eee
N: Which friends?
T: (gestures "anyone")
N: *You* can recommend the City!
T: (nodding) Eee!
N: For people have the dysphasia like you? Yeah?
T: Yeah!
      (expansive gesture; nodding)
N: I understand what you mean. That's it; all
      right.

Reassembling language and identity: A longitudinal programme involving psycholinguistic and social approaches in the life of a young man with aphasia

Claire Gatehouse and Liz Clark

INTRODUCTION

This chapter reports a course of speech and language therapy (SLT) provided to WL, a young dysphasic man, over the period of 18 months post-onset. The SLT took place in two different clinical settings and involved two different speech and language therapists with quite different emphases. As a result, the chapter will be divided into two sections. Section One will cover the SLT that WL received in the first 7 months post-onset. In this section the major emphasis will be on impairment-based intervention. Nevertheless, this section will conclude with reference to the ongoing psychosocial difficulties that WL experienced and some wider "political" issues. By leaving issues concerning WL's disability and handicap until the end of Section One, it is hoped that these issues will dovetail into Section Two, where intervention has been primarily directed at WL's self-advocacy and return to employment.

SECTION ONE

Background

WL is a young black man in his late twenties, who was working as a GP practice receptionist at the time of his stroke. At that time he was living with his brother in a council flat on a Hackney housing estate. WL has two children who live nearby with their respective mothers and has a large extended family in his local area. WL's social situation and local community was found to both help and hinder his ability to cope with his aphasia. These issues will be discussed later.

WL was admitted to his local hospital on 29 January 1997 with right-sided weakness and unable to speak. While waiting in casualty his right-sided weakness began to resolve. However, he was admitted to hospital for investigations. A left MCA infarct, affecting the temporo-parietal lobe, was later diagnosed on MRI scan.

WL was transferred to a specialist neurological hospital for further investigations, where he was first seen by the first author.

Initial speech and language therapy assessment

An SLT assessment at his local hospital some days following his stroke found him to have "severe expressive language problems (resolving) with severe word-finding difficulties". He was "unable to write and was struggling to copy written words".

At initial informal assessment by the first author, at 13 days post-onset, he presented as a cheerful, co-operative, fully mobile young man with fluent aphasia. His sentences began with ease but when specific content words were required output quickly degenerated into neologistic errors or pauses and attempts at repair. WL's comprehension in conversation appeared good, which contrasted markedly with his frequent requests for repetitions on informal single word assessments. These assessments revealed that WL was unable to name pictures or be cued to name them; he was unable to repeat and unable to write picture names. However, functionally, written errors on family names bore some relationship to the target. In terms of facilitating communication, WL was able to choose between close semantic alternatives both written and spoken. WL appeared to use his communicative resources extremely well. He acted, gestured, and circumlocuted as effectively as possible although he did not attempt to write or draw. An example of WL's communication is given in Figure 3.1.

At the end of the first session a Personal Dictionary was started and a "total communication" approach was encouraged with WL and his partner J. However, since WL's medical investigations were complete, no medical cause of his CVA had

---

FIGURE 3.1

WL: "yeah, but then I, then I went back so I could,...um..go..um..to the /koupl?/...you know, um, I went to, so I could (*gets money out of pocket*)"

Therapist: "Bank?"

WL: "no, no, so I /kot I?/ the man, so I could say to the man what I want, 'there you go mate' so I can go where I wanna go"

Therapist: "ticket, on the bus"

WL: "yeah! what! the geezer just looked at me like I was crazy. If I, if I, if I...look this is alright 'coz I've got the same....I've got the same thing (*points to money*) but if it's not the proper thing, What! the geezer was looking at me like I was crazy. What's the matter with you. What's the matter with you?"

WL describing a communication difficulty.

been found, and he had no residual physical or perceptual difficulties, he was discharged from hospital the next day. Unfortunately, WL's local hospital did not provide SLT to adults with acquired disorders in the community, since the community NHS Trust had opted not to purchase the service from the local hospital trust for financial reasons. In light of WL's age and social situation, the specialist neurological hospital where the first author worked made an exception to its current "no outpatients" policy and WL continued to be seen on a once a week basis. This difficult situation will be discussed later under Political Issues. At present, however, it must be borne in mind that SLT time was exceedingly limited.

SLT assessment and intervention

WL did not find a Personal Dictionary useful but continued to communicate in his own, relatively effective, way. Since time was exceedingly limited and his overall communicative effectiveness was judged to be good, functional communication was not directly targeted in SLT sessions. Instead, the initial emphasis was on identifying and treating his underlying language impairments, alongside providing psychological support. The latter area ran parallel to all impairment-based work and at times assessment and treatment plans had to be abandoned in order to deal with these more pressing issues. However, responsiveness to WL's emotional needs inevitably placed limitations on applying some aspects of single case study methodology in the clinical setting, such as repeated baseline measures.

Hypothesis formation

A short range of single word production tasks were evaluated in WL's second SLT session, using a small number of items from the Psycholinguistic Assessment of Language Processing in Aphasia (PALPA; Kay, Lesser, & Coltheart, 1992). The results of these assessments are given in Table 3.1. Although WL failed to correctly produce any items, the severity of his disorder in reading aloud and naming was particularly striking, since errors deviated so clearly from the target. This contrasted somewhat with repetition where, although

TABLE 3.1

PALPA 53: 10 items on repetition, reading aloud, and naming tasks

Tasks	Score	Errors
Oral naming	0/10	*kuz* (comb), *kon* (horse), *wun* (glove), *komishen* (bear)
Reading aloud	0/10	*vatch* (comb), *frunt* (belt)
Repetition	0/10	*glark* (glass), *darrow* (arrow), *ka* (iron), *kowsower* (elephant)

he was still unsuccessful, errors were more closely related to the target.

With reference to spontaneous speech, it was noted that despite his language being relatively empty and displaying unrelated neologisms, WL's output did not descend into extended neologistic jargon. Indeed, his frequent pauses and attempts at repair suggested that he was both monitoring and inhibiting his errors at times. In addition, he responded quickly to the listener's provision of the target word, nearly always knowing if their guesses were right or wrong, although almost always unable to then reproduce the target himself.

It appeared that WL could be broadly described as a conduction-type aphasic. His output was fluent but with frequent hesitations, his comprehension was functionally good, and he was surprisingly communicatively effective considering the severity of his output deficits (Kohn, 1989). Somewhat atypically, his errors were not clearly phonemically related to the target and he did not demonstrate *conduit d'approche* (sequences of phonemic approximations) in spontaneous speech (Joanette, Keller, & Lecours, 1980). However, later these characteristics were to emerge. This broad label of conduction-type aphasia was useful merely in terms of helping the author to hypothesise that a severe phonological difficulty might underly WL's language deficits (Caramazza, Basili, Koller, & Berndt, 1981). Traditionally this "syndrome" was viewed as a "disconnection syndrome" characterised by intact comprehension, selectively impaired repetition, and *conduit d'approche* (Carramazza et al., 1981). However, Shallice and Warrington (1977) drew a helpful distinction between *repetition conduction aphasia*, resulting from impaired auditory short-term memory, and *reproduction conduction aphasia*, resulting from impaired phonological output processes. In light of WL's severe impairment in all output modalities, it was hypothesised that his disorder could broadly be described as reproduction conduction aphasia. Wilshire and McCarthy (1996) describe this as "an aphasic disorder in which the ability to encode phonological information is selectively impaired, characterised by the production of phonological errors in spontaneous speech and on a range of single word production tasks" (p. 1059).

An interesting insight into WL's repetition disorder was given by an informal assessment of phrase repetition, reported in Table 3.2. In phrase repetition, it appeared that WL could preserve the broad meaning of the phrases, although not the precise lexico-semantic items. It was hypothesised that WL could access the semantic information of the heard phrases but that the input phonological representations quickly became degraded. As a result, WL was unable to access the precise lexical items for output and relied on semantics alone for access to the phonological output lexicon. Consequently, he was only able to produce appropriate, but not identical, short and highly frequent words to replicate the phrases. This finding suggested that, in keeping with Wilshire and McCarthy's (1996) explanation of reproduction conduction aphasia, WL's ability to encode phonological information was selectively impaired.

Further formal assessments of WL's semantic comprehension were undertaken to confirm that his phonological deficit was truly "selective". His results from semantic subtests of the PALPA (see Table 3.3) indicate that although WL would appear to have an abstract semantic comprehension deficit (77% on low imageability synonym judgements), high imageability synonym judgements (93%) and word to picture matching tasks (98%+) suggest that WL's semantic abilities were more than adequate for concrete word-finding (lexical access).

TABLE 3.2

Repetition of high frequency phrases (examples): none were accurate but all had semantic content well preserved

Stimulus phrase	Response
Where are you going?	Where am I going?
I don't know	I do know when its gonna be
I see what you mean	I know what you mean

TABLE 3.3

Summary of tests of WL's semantic comprehension

Tasks	Score	Errors
PALPA word-to-picture matching		
Auditory	38/40	saddle > stirrup, lobster > crab
Written	39/40	lobster > crab
PALPA synonym judgements		
Auditory	28/30 (93%)	
High imageability	28/30 (93%)	
Low imageability	23/30 (77%)	
Total	51/60 (87%)	

It was therefore necessary to establish the extent of any phonological input deficit. Thus PALPA auditory same–different judgements, auditory short-term memory span, and lexical decision tests were conducted. The results of these assessments are given in Tables 3.4 and 3.5. WL's good lexical decision performance in both modalities suggested good access to both phonological and orthographic input representations. However, 82% on real-word and 75% on non-word same–different judgements were interpreted as constituting a significant impairment (Morris, Franklin, Ellis, Turner, & Bailey, 1996). In addition, WL's auditory short-term memory span was found to be unreliable even at the two-item level (80%). This finding was in keeping with a number of patients in the literature and has been consistently associated with disorders of phonological encoding (Shallice & Warrington, 1977; Strub & Gardner, 1974). Indeed, Allport (1984) goes so far as to argue that there is "a central

phonological code used in both speech production and perception", which when impaired might account for the pattern of deficits observed in conduction aphasia. Unfortunately, at the time of this treatment programme there was no literature which addressed whether this central phonological code could be remediated in any way. As Pierce (1992) points out, there is a dearth of literature on the treatment of phonological errors as compared with that on treating speech dyspraxia. However, Morris et al. (1996) have shown that therapy tasks can improve auditory same–different abilities in patients more severely affected than WL and this provided a pointer for therapy.

It was hypothesised that an improvement in WL's phonological input abilities would be beneficial for two reasons. First, because it should improve WL's repetition which, although not of any functional significance, constituted his only output strength. Second, and more importantly, WL would need good input abilities if he were to be able to correct his own non-word (neologistic) errors. Of course, there is evidence that good auditory discrimination abilities alone do not automatically guarantee a dysphasic person's ability to correct their own neologistic errors (Marshall, Robson, Pring, & Chiat, 1998). However, since WL was already showing good monitoring of his own errors, it seemed an important next step for him to be able to identify how errors differed from the target before he might go on to correct them.

Auditory discrimination therapy

With the short-term goal of establishing reliable auditory discrimination and phonological segmentation and the long-term goal of enabling WL to correct his own errors, he and his partner J were given a homework programme at the end of the second session. The instructions for homework are given in Figure 3.2.

Reassessment on same–different judgements the following week (26th February) revealed no improvement in real words but non-word judgements had risen from 67% to 83%. J and WL were asked to continue with this work and after two more weeks (12th March) J reported a surprising

---

TABLE 3.4

Assessments of WL's auditory processing

PALPA 1 & 3: Auditory same–different judgement

Real words	59/72 (82%)
Non-words	54/72 (75%)

PALPA 13: Auditory digit matching span

# digits	Score	Errors
2 digits	8/10	2 false positives
3 digits	7/10	3 false positives
4 digits	0/3	3 false positives

TABLE 3.5

PALPA 5 & 25: Lexical decision tests

Modality	Score	Percentage correct
Auditory	72/80	90
Visual	56/60	93

FIGURE 3.2

Step 1.

J says two (short) words that differ either at the end, (e.g. dog – doll) or the beginning, (e.g. dog – log)

Step 2.

WL has to listen to the pair and indicate whether they differ at the beginning or the end, by pointing to the diagrams below;

Beginning _ _
　　　　　 _ _ End

Repetitions are allowed although WL should try and have a go first time.

Instructions for listening homework.

TABLE 3.6

Repeated measure of repetition of nine CVC words over 4 consecutive weeks

	Date	Correct	Single phoneme errors
Pre-therapy	19 Feb	1/9	2
Therapy, week 1	26 Feb	1/9	1
Therapy, week 2	5 March	3/9	N/A
Therapy, week 3	12 March	5/9	3

finding. As well as repeating, WL could now write some words to dictation during the homework task. An informal repetition task that had been conducted each week appeared to confirm this. The repetition task comprised the first word from the first nine items of the PALPA real word auditory same–different task. These items were chosen because WL had judged these items correctly when assessed on 19th February.

The results of this admittedly very small repeated measure are given in Table 3.6. It can be seen that over the 3 weeks of therapy, performance rose from 11% to 55%. In terms of clinical significance, WL's improvement in repetition and the emergence of his writing to dictation suggested that that his phonological input processing had improved. Unfortunately, at the time WL's auditory discrimination was not reassessed since time was severely limited and priorities were governed by clinical relevance. However, phonological segmentation therapy would appear to merit further investigation in clients with phonological deficits. Indeed, a study conducted by David Howard and colleagues (personal communication, July 1998) also found that improving conduction aphasics' input processing resulted in improved spoken output.

Further assessment

The priority for further assessment at the time became a thorough evaluation of WL's written as well as spoken output abilities. He was therefore assessed on the 40-item PALPA 53 subtest in written naming, writing to dictation, repetition, oral naming, and reading aloud. The full 40 items were tested in all but repetition, using a modified Latin Square design over four sessions, thus ensuring that baseline measures were stable and consistent across tasks, prior to therapy. Repetition was only assessed on the first 20 items due to time constraints. The results of all these assessments are given in Table 3.7.

Written output was found to be superior to spoken output. In terms of correct items, written naming (52%) and writing to dictation (50%) do not significantly differ from each other and neither are significantly superior to repetition (35%) (p = .0835 and .09, respectively). However, all are significantly better than spoken naming (5%) and reading aloud (2.5%) (p < .001). Error analysis in both of the writing tasks and in repetition reveals a high number of closely related errors. This was especially striking in writing to dictation, where close errors formed 90% of all errors, most of which were assembly errors. "Close errors" were classified as those in which all but one phoneme/grapheme were correct or where all phonemes/

TABLE 3.7

PALPA 53: Comparison across tasks

	Correct	Single item or assembly errors
Written name	21/40 (52%)	68%
Write to dictation	20/40 (50%)	90%
Repetition	14/20 (35%)	65%
Spoken name	2/40 (5%)	18%
Reading aloud	1/40 (2.5%)	58%

TABLE 3.8

PALPA 39: Letter length spelling

# letters	Score
3 letters	6/6
4 letters	6/6
5 letters	3/6
6 letters	2/6
Summary	17/24 (71%)

Significant trend, $p < .01$. Error analysis: 38% single letter errors, 48% assembly errors.

TABLE 3.9

Analysis of repetition (PALPA 53) re phoneme number

# phonemes	Score	Percentage correct
3 phonemes	11/18	61
4 & 5 phonemes	2/18	11

$p < .01$. Error analysis: 57% single phoneme errors, 7% assembly errors.

graphemes were correct but in the wrong order (assembly errors).

The nature of errors in both repetition and writing tasks suggested that WL had assembly difficulties in both graphemic and phonological output. To explore this, WL's writing to dictation was assessed on PALPA 39, letter length spelling, which includes items from three to six letters in length (see Table 3.8). To cut down on assessment, his repetition responses on the PALPA 53 were analysed in terms of number of phonemes (see Table 3.9). Statistical analysis confirmed significant length effects in writing to dictation (Jonckhere Trend test, $Z = 2.75$, $p < .01$) and repetition (Fisher Exact, $Z = 2.74$, $p < .01$).

The significant length effects in repetition suggested that WL's disorder resulted "not from an impairment in the ability to retrieve stored lexical phonological forms but in the ability to process that information subsequent to retrieval" (Wilshire & McCarthy, 1996, p. 1060). The pattern of WL's spoken output deficit, whereby repetition is significantly superior to naming and reading aloud, mirrors Wilshire and McCarthy's patient RN, although RN was only very mildly impaired. They suggested that in repetition the "phonological information provided in the auditory stimulus can assist during output phonological processing" (p. 1070). It was therefore hypothesised that WL had a severe phonological assembly deficit that could only be overcome if

additional input phonology was available. While this was available in repetition it was not available in reading aloud or naming.

Significant length effects in writing to dictation indicated graphemic assembly problems similar to, but less severe than, those in phonological assembly. Fortunately, WL's relatively good written naming performance suggested good access to the orthographic output lexicon, in contrast to lexical access in spoken naming.

Summary of impairments

WL had been found to have intact concrete semantic comprehension. Writing tasks had demonstrated good access to orthographic output representations on the basis of auditory (dictation) or picture input (oral naming). Unfortunately, subsequent graphemic assembly problems were evident, characterised by graphemic order-ing errors and word length effects. Spoken output tasks revealed a similar but more severe phono-logical assembly impairment.

These disorders of phonological and graph-emic assembly (or encoding) are thought to occur after the stage of lexical retrieval. Kohn (1989) describes phonological encoding as "the stage at which the lexical (phonological) representation is transformed into a string of (phonemic) segments before it can be phonetically encoded for eventual articulation" (p. 209), and that it is at this post-lexical level that conduction-type aphasics often reflect a breakdown. Orthographic repre-sentations are thought to be "transformed into a graphemic string in a manner analogous to the stage of phonemic string construction in spoken output" (p. 211).

WL's phonological impairment was therefore assumed to be at the level of the segment-to-frame association process of Levelt and Wheeldon (1994) or in Butterworth's (1992) phonological assembly subsystem with an analogous disorder in graphemic assembly. It appeared that WL's phonological assembly disorder could be ameli-orated to some degree by additional phonological input (in repetition), but that semantics (in nam-ing) or orthography (in reading aloud) alone were insufficient to support phonological assembly.

Graphemic assembly therapy

WL's profile of impairments suggested that his graphemic assembly deficit would be most use-fully targeted in the next stage of therapy. The rationale for this decision is outlined in Figure 3.3. The final hypothesis in Figure 3.3 concerns potential generalisation of improved assembly abilities from written to spoken output. This was based on two factors. First, previous experience of clients with phonological problems who could read aloud better than they could repeat or name suggested that orthographic representa-tions could provide stable, non-temporal infor-mation that could help overcome phonological assembly deficits. Indeed, Nespoulous, Joanette, Ska, Caplan, and Lecours (1987) have reported an advantage in four conduction aphasics' oral reading compared to other spoken tasks. They argued that this resulted from the visual stimulus providing constant "external reinforcement" and so allowing them to access their visual-verbal sys-tem. Second, since reproduction conduction aphasics "have been found to produce qualita-tively similar errors in speech and writing tasks" (Wilshire & McCarthy, 1996, p. 1060), it was hypothesised that a common underlying deficit may be involved.

A number of authors have argued for a com-mon underlying deficit in spoken and written

---

FIGURE 3.3

1. Whenever possible or relevant, therapy should target a patient's strengths, i.e., WL's written output and good lexical decision.

2. Treatment can only be undertaken in a modality that can be facilitated in some way, which ruled out naming or reading aloud.

3. WL could work on writing as homework, without relying on anyone else, unlike repetition.

4. Treatment could be pitched at a level that would ensure maximal success and minimise errors.

5. Writing had a direct communicative relevance whilst repetition did not.

6. WL's job relied heavily on orthographic skills and writing was a pre-morbid strength.

7. Improved graphemic assembly might generalise to phonological assembly.

Rationale for graphemic assembly therapy.

output in conduction aphasia. Hecaen and Albert (1978; cited in Caramazza et al., 1981) accounted for the repetition deficit and other symptoms in conduction aphasia as the result of a disturbance of "first articulation"—a kind of inner speech, translating abstract representations into forms that guide all output processes. Similarly, Kohn (1989) explains the similarities in her patient CM's oral and written output as "consistent with the interpretation that CM's orthographic difficulties could involve interference from his deficit in phonemic string construction" (p. 222). Interestingly, the implication here is that an improvement in CM's phonemic deficit would lead to an improvement in his writing. However, it was hoped that the reverse would be true for WL. Kohn makes the assumption that writing is dependent on phonology. If this were the case it would be difficult to explain WL's writing superiority. In contrast to Kohn (1989), Caramazza and Miceli (1990), on the basis of disassociations, argue for "orthosyllabic structure" in written word production that is very similar to, but independent of, phonology. This would appear to be more consistent with WL's profile.

In conclusion, the theoretical relationship between phonological assembly remained debatable but it seemed clinically reasonable to hope that an improvement in one assembly subsystem, in this case graphemic, would aid another assembly subsystem, in this case phonological.

Therapy task

Treatment materials were presented on a sheet of A4 paper. On the left-hand side of the page, typed words were presented as if for a lexical decision task (half were real words and half non-words). All non-words were anagrams of real words. On the right-hand side of the page the correctly ordered targets were presented. When given to WL, the sheet of A4 was folded in half lengthways, so that WL could only see the left-hand column of real and non-words. He was first required to look at each item and decide if it was a real word or not. This lexical decision component was included to "force" WL to utilise access to his intact orthographic input lexicon. (However, since it was so easy for him this step was

quickly removed so that all items were non-word anagrams of real words).

The next step required WL to turn over the sheet to view the correct target. He was required to commit the correct letter-order to visual memory, then turn back to the original item and write it next to the anagram. If he had difficulty he was encouraged to look back at the target as often as he liked, but was asked not to simply open out the A4 sheet and copy the word. Finally, he was asked to check his answer against the target to ensure that it was correct. This procedure is summarised in Figure 3.4.

FIGURE 3.4

Example of treatment materials

KYE	KEY
BED	BED
SYK	SKY

Procedure

1. Sheet folded in half with left-hand side visible.

2. WL views real & non-words and judges if real word or not.*

3. If not real word WL must look at target on reverse side of paper.*

4. WL turns over answer and writes from memory*. If not sure he looks again.

5. Once word finished check against answer and correct.

* Steps 2 and 3 and the first part of step 4 were eliminated once WL's confidence grew.

Hierarchy

Stage 1	3 letters
Stage 2	3 & 4 letters
Stage 3	4 & 5 letters
Stage 4	5 & 6 letters

Example of WL's homework sheets and procedure.

A treatment hierarchy was constructed on the basis of number of letters. The first level comprised 3-letter words. Once WL was proficient at these, 4-letter words were introduced but mixed-up with the 3-letter words. Once 4-letter words were easy for WL, the 3-letter words were dropped and 5-letter words were introduced, and so on. In this way, therapy items always included items that WL could succeed on so he was always working just within his level of ability. This hierarchy is summarised in Figure 3.4.

Treatment items were taken from PALPA 39, letter length spelling, plus other concrete words that were chosen to conform to letter length hierarchy. However, these extra items never comprised items from PALPA 53 since these items were acting as untreated controls.

WL was provided with two sheets for each stage (12 items per sheet). He was asked to repeat the same exercise each day, cutting out his look at the target before attempting to answer as his ability grew (i.e., on the shorter words). However, the items were always pitched within his level of ability and WL was encouraged to use as much assistance from the correct target as possible to try to ensure errorless responses. This treatment programme was conducted partly as a homework programme and partly in sessions with a student speech and language therapist, from 16 April until 8 May. Six sessions were conducted in the clinic and WL's compliance with homework was variable. The most he ever completed was three sets of homework in a week. At the time WL was also experiencing quite a lot of emotional difficulties and these diverted the treatment programme at times. Reassessment began on 8 May because WL was no longer complying with the homework.

Reassessment of writing tasks

Writing to dictation was reassessed on PALPA 39, letter length spelling (treatment items), and both writing to dictation and written naming were reassessed on the 40-item PALPA 53 subtest (untreated control items). These results are summarised in Tables 3.10 and 3.11, respectively.

The results of the reassessments were impressive. Changes in writing to dictation from 71% to

96% and from 50% to 96% were highly significant (McNemar, $p < .01$ and $< .001$, respectively), and a change from 52% to 85% in written naming (with parallel qualitative improvements) was also significant (McNemar, $p < .001$). Unfortunately, it was not possible to unreservedly assign these changes to the effects of therapy since the absence

TABLE 3.10

PALPA 39 letter length spelling: Assessment of writing to dictation of treatment items pre- and post-writing therapy

	14 April (pre-therapy)	*8 May (post-therapy)*
3 letters	6/6	6/6
4 letters	6/6	6/6
5 letters	3/6	6/6
6 letters	2/6	5/6
Totals	17/24	23/24*
Percentage totals	(71%)	(96%)

* Significance level, McNemar, $p < .01$.

TABLE 3.11

PALPA 53: Assessment of untreated control items pre- and post-therapy in written naming and writing to dictation

	March–April (pre-therapy)	*May (post-therapy)*
Written naming		
Correct	21/40 (52%)	34/40 (85%)*
Close errors	58%	80%
Writing to dictation		
Correct	20/40 (50%)	38/40 (96%)*
Close errors	90%	85%

Significance level, McNemar, $p < .001$.

of more than one pre-therapy baseline means that the possibility of changes occurring regardless of therapy could not be ruled out.

These methodological problems arose from trying to conduct a well-controlled treatment study in a (difficult) clinical setting. At the time, repeated measures could not be a priority in light of WL's many needs. Unfortunately, this made interpretation of results difficult. It was therefore necessary to seek converging sources of evidence that might support a direct therapy effect. The first source of evidence involved an evaluation of generalisation to spoken output tasks (where repeated measures had been made) and the second was an assessment of all tasks 3 months post-therapy.

Generalisation to spoken output tasks

It will be remembered that WL's repetition had been found to be improving in the first 3 months post-onset, prior to this therapy programme beginning. It can be seen in Table 3.12 that in February he was unable to repeat, although errors were close, whilst in March performance had risen to 35%. After the period of writing therapy, repetition appeared to have continued on its improvement trajectory, but not to have been accelerated by therapy. The rise from 35% to 52% just escaped significance ($p = .0592$).

Repetition contrasted strongly with spoken naming and reading aloud. These latter two tasks showed no signs of recovery in the first 3 months post-onset (see Table 3.12). In February, WL was unable to read any words aloud and immediately prior to therapy he managed to read 1/40 PALPA items. Similarly, his spoken naming only changed from 0/10 in February to 1/24 prior to therapy. Considering that these repeated measures occurred in the period that has often been identified as that of greatest spontaneous recovery it seems fair to conclude that pre-therapy spoken output baselines were more or less stable (although some qualitative changes in errors were observed). It was therefore striking to find that both of these tasks improved significantly after writing therapy (see Table 3.13). Spoken naming rose from 5% to 45% (McNemar $Z = 2.47$, $p < .001$) and reading aloud from 2.5% to 50% (McNemar $Z = 2.85$, $p < .001$).

It must be remembered that these items from the PALPA 53 subtest were not used in therapy and so constitute untreated control items. Therefore, following a period of therapy targeting written output, WL's spoken naming and reading aloud of control items had improved significantly and had been brought into line with his repetition ability.

Three months post-therapy follow-up

Three months after graphemic assembly therapy ceased, WL was reassessed on PALPA 53 in

---

TABLE 3.12

PALPA 53: Comparison of performance on spoken versions pre- and post-writing therapy

Tasks	February	March/April (therapy)	May
Repetition			
Correct	0/10	14/40 (35%)	21/40 (52%)
Close errors	60%	50%	42%
Reading aloud			
Correct	0/10	1/40 (2.5%)	10/20 (50%)*
Close errors	20%	58%	60%
Spoken naming			
Correct	0/10	2/40 (5%)	9/20 (45%)*
Close errors	0	22%	27%

* Comparison of pre- & post-therapy measures, McNemar significance level, $p < .01$.

TABLE 3.13

PALPA 53: Repeated measures of in five modalities demonstrating treatment effects and maintenance

Task	Feb	Mar–April	May (therapy)	Aug–Sept
Written naming		21/40 (52%)	34/40 (85%)	28/40 (70%)**
Reading aloud	0/10	1/40 (2.5%)	10/20 (50%)	10/20 (50%)
Spoken naming	0/10	2/40 (5%)	9/20 (45%)	12/20 (60%)
Repetition	0/10	14/40 (35%)	21/40 (52%)	28/40 (70%)*
Writing to dictation		28/40 (71%)	38/40 (96%)	33/40 (83%)**

* Significant improvement, McNemar $p < .001$.
** Significant decline, McNemar $p < .05$.

all output tasks (see Table 3.13). Reading aloud remained unchanged at 50%, therefore maintaining the treatment effect but making no further gains. WL's spoken naming had also maintained but failed to improve further (statistical analysis of the same 20 items, McNemar $Z = 0.76$, $p = .227$). In contrast, repetition had continued to steadily improve, maintaining the same significant trajectory already observed (Jonckhere trend test, $Z = 3.954, p < .001$).

Interestingly, those areas directly targeted by therapy and which had shown significant improvements immediately post-therapy were both found to have declined. WL's written naming had fallen significantly from 85% to 70% (McNemar, $Z = 2.04, p < .05$), although this still remained significantly higher than his 52% prior to therapy ($Z = 1.66, p < .05$). His writing to dictation had also dropped significantly from 96% to 83% (McNemar, $Z = 1.79, p < .05$), which was nevertheless also significantly superior to his ability (71%) prior to therapy (McNemar, $Z = 3.1, p .001$).

Interpretation of converging sources of evidence

The full set of results presented in Table 3.13 support a number of conclusions.

1. Changes in written output were the direct result of therapy. Significant improvements were found to correspond with the therapy programme and without therapy these improvements fall off significantly. This "fall-off effect" discounts spontaneous recovery from accounting for the initial therapy effect.

2. Therapy did not impact on repetition. The statistically significant recovery trend in WL's repetition was neither affected by the initiation nor the cessation of the therapy programme.

3. Well-maintained gains in reading aloud and spoken naming can be directly attributed to graphemic assembly therapy. Stable pre-therapy baselines, significant improvements when therapy occurred, and the absence of further improvements when therapy ceased all support this conclusion.

DISCUSSION OF SECTION ONE

Whilst repeated pre-therapy baselines would have been preferable, repeated post-therapy measures have been shown to be useful in demonstrating therapy effects and may provide a useful alternative for the busy clinician.

Graphemic assembly therapy, targeting WL's strength in writing, resulted in significant gains in two writing tasks and two out of three spoken output tasks. However, an important question remains unanswered. How did therapy targeting the graphemic assembly subsystem have an effect on WL's spoken naming and reading aloud?

I would like to argue that there is an intimate relationship between written and spoken assembly subsystems, which has not been previously well explored, and that this can account for the results of the therapy study. It will be remembered that Caramazza and Miceli (1990) found dissociations between orthography and phonology in their patient LM and therefore argued for separate assembly systems. However, they claimed that consonant, vowel, and syllable representations also exist in orthographic representations. Although it is not discussed, it seems that these "phonologically" based representations must have originated (developmentally) within the phonological system and so orthography cannot be quite so easily divorced from the phonological system as they would like to suggest. A second issue to bear in mind is that once the language processing system becomes disrupted after brain damage we cannot assume that it will function in as sophisticated or implicit a way as premorbidly. I would argue that a common assembly system for orthography and phonology is crucial in written language development. Indeed, Goswami and Bryant (1990) state that whereas they were unable to find any eveidence that children use phonological awareness in reading tasks, they found "abundant evidence that children depend on a phonological code when they are working out how to spell a word" (p. 61). In addition, Goswami and Bryant emphasise the importance of phonological segmentation skills (most especially of onset and rhyme) as a precursor to the development of writing. This neatly parallels the phonological segmentation skills targeted in WL, which appeared to provide a precursor to the emergence of writing as a useful output modality.

This hypothesised "common assembly system" may well become redundant in the mature, lexically orientated adult language system. However, once this mature system is disrupted in aphasia, these common assembly processes could become re-accessed and could be utilised in therapy programmes such as WL's.

Whereas Kohn (1989) argues that graphemic assembly is dependent on phonological assembly, a more two-way relationship is suggested in an earlier Caramazza paper. Caramazza, Berndt, and Basili (1983) argued that for their patient JS, "the graphemic representation in the output buffer decays very rapidly but can be refreshed through a phonological 'rehearsal' loop" (p. 153). However, JS's additional phonological processing disorder meant that the graphemic output buffer could not be refreshed in writing. Caramazza et al. therefore argued for a direct "refreshing" role between buffers, with the superior buffer refreshing the inferior.

Based on the assumption that there is a potential two-way, "refreshing" relationship between graphemic and phonological assembly, it can be argued that WL's graphemic assembly therapy resulted not only in an improvement in writing but also in spoken output. Prior to therapy, WL's graphemic assembly was too impaired to be of any benefit in refreshing his phonological assembly deficit. After therapy, WL became able unpack and assemble graphemic representations more effectively and so this serially ordered information could then "refresh" phonological processes in reading aloud and naming, thus compensating for rapid decay in the phonological output buffer. Importantly, this explanation would account for the finding that the written word form (in reading aloud) did not aid spoken output prior to therapy: Until WL could process a written word as an ordered string of graphemes, the written word was of no use to his disordered phonological assembly system; it was merely a whole lexical item that could not be unpacked/encoded into its constituent parts. However, after therapy the graphemic representation could be "unpacked" and reading aloud improved by virtue of the "refreshing" relationship between graphemic and phonological output buffers.

The effect of graphemic assembly therapy on spoken output was not one of direct remediation of phonological assembly but an indirect effect, counteracting WL's rapid decay in the phonological output buffer. This argument would also explain why repetition made no additional benefits from therapy. Because (after the initial input therapy) the phonological input representation was available to refresh the phonological output buffer in repetition, the improved availability of graphemic information would be redundant. However, repetition benefited from ongoing (spontaneous) recovery of phonological assembly and, since it did not rely on graphemic support, no actual therapy effect was found. The contrasting drawing-to-a-halt of further gains in reading aloud and naming once therapy ceased can be accounted for by the decline in the graphemic assembly system, which remained essential to both tasks. No actual decline was observed in naming and reading aloud since phonological assembly had made some spontaneous recovery, counterbalancing graphemic decline.

Conclusions for graphemic assembly therapy

Despite the difficulties that arose in trying to employ single case study methodology in a weekly, out-patient setting, it has been possible to demonstrate significant effects of graphemic assembly therapy. Converging sources of evidence were sought, which included generalisation to spoken output tasks and patterns of maintenance once the therapy programme had ceased.

It is concluded that improvements in four out of five tasks occurred as a result of graphemic therapy. These improvements involved generalisation to untreated items and to spoken tasks. WL's performance remained significantly superior to pre-therapy levels in all tasks, 3 months after therapy ceased. In addition, therapy took place after what is often cited as the period of greatest spontaneous recovery (Basso, 1992). All this information meant that these findings could be later used to support the argument that WL's NHS Trust should fund further SLT.

Finally, a theoretical explanation has been arrived at, which, if supported by further research, may provide an illustration of how therapy can inform theory and not simply the reverse.

Carry-over of language skills and functional relevance

The vexing question as to whether changes at the impairment level affected changes in real-life communication inevitably rears its head in all impairment-based treatment programmes. In terms of functional writing, no pre-therapy assessments were made although WL's use of

writing as a functional strategy increased in parallel with his abilities. However, there was a short period after writing therapy when WL did need reminding to try writing words in order to overcome his word-finding difficulties. Soon after the therapy programme ended, WL's ability to write sentences was assessed, using the test of Thematic Roles in Production (Whitworth, 1996), and it was found that WL's sentence production was relatively good post-therapy. His ability to write a description of the Cookie Theft Picture was also assessed very soon after therapy and revealed greater difficulties, and his ability to write propositionally was found to be virtually nil. Writing was therefore targeted in the next phase of SLT and, while it is not to be reported here, WL's written Cookie Theft Picture description rose from 52% correct in June to 81% correct in September 1997.

In terms of spoken communication, WL was quite typical of many "conduction-type" aphasics, in that his communicative performance was always equal to his actual competence. Thus, the therapist had little to "teach" him. In terms of objective measures, "The Story of Cinderella" and conversations were videoed at regular intervals and illustrate WL's functional improvements (but have not been formally analysed). Indeed, in his fifth and final Story of Cinderella assessment with the second author, WL comments with great enthusiasm on the improvements he has made in the task. So whilst some SLTs may have objections to this measure, it was of benefit to both SLTs and WL himself.

Handicap and emotional issues arising from it

Although the emphasis in this section has been on WL's impairments and the therapy directed at them, his psychological adjustment was also a constant area of therapist involvement. From our fourth session onwards WL reported feelings which suggested that he was experiencing an acute sense of loss. Factors that related to WL's psychosocial adjustment are summarised in Figure 3.5.

WL's partner, J, was initially very involved with him. She attended SLT sessions and supported him in the community. Unfortunately, she bore

FIGURE 3.5

Primary factor:

• WL's aphasia and its direct effects

Sense of loss of:

• a job he enjoyed and career prospects
• the ability to be a father and provider
• social status in his community and peer group
• attractiveness to women

Exacerbating factors:

• WL's personality & coping strategies
• WL's social circumstances
• WL's difficulties coping manifested in angry outbursts, social withdrawal and general symptoms of depression

Management made more difficult by:

• the distance of NHNN from WL's local community
• only one session a week
• the lack of active family involvement
• WL's anger/emotional reaction

Factors related to WL's emotional difficulties.

the brunt of his anger and their relationship deteriorated over the first couple of months and became very "on–off". WL became increasingly concerned about his ability to act as a father, particularly to his 7-year-old son. This caused him feelings of humiliation and anger.

A number of WL's family members attended SLT sessions, some of whom were also quite angry about WL's circumstances. Sometimes this was manifest as anger towards the therapist. Unfortunately, other than J, no one ever attended SLT more than once, and no family member ever contacted the therapist to discuss WL nor did they take up any invitations, advice, or suggestions given. WL appeared to feel very let down by his family at times. He complained that they all did a lot of talking but never did anything else to help him.

Work issues

WL's main goal was to get back to work. Unfortunately, his work as a GP practice receptionist involved the comprehension and production of very specific language such as names, times, dates, and test results.

Initially, WL's employers agreed to keep his job open for him for 3 months, which WL accepted. However, it seems probable that he was anticipating a quick resolution to his aphasia and thus a quick return to work. As time passed and changes were slow, work became a bigger and bigger issue for WL.

Eventually, WL's employers were forced to take on a replacement and so stop paying him. Nevertheless, the appointment was made on a 6-month contract in order to allow WL the opportunity to return at the end of the year if he was able.

WL was referred to the occupational therapy (OT) department at the neurological hospital in March, due to some subtle disturbance in his right hand function. The OT then involved the Disability Employment Officer (DEA) at WL's local job centre. Unfortunately, WL's initial appointment with the DEA (in late June) went badly and so this potential source of help was lost. The DEA was concerned that WL's difficulty controlling his anger meant that it would be difficult to recommend him for employment. At the time, WL was still awaiting an appointment with a cognitive-behaviour therapist at the neurological hospital, who, it was hoped, would be able to help WL control his angry outbursts.

In the meantime WL was encouraged to consider what alternative work he might pursue, utilising his strengths. He was able to do DIY at home, which he enjoyed, but he was very concerned that he would be forced into working as a manual labourer, which he was very reluctant to do. He felt proud of the fact that he had made something of his life, having had a rather chequered record at school, and was despondent to be back to square one. He liked art and was also interested in working with disabled people. Opportunities at his local adult education college were investigated but WL was not keen to pursue any of the courses.

"Political" issues

Finally, it is interesting to consider some of the wider "political" issues raised by a case such as WL. As an SLT I found myself in the position of objecting strongly to the failure of WL's local SLT service to provide for him. In addition, I was unclear as to whether or not it was professional to encourage and assist a client to make complaints about another SLT service. However, I felt that factors such as cultural and educational background made it difficult for WL's family to become actively involved in advocating on his behalf. I also felt acutely aware that by agreeing to see him at a specialist hospital I was shoring up this inadequate local service. This presented a professional dilemma; balancing the needs of the individual against wider service provision issues. Communicating Quality 2 (RCSLT, 1997) states that "The speech & language therapist should aim to educate professionals, employers and others in positions of social significance in order to increase their understanding of aphasia". However, our role as advocate is not directly mentioned. I tried to reconcile this by taking a number of steps summarised in Figure 3.6.

Despite the fact that WL had to wait an interval of many months, his referral to the specialist dysphasia centre described in Section Two proved to be an invaluable next step.

SECTION TWO

Background

This section attempts to continue to describe and discuss the therapy and therapeutic process conducted with WL. It follows the therapy described by the first author and tracks subsequent therapeutic involvement in the management of this person with aphasia. Whilst the therapy conducted previously had addressed aspects of disability and handicap, it focused primarily upon impairment-based therapy utilising the period of the client's maximum potential for spontaneous recovery.

In contrast, the therapy described in this section was done almost 1-year post CVA. Hence, the

---

FIGURE 3.6

Initial report measure

Specified that WL would only be seen as a temporary measure and urged all professionals (e.g. GP) to complain to his NHS Trust. Also advised family to complain to Trust, GP, MP etc. but they did not do so.

Contacted ADA

Wrote to ADA (Speakability) asking for their support for WL and his family.
a. ADA wrote to Chief Executive
b. ADA drew up standard letters of complaint for family (which family never used, which angered WL)

Contacted Royal College of Speech Language Therapists

Asked for professional guidance, which resulted in:
a. practical advice
b. "it would be inappropriate for you to act as lobbyist on this occasion but client/carers could be pointed in the right direction"

Patient advocate

In last few sessions helped WL to write a letter, outlining his predicament.
- we discussed
- I drafted
- we discussed and he edited
- we circulated to family
- (no feedback)
- we finalised and sent to 15 agencies
- WL did not want to involve Press

Other resources

a. SLT student: a student SLT sought from university for a 5-week block in order to provide intensive SLT
b. Referral to specialist dysphasia group: referred WL almost 6 months to the day post-onset (= referral criteria). The following issues were highlighted:
- difficulty fulfilling role as father
- unable to return to work
- difficulty socialising

Summary of action relating to "political" issues.

---

intervention primarily focused upon disability issues taking into account a social model approach to working with aphasia. The prospect of specific impairment-based therapy, however, was not excluded. The intervention with WL outlined in this chapter describes initial therapy and the ongoing "work in progress" that was being conducted at the time.

The philosophy

LeDorze and Brassard (1995) linked the World Health Organisation's models of Impairment, Disability and Handicap (1980) to descriptions of aphasia, thus supplying a framework in which to describe therapies beyond the level of the language impairment.

The disability movement has been a key driving force in the development of the social model of disability (e.g., Lenny, 1993; Oliver, 1987), which states that disability does not stem from the functional limitations of impaired individuals but rather from the failure of the social and physical environment to take account of disabled people's needs.

A social model approach considers the perspective of the disabled individual's experience rather than that of the health professional. This is set within a framework of gaining a positive disabled identity, identifying and dismantling the barriers that aphasic people face in their everyday lives (Pound, 1998).

Whilst the therapy described within this chapter addresses some of the issues associated with identity and barriers, it is by necessity from the perspective of the author as a speech and language therapist, rather than from that of the person with aphasia themselves.

Initial interview

WL was initially assessed in December 1997, having not received SLT intervention for 3 months. He attended the appointment with his girlfriend J. The purpose of the initial assessment, like most initial sessions, was to become acquainted with the client and vice versa, to investigate the nature of the communication impairment and any changes from the time of referral, and to determine whether attendance at the clinic might be appropriate and beneficial.

On initial impressions and informal assessment, WL's communication abilities were broadly similar to those described by the first author and WL was able to express many of his ideas.

However, as a therapist, the overriding amount of effort and work associated with that first session was trying to manage WL's frustration and anger. He had not received speech and language therapy since being discharged from the tertiary hospital facility as there was no adult SLT service available for him within his local borough.

Throughout the session, WL became increasingly agitated, particularly with his girlfriend, who at the time of the appointment was pointing out to him that he had to "help himself". The session ended with WL swearing and walking out of the clinic, having had a row with his girlfriend. At that point the only thing I, as a therapist, was able to do was to offer WL, via his girlfriend, an appointment for the following week. It later transpired that the emotions displayed in that session were somewhat typical of an initial interaction of WL with anyone who represented part of an establishment or official body (e.g., occupational therapist, Disabled Employment Office, member of Different Strokes).

It could have been at this point that WL failed to access further speech language therapy and hence a source of support that could be providing input to address his difficulties. Typically, speech and language therapists are under pressure to allocate resources to those who will benefit from intervention quickly (demonstrating a measurable outcome) and within a potentially limited contract. WL was someone who quite clearly had significant psychosocial needs and the picture was unclear as to whether he would benefit or even attend therapy sessions. On the other hand, here was someone who had obviously benefited from input in the past and had shown significant improvement.

WL arrived for his appointment the following week and never subsequently displayed the behaviour evident on the first appointment, although he was often frustrated and angry.

Initial assessment

Initial sessions were spent establishing, from WL's perspective, his experience and difficulties resulting from his CVA and aphasia. This included not only identification of barriers, but also language assessment. This enabled WL to demonstrate his language abilities and feel understood and heard about his difficulties. Perhaps it also provided a structure and safety net for the therapist and client as the in-depth impact of aphasia was investigated.

Identity and roles

As a result of his stroke and subsequent aphasia, WL had experienced a significant loss of many roles within his life, culminating in an overall loss of his sense of his former self (Brumfitt, 1993).

These included loss of:

- financial income as a full-time employee
- social life within a young, fast-moving crowd
- feeling like an authority figure and protector of his children
- image through loss of pride and ability to participate in his own culture
- relationships with his partner, brother, and family, to varying degrees.

Barriers

Barriers experienced by a person with a disability can be described in terms of environmental, structural, attitudinal and informational. Some of the barriers WL was experiencing are described below.

Environmental

These are the difficulties the environment presents in allowing an individual to be able to participate equally in communication.

- WL's social life consisted of attending raves and social occasions that were noisy, involved many people talking, and also involved a "street" language of their own.
- The workplace where WL was employed at the time of his stroke was a busy, crowded, but friendly GP surgery. He worked there as a receptionist. Again, this was noisy environment that demanded fast and effective communication skills both in written and spoken language.

Structural

Structural barriers include the inability to access social services and other services effectively in order to gain the necessary support required.

Upon investigation, this barrier was all too evident. WL's inability to read or use the telephone effectively proved a huge disabling effect in trying to access services. Help was not available as his relationship with J, his girlfriend, had broken down and his brother was no longer living with WL in his flat. Examples include:

- As a result of the letter jointly written by the first author and WL, which complained about the lack of SLT service in his local borough, WL received a letter from the chief executive explaining why there was no service. Unfortunately, this consisted of a two-page, small print letter explaining the finer details of London Inner Zone funding and the prioritisation system within the Health Authority. WL's MP also responded to his letter, enclosing a copy of the same letter written by the chief executive.
- At the time of an initial social services assessment, J had been identified as the main carer and was in receipt of some benefit. After the break-up of their relationship, J continued to receive money and it was extremely difficult for WL to understand the system and identify benefits that he was entitled to. This also meant a huge loss of independence and privacy as he was forced to declare all earnings and benefits, etc., not only to Social Services, but also to other professionals who could potentially advocate on his behalf.

Attitudinal

Attitudinal barriers include perceptions of others about aphasia and its impact. For WL, these have included the following.

- Difficulty communicating with a wide network of friends who did not understand WL's reluctance to speak.
- Conflict between WL and his father, who believed WL should simply accept his disability and seek non-communication-based employment and leisure activities. "Can't you just tell him to take up pottery classes or something?"
- Difficulties in his relationships in communicating with his children. WL described his

loss of his role as a father. In particular, he felt unable to help his 8-year-old son with his homework.

- Potential barriers in meeting WL's wish to return to work. Did his colleagues still view him as a competent individual with skills to offer?

Informational

These include barriers concerning access to information as well as difficulties communicating information.

- Difficulties in processing and utilising information essential to gaining support (e.g., letters from social services, information from the Stroke Association).
- Difficulties in being able to select and express relevant information that would assist potential advocates whilst not compromising personal confidentiality. This was particularly evident in disclosing information on finances.

As a result of the above, intervention with WL addressed identity and barrier work within the context of WL's aphasia. To give the impression that WL's therapy was a seamless service addressing all things social and psychological would be greatly misleading. Input was never a question of merely providing a few communicative ramps in order to overcome some simple and clearly defined obstacles. Instead, it entailed a somewhat complex process through largely uncharted territory. However, a fundamental aspect of the management of therapy sessions was juggling the complexity of the situation and being able to respond to the priorities at any one given moment, whilst still trying to maintain sight of planned therapy goals.

The intervention described below is not listed in chronological order, but rather tries to pull out the themes of identity and barrier work that was an integral part of WL's therapy. It is based very much on WL's personal experience of his aphasia, and attempts to promote an appreciation of WL's skills and self-worth alongside attempts to dismantle some of the barriers that he was and continues to face. It should also be acknowledged

that the headings which describe the therapies are included for the sake of structure and organisation. In reality, the therapies interlinked and frequently the outcome of one idea became the inspiration and logical step to the next.

Returning to work

Very shortly after WL had begun to attend City Dysphasic Group (CDG), in London, the practice manager from the surgery where WL had worked contacted the clinic asking for a professional opinion as to whether WL would be able to return to work. WL's job had officially been kept open for a year, but his employers had reached the stage where they were reluctant to keep his job open any longer without an assurance of an ability to return to work.

Rather than stating categorically whether WL could return to work, the nature of WL's communication disability was explained and discussion took place about which tasks within the workplace would still be possible, which had potential, and which were likely to be very difficult to achieve.

A visit to the surgery was arranged whereby the practice manager, SLT, and WL identified tasks that WL would be able to continue to do. These included filing, recording of blood and urine samples sent off for analysis, giving out prescriptions that patients came to collect, and checking in orders such as stationery. Tasks WL felt he was no longer capable of doing were the more front-line tasks of answering the phone, talking with patients, and booking their appointments.

These tasks, both ones WL could do and ones he had doubts about, were then simulated in therapy. WL was very accurate at predicting tasks he was still able to fulfil. The one exception to this was in giving patients prescriptions. Whilst entirely accurate in checking the patients' details against the prescription form, WL was unable to reliably ask for a person's date of birth or address. Specific impairment-based language work to help WL on this task was therefore conducted.

As a result of the above, WL's prospects for future employment were opened up. WL was taken on for a trial part-time period of

3 months, working 9 hours per week so as not to jeopardise his benefits. SLT input took the form of offering training for staff about the nature of aphasia, regular reviews, and an undertaking to link therapy tasks to relevant work tasks.

Since commencing work, WL's contract was expanded and increased to to 21 working hours per week; a level that enabled him to come off income support. Instead, WL was employed under a supported placement scheme in recognition of the need for him to have potential in his career and with a view to expanding his work opportunities. The GP practice also took financial advantage of a government "New Deal" scheme at that time.

Whilst WL is not doing the job he was doing previously, he nevertheless has re-accessed some employment that has credence and some status, and the practice has shown a willingness to consider ways of expanding WL's role that are not so dependent upon receptionist duties.

In my opinion, throughout this process there were two major obstacles to overcome, neither of which were fully negotiated.

- The Social Services benefits system had been a logistical nightmare for WL's employers to understand and negotiate. It is the opinion of the author that had it not been for the practice manager's commitment and willingness to step outside his usual role, re-accessing employment in a realistic way for WL might have failed.
- Having got over the euphoria of returning to work on a part-time basis, WL was often frustrated by his limited role at the surgery. This meant that at times there were fears that the emotional effects of WL's stroke, set against his personality, might have jeopardised WL's ability to act appropriately at work. However, those fears turned out, eventually, to be unfounded.

Was this being paternalistic and overprotective? If therapy is viewed as a partnership, should there have been more trust in WL's commitment and ability? Interestingly, the practice manager expressed similar fears, but then qualified his comment:

There have been times when WL has inevitably got quite frustrated with the situation and that has been expressed in very obvious ways, like he's walked out a couple of times and just gone down the road for a bit, which obviously is not how you'd normally deal with that situation. Having said that, every member of staff occasionally gets frustrated and perhaps just goes out of the room for a few minutes. I mean it's nothing that we can't cope with.

(Self-) advocacy—teaching other people about a new disabled identity

Aphasia is not apparent to others until the aphasic person tries to communicate, and this may make the disorder less readily comprehensible than more visible impairments such as paralysis. (Jordan & Kaiser, 1996)

During the early part of therapy at CDG, the Action for Dysphasia Adults (ADA) video "Dysphasia Matters" had been shown to WL in order to assist in his understanding of aphasia and its impact on people. This commercially available video was particularly poignant, as it used people who had aphasia to explain the manifestation and impacts aphasia. Following the success of using this video with WL, coupled with its original purpose to train health professionals, we combined the "Dysphasia Matters" video with a self-made video to use as a training tool for WL's colleagues at the surgery. Staff at the surgery included the receptionists, the practice manager, the doctors, and practice nurses. It was important that the training was accessible to all and video format was ideal in achieving this. By alternating the formal ADA video with pre-recorded clips of WL's descriptions of his own aphasia, it was possible to give a clear account of his abilities.

This was then followed by an open discussion, facilitated by myself, in which staff were able to ask WL questions about his communication that he was able to respond to "on-line".

The rationale behind this training session and the use of video as a means of presentation was threefold:

- to heighten awareness of WL's aphasia and its impact for his work colleagues
- to enable an open discussion between WL and his work colleagues about ways of reducing barriers of communication in the workplace
- to enable WL to have a "voice" and therefore advocate for himself without the pressure of "on the spot" explanations.

The session received positive feedback from all concerned, and WL reported greater opportunities for communication and equal discussion. With the benefit of hindsight, it would have been ideal to measure the benefit of this approach more formally. Set against a health culture of demonstrating quantitative outcomes, we should strive for more concrete ways of demonstrating benefits and change, based not only upon quantitative but also qualitative information in order to add credence and value to "less traditional" approaches.

I believe that preparing for and participating in this session had many therapeutic benefits for WL They included:

- identification with others with aphasia
- providing the opportunity for self-expression and disclosure
- revealing WL's communicative competence by having him serve as an expert to train others.

Interestingly enough, WL also chose to use those tapes to show his family. I was not involved in this apart from supplying the videos. Thus, WL advocated for himself about his communication disability. Was another outcome, therefore, that WL had found a means by which to advocate for himself?

Promoting a positive identity—improving self-confidence and self-worth

Throughout both authors' discussions, we have made reference to some of the emotional and psychological aspects that have been an integral part of SLT management. Whilst in therapy, WL was referred to our stroke counsellor who had personal experience of stroke and dysphasia. WL attended a few sessions, but felt that counselling

was not a useful source of support for him. "Well, I've told him all that there is now." I had naturally assumed that counselling would be a solution for WL. In reality, some people, including WL, are reluctant to take up counselling, even with an experienced counsellor who had insight into communication disability.

A set of pictures of "blobby men" (Wilson, 1992) were used as a visual means of self-expression requiring WL to plot his emotional reactions to intervention. This also proved useful as a means of acknowledging his experiences and adjustment to date.

Later on in therapy, WL was shown some personal portfolios completed by other people with aphasia. In their document "Self Advocacy at Work" (EMFEC, 1991), the authors describe a "portfolio" as a collection of information about an individual's past, information and examples of what is happening in the present, and plans, ideas, and dreams for the future. The purpose behind developing a personal portfolio includes:

- as a means of seeing oneself and building self-identity and self esteem
- to see oneself in relation to other people
- as a focus for developing skills including making choices and decisions, being assertive, and representing oneself
- for progression to education, training, employment
- to record what has been achieved and to gain credit.

Again, WL was fascinated and also intrigued at how the people concerned had managed to compile their portfolios when they had aphasic language difficulties. WL had expressed a desire to write a book "when I get better". I considered that a portfolio might be a way of meeting that desire to some extent, and at the same time facilitating a concept of alternative ways of expressing oneself. Portfolios had also been used very successfully with a high-level language group at CDG.

We hit a stumbling block when pursuing this project. Despite expressing a desire to return to life as it was before the stroke, WL had difficulty in identifying positive life events and achievements from the past. The idea of a portfolio was abandoned with the proviso of reinstigating it in the future and including a retrospective look at achievements since WL's stroke. It is possible that portfolios work best within a group context, allowing group members to support each other

Conclusions

Therapeutic intervention with WL did not only focus upon the disability therapies described above. It included tasks directly related to communication, including strategies for accessing written information (e.g., key word reading) and dealing with numbers, particularly finances. Ideas for therapeutic input in the future included a video diary as a means of continuing to establish a positive identify, facilitating access to adult education or employment-related training, and the possibility of some further specific impairment-based work.

The input described above complements the impairment-based therapy outlined by the first author. Neither approach is mutually exclusive, and the therapeutic approaches adopted were designed to meet WL's different needs at different times.

REFERENCES

Action for Dysphasic Adults. (1997). *Dysphasia matters: Training for medical staff*. Videotape.

Allport, A. (1984). Auditory-verbal short-term memory and conduction aphasia. In H. Bouma & D.G. Bouwhuis (Eds.), *Attention and performance 10: Control of language processes*. Hillsdale, NJ: Lawrence Erlbaum Associates Inc.

Basso, A. (1992). Prognostic factors in aphasia. *Aphasiology, 6*, 337–348.

Brumfitt, S. (1993). Losing our sense of self: What aphasia can do. *Aphasiology, 7*, 569–575.

Butterworth, B. (1992). Disorders of phonological encoding. *Cognition, 42*, 261–280.

Caramazza, A., Basili, A., Koller, J., & Berndt, R. (1981). An investigation of repetition and language processing in a case of conduction aphasia. *Brain and Language, 14*, 235–271.

Caramazza, A., Berndt, R., & Basili, A. (1983). The selective impairment of phonological processing: A case study. *Brain and Language, 18*, 128–174.

Caramazza, A., & Micelli, G. (1990). Orthographic structure, the graphemic buffer and spelling process. In C. von Euler, I. Lundberg, & G. Lennerstrand (Eds.), *Brain and reading*. Macmillan/Wenner-Gren International Symposium Series. Basingstoke, UK: Palgrave Macmillan.

EMFEC. (1991). *Further education, training and support. Self advocacy at work. Training materials for people involved in supporting others to represent themselves*. Nottingham, UK: Print Partnership.

Franklin, S., Buerk, F., & Howard, D. (2002). Generalised improvement in speech production for a subject with reproduction conduction aphasia. *Aphasiology, 16*, 1087–1114.

Goswami, U., & Bryant, P. (1990). *Phonological skills and learning to read*. London: LEA.

Joanette, Y., Keller, E., & Lecours, A.R. (1980). Sequence of phonemic approximations in aphasia. *Brain and Language, 11*, 30–44.

Jordan, L., & Kaiser, W. (1996). *Aphasia, a social approach*. London: Chapman & Hall.

Kay, J., Lesser, R., & Coltheart, M. (1992). *Psycholinguistic assessment of language processing in aphasia*. Hillsdale, NJ: Lawrence Erlbaum Associates Inc.

Kohn, S. (1989). The nature of the phonemic string deficit in conduction aphasia. *Aphasiology, 3*, 209–239.

LeDorze, G., & Brassard, C. (1995). A description of the consequences of aphasia on aphasic persons and their relatives and friends, based on the WHO model of chronic diseases. *Aphasiology, 9*, 239–355.

Lenny, J. (1993). Do disabled people need counselling? In E. Swain, V. Finklestein, S. French, & M. Oliver (Eds.), *Disabling barriers, enabling environments*. London: Open University Press.

Levelt, W.J.M., & Wheeldon, L. (1994). Do speakers have access to a mental syllabry? *Cognition, 50*, 239–269.

Marshall, J., Robson, J., Pring, T., & Chiat, S. (1998). Why does monitoring fail in jargonaphasia: Comprehension, judgement and therapy evidence. *Brain and Language, 63*, 79–107.

Morris, J., Franklin, S., Ellis, A., Turner, J., & Bailey, P. (1996). Remediating a speech perception deficit in an aphasic patient. *Aphasiology, 10*, 137–158.

Nespoulous, J.-L., Joanette, Y., Ska, B., Caplan, D., & Lecours, A.R. (1987). Production deficits in Broca's and conduction aphasia: Repetition versus reading. In E. Keller & M. Gopnik (Eds.), *Motor and sensory processes in language*. Hillsdale, NJ: Lawrence Erlbaum Associates Inc.

Oliver, M. (1987). Re-defining disability: Some issues for research. *Research Policy and Planning, 5*, 9–13.

Pierce, R. (1992). Apraxia of speech versus phonemic paraphasia: Theoretical, diagnostic and treatment considerations. In D. Vogel & M. Cannito (Eds.), *Treating disordered speech motor control: For clinicians by clinicians*. Austin, TX: Pro-Ed.

Pound, C. (1998). Therapy for life: Finding new paths across the plateau. Clinical Forum, *Aphasiology, 12*, 222–227.

RCSLT. (1997). *Communicating quality 2: Professional standards for Speech Language Therapists*. London: Royal College of Speech and Language Therapists.

Shallice, T., & Warrington, E. (1977). Auditory verbal short-term memory impairment in conduction aphasia. *Brain and Language, 4*, 479–491.

Strub, R.L., & Gardner, H. (1974). The repetition deficit in conduction aphasia: Mnestic or linguistic? *Brain and Language, 1*, 241–255.

Van der Gaag, A. (Ed.) (1996). *Communicating quality 2*. London: Royal College of Speech and Language Therapists.

Whitworth, A. (1996). *Thematic roles in production (TRIP): An assessment of word retrieval at the sentence level*. London: Whurr.

Wilshire, C., & McCarthy, R. (1996). Experimental investigations of an impairment in phonological encoding, *Cognitive Neuropsychology, 13*, 1059–1098.

Wilson, P. (1992). *Games without frontiers: Fun, growth and development games for group workers (1988)*. London: Marshall Pickering.

4

Beyond the simple sentence level: A case study of a client with high level aphasia

Debbie Graham

This is a report of a therapy programme provided to KB, a 56-year-old man with dysphasia. The therapy was administered in three phases. Initially, from 6 months post onset, the emphasis of therapy was on syntax, phonology, and morphology. We then moved on to a therapy that involved monitoring strategies for dealing with on-line processing, complex sentences, and low frequency verbs. In the final stage we embarked on therapy to address organisational skills, in an attempt to improve KB's cohesion of ideas. Throughout all the therapies we worked to help KB to develop realistic expectations so that he could come to terms with his aphasia. Before describing the therapy programmes in detail, I will provide some background information about KB.

BACKGROUND

KB was 56 years of age and married with three children, two grown-up and one just beginning secondary level education. Prior to his CVA, he worked as a Finance Director for a local transport company. KB had worked for various accountancy companies throughout his career, after graduating from Durham University aged 22 with two degrees (maths and economics). Work constituted a large part of KB's life. He would often spend 12 or more hours a day at the office in the week. KB's wife worked part-time as a bank employee. They both enjoyed an active social life, mainly centred around their local Methodist church, where KB held a key role as a preacher at the Sunday Services and enjoyed the annual review, where he always excelled as the "compere". KB was a very private person and he was not comfortable sharing feelings openly. He had a wonderful sense of humour and enjoyed good conversation.

KB was admitted to hospital, presenting with a left CVA and right hemiparesis. He had a history of hypertension, and a carotoid scan revealed a 50% stenosis in the left internal carotid artery.

ASSESSMENT

Several assessments were done, one initially at the hospital, an in-patient one done by another therapist, and a second when KB was transferred to the rehabilitation unit. A summary of those combined results revealed the following.

Initial evaluation results, in the hospital, immediately post-stroke

- KB was able to comprehend social questions, but was inconsistent in following verbal commands
- he had mild right sided facial weakness
- no appropriate verbal output
- KB's attempts at speech led to non-words and "dyspraxic" type groping
- he was very agitated and obviously frustrated.

Results from an assessment at the Rehabilitation Unit

These tests were administered approx 6 months post onset when he was transferred to residential rehabilitation unit.

Single word and sentence level investigations

A combination of formal and informal measures were used to examine levels of functioning, based on the cognitive neuropsychological principles of language processing (Garrett, 1980; Kay, Lesser, & Coltheart, 1992).

It became evident that KB had difficulties at a number of different levels of processing (semantic, syntactic) that continued to affect both written and verbal fluency. He also had difficulties with low frequency verb access, struggling with tasks such as those following.

Lexical semantic anomalies
"The barber *captured* the razor." (KB accessed, from a written choice, closely related verbs, trimming, cutting, but knew they were incorrect.)

Verb synonyms
"The chimney *produced* thick smoke."

Noun access
Good high frequency noun access but reduced access to low frequency items.

Phonological/phonetic accessing difficulties
KB struggled with:

- Syllabification: He struggled to internally segment multisyllabic words.
- Unable to convert written vowels to spoken ones.
- Sound substitutions, "false starts", particularly with words of increasing length.

Morphology access
Difficulties with tense agreement across sentences evidenced in written sentence completion tasks.

Argument structure access
Once the verb was accessed, KB appeared to have appropriate access to the argument structure and mapping.

Syntax
Input syntactic knowledge was accurate.

Conversation
A conversational sample of KB's response to a question "What have you been doing this morning?" and to the Cookie Theft picture is transcribed in Appendix 4.1. Analysis of the sample indicated the following pattern of performance:

- verb accessing problems
- hesitant effortful output

- some aborted sentences
- starts by slotting a lexical item into the correct thematic role, but then self-corrects, e.g., the "kitchen is in a"
- difficulty in accessing syllable initial phonemes and repetitions
- some use of sentence co-ordination but no use of complex connectives or causal information
- content limited and little elaboration of ideas
- struggling to access semantics
- perseveration
- limited range of tenses and verb structures
- occasional vowel error.

Boston Naming Test (Goodglass & Kaplan, 1972)
KB scored 54/60; errors were length effects and phonetic errors.

THE FIRST PHASE OF THERAPY: SYNTAX, PHONOLOGY, AND MORPHOLOGY (6 MONTHS POST-ONSET)

KB was seen from four to five times per week during his 6-month stay as an in-patient at the unit. He returned home on the weekends. Each session lasted around 45 minutes. The focus of therapy at the early stages was to address the underlying language impairment, basing my approach on cognitive neuropsychological principles.

Aims of the phase one therapy
1. To improve wider access to the lexicon (particularly low frequency items) across different word groups.
2. Increase access to morpho-syntax, both verbally and in the written format.
3. To improve phonological/phonetic processing, particularly for words of increasing length, and to develop phoneme-to-grapheme link for vowels.
4. To improve access to tense markings across sentences.

This therapy focus continued for 7 weeks. The tasks themselves, as well as conversational exchange, were used as measures of change. With the increase in the amount of written work we were doing, KB moved onto using a word processor, which overcame both the fatigue and the physical factors affecting his written output. His right hand still had no functional use in either the wrist or selective finger movements. KB remained highly motivated during therapy, and was given tasks each time he was seen to complete outside of each session.

Therapy methods
The following is a summary of the whole range of therapy tasks and activities that KB undertook:

- given a set of verbs within the same semantic field KB was asked to put them into simple sentences
- KB replaced low frequency verbs in a given sentence structure with a synonym
- given a verb category, KB was asked to access a range of verbs within the category and then put them into sentences (all tasks were completed with both verbal and written output)
- KB provided a synonym for a given adjective
- KB identified a correct/incorrect verb particle in a given sentence
- KB selected an appropriate verb to fit into given sentence structure
- KB put one verb plus a variety of particles linked to that verb into appropriate sentences
- KB identified tense errors in simple and complex sentences
- KB used his own sentences with errors as a source of material for him to analyse and correct
- KB put written sentences into past, future, and passive sentences
- KB gave a verbal description of sequencing cards using different tenses
- KB manipulated sentence structure, e.g., he transformed statements into questions
- KB "unjumbled" complex sentences verbally and then wrote them down
- KB segmented single words into separate consonants and vowels

- KB practised with comparative and superlative adjectives by generating them from a given root and then generating a sentence around them
- KB performed tasks building on earlier grapheme-to-phoneme tests, e.g., reading aloud nonsense syllable chains such as nin wandat.

Progress

At the end of therapy, KB showed improvement in many areas. These included identifying tense errors and phonological processing skills. He was able to identify and segment syllable structures and his reading aloud was highly fluent. There was a reduction in struggle behaviour, experienced previously with polysyllabic production. KB was beginning to notice some errors in his own conversation and to correct himself. Although he was highly functional and coping well with the demands of most everyday conversation, there was still evidence of word-accessing difficulties affecting his planning of sentence structure and ultimately his fluency.

While his core skills had improved, he was still vulnerable to language breakdown in "on-line processing"; it appeared that processing overload, fatigue, and word-finding difficulties for low frequency words were all continuing to affect his overall fluency.

KB continued to have high expectations of himself. At this stage, he wanted to resume full-time work. We spent a great deal of time debating this issue and discussing whether his goals were realistic. As a clinician, I was challenged to consider what the future goals would be. Were we aiming for grammatical/semantic completeness? Were we aiming for greater communicative competence, which would essentially still leave him with aphasic language? KB's pre-stroke sophisticated use of language was a major part of both his work and social life. He viewed himself as being a fluent, confident speaker who, prior to his CVA, enjoyed taking centre stage; for example, regularly giving sermons in his local church or acting as compere at church variety productions. As his therapist I felt that I should try to maximise his communicative potential even though I

could not be sure that further progress would be made.

My sense was that, if we could address processing of language off-line by bringing the impact of processing overload to a "conscious" level for KB and increasing his awareness of the planning skills involved in the integration of semantic/syntax and cognition, then we might see a transfer into on-line processing. At the same time we could continue to improve low frequency word access.

THE SECOND PHASE OF THERAPY: ON-LINE PROCESSING, COMPLEX SENTENCES, LOW FREQUENCY VERBS

Aims of phase two therapy

1. To build KB's self-monitoring and awareness of being too apologetic (he was constantly saying sorry when he had word-finding difficulties).
2. To encourage him to reduce his rate of speech and give himself more time to plan syntactic output.
3. To bring to a conscious level lexical access and mapping of thematic roles onto syntactic structure.
4. To improve word-finding skills for low frequency verbs.

Therapy methods for phase two therapies

Although the following tasks were actually well within his capabilities, I felt that, by carrying them out, I was in essence getting him to think about the structure of the sentence—that is, the principles behind how to process a sentence for output. By bringing the process to conscious awareness, we might see some generalisation into conversation.

- Mapping task: For low frequency verbs such as "examine", "incinerate" before moving on to verbs that lead to more a complex clause structure, for example, "feel", "believe", "perceive", "think".
- Following this, KB had to access verbs within

a given category without support and then carry out the mapping task above.

KB was asked to determine the number of thematic roles that need to go with each type of verb, e.g., who, what, why, where?

We examined optional versus obligatory thematic roles such as temporal aspects and causal information. These were then built into spoken sentences, tape-recorded for evaluation by KB, and transferred into written output for practice outside of the session.

Letter of complaint

KB was asked to write a letter of complaint to British Gas regarding a faulty gas fire. When asked to describe the component parts of the letter, KB exhibited slow processing, but when he gave himself planning time he produced some clear sentence structures. He also had difficulty recognising when his ideas could be combined using more sophisticated structures. Finally, KB had some trouble with the use of connectives between sentences.

I felt that I needed to assess other types of discourse that would highlight KB's ability to use complex and varied structures as well as to provide information on his ability to cope with the increasing cognitive demands that these tasks would entail. Although conversation is unpredictable, it generally comprises shorter segments, therefore giving fewer opportunities to use complex structures than in other types of discourse (Freund, Hayter, MacDonald, Neary, & Wiseman-Hakes, 1999). The following tasks were therefore chosen to assess his discourse skills.

Assessing procedural discourse

"Describe how to sharpen a pencil". KB would have to provide simple syntactic structures that were temporally and hierarchically related

Assessing narrative discourse

Story-telling was used as an assessment tool for analysing KB's syntax and cohesive devices. A story is obviously centred around events and characters, so cohesive devices are critical to provide meaning throughout the text. As cohesion relies heavily on cognitive skills, I felt this task would also highlight any deficits in this area. KB was given characters and a basic setting to build a story around. He produced stories in written format using a word processor (see Appendix 4.2). The following tasks were designed to encourage him to recognise when and how to use a wider variety of clause structure aiming to achieve a more sophisticated cohesive output.

Complex sentences

KB was asked to combine two given sentences into one by identifying redundant information and using embedding.

He was also given a series of short simple sentences and asked to make the information more sophisticated by joining the sentences using appropriate connectives. Below is an example, and KB's response:

The sentences:
Pam fell last week. The fall occurred outside King's Cross Station. She cut her knee badly. No-one helped her.
KB's response:
Pam fell last week outside King's Cross Station, but cut her knee badly and no-one helped her.

Further, KB was asked to use sequential and composite pictures to generate coordinating/subordinating sentence structures. I felt this task was important because it gave us insight into his ability to gain a perspective on an event and its subsequent implication for his language access. With the picture material he had to decide where he was going to begin and what angle he would take. He was able to link sentences verbally (although they were slowly executed) with the appropriate connective. However, with more composite type pictures where the number of possible perspectives increased and were more intertwined, there was a noticeable deterioration in his output.

KB was then asked to formulate a short story from a set of written short simple sentences. The task involved linking the sentences with appropriate connectives.

For example:

Mary and Bill went into town. Bill went to purchase a new jumper.

Mary went to have a cup of tea. Mary did not return to the meeting point. Bill decided to go and look for her.

KB's response:

Mary and Bill went to town. Bill went to purchase a jumper whilst Mary went to have a cup of tea. Mary didn't return to the meeting point so Bill decided to go and look for her.

The picture material revealed KB's difficulties in drawing together a number of different perspectives on an event and linking to the appropriate language. How would this then affect his ability to sequence and summarise written information, particularly if the ideas were totally self-generated? In order to determine this, I asked him to generate a series of short sentences about an activity that happened over the weekend and then to link them into cohesive narrative text. For example, he said:

> Sunday morning L was ill. K looked after her. L had an ear ache. Sunday afternoon S and K went out. Went to Colne. Visited a church St. Barthols. 500 years old. Found Colne Library.

THE THIRD PHASE OF THERAPY: ORGANISATIONAL SKILLS AND DISCOURSE COHESION

When KB had to gather together a number of different perspectives and link them appropriately to language his performance markedly decreased. The more information he had to summarise, the more muddled his output became. KB was unaware of this even when it was pointed out to him. He would say "Well I wouldn't have done it like that before my stroke".

These tasks were making increasing demands on his cognitive skills and I felt that if we were to improve his ability to gather ideas together

cohesively, we needed to address organisational skills by using an external strategy. We achieved this through simultaneously working on low frequency word-finding tasks and getting KB to summarise information into key words, particularly related to events.

Therapy methods for phase three therapies

- KB was asked to summarise information by thinking of a single word to describe the following event, e.g., There's an ambulance. Nearby is a lady lying in the road. Near to her is a car with a smashed headlamp.
- He was also asked to think of synonyms for low frequency adjectives/adverbs (e.g., upset, sad) linking to each event.
- Creating an account of an historical incident. This demonstrated that he was beginning to show improved planning and execution of original ideas with detailed content but he still had some difficulty trying to bring together too many ideas into one sentence. (This was produced following the use of the narrative discourse structure framework to encourage better planning and organisation of ideas.)

It became clear that, when KB was given a structure to follow, his ability to organise his ideas and process them into language improved. However, he still had difficulties in manipulating language and summarising information; I felt this was due to increased cognitive demands. Also, his recognition skills at this level were very poor so that he was not able to reflect on what he had written.

I would have liked to have explored this therapy focus for longer than I was able, linking more closely to his work and social needs, and looking more closely at the area of taking a "perspective" on events. Perhaps I could have worked on where to start in conveying an event and perspective through using picture description tasks rather than just with the verbal and written tasks. Perhaps this would have had a carryover effect on his spoken and written skills.

SUMMARY

I felt the therapy programme had moved through three set phases. Initially we had concentrated on the simple sentence level, addressing simple semantics and syntax, before moving on to more complex sentences and increasing KB's self-monitoring skills. Finally, we had embarked on therapy to address organisational skills in an attempt to improve the cohesion of ideas.

Despite continued progress, KB still had aphasic language and he found this very difficult to accept. He still had inconsistent difficulties with word-finding, noticeable in tasks that demanded a high semantic or cognitive load (in written text and in on-line spoken processing). If he was overloaded or fatigued, his dysfluency increased, with back-tracking and hesitations. However, overall his language structure was more sophisticated, with an increase in the variety and type of complex clauses used. Written output continued to be superior to his spoken output, due to planning time and, of course, the opportunity to edit. He did not feel confident enough at this stage to resume his role in the church.

KB was a very rewarding person to work with for me personally because of his excellent metalinguistic skills, enthusiasm, and motivation throughout therapy. He also challenged me immensely because he was the first client I had worked with who had so much language available to him but still wanted to work to improve it, as it did not meet his personal expectations.

I think working with a client like KB raises many clinical and managerial issues. First, it can often be difficult to adequately baseline this type of client, who does not fit neatly into clinically available models of language processing because their difficulties predominantly appear in tasks where there is an integration of all knowledge sources. Therefore clinicians have to bring their own knowledge and thinking into devising appropriate assessment tasks that will provide the client with opportunities to use different language structures. This will enable clinicians to look for patterns of language difficulty and to select appropriate therapy goals. Many formal measures tend to examine discrete processes that may not reflect what goes on in the multicomplexity of on-line processing. The clinician is faced with trying to find satisfactory measures. I found that the therapy tasks themselves became the measure of progress, along with some of the more formal replicable assessments.

Second, it can be difficult to locate therapy resources at this level. There are many resource packs readily available for semantic/phonological processing. However, after having worked with KB, I now feel that there may be a wealth of resources in English workbooks for secondary level pupils that may have been appropriate.

When should we consider discharge for these clients with so called "higher level difficulties"? The client's aspirations surely need to be considered in the decision-making process and yet, with ever increasing pressures on therapy services, clinicians may be faced with the problem of whether they have the resources to treat clients who appear to have less severe aphasia.

Following discharge from the rehabilitation unit, KB continued to have speech and language therapy once a week by my colleague on an outpatient basis. The therapy continued to focus on further low frequency word-finding tasks, particularly with verbs and adjectives, manipulation of grammatical constructions in speech, creative use of language, functional written output for grammar and style (reports/letters), continued self-monitoring, and awareness of normal speech errors.

KB made steady progress during this later period, achieving increased verbal fluency, but he still remained vulnerable to fatigue factors. He decided that he may wish to return to part-time employment in the future but wanted to consider any plans alone. The speech and language therapist felt he would now be able to return to his professional work if he could find a supportive employer. KB was seen on a review basis for support before being finally discharged.

ACKNOWLEDGMENTS

I would like to thank KB for his enthusiasm and commitment throughout the therapy process. Many thanks to Eirian Jones for her inspirational ideas, materials, and helpful advice, and to Sian Davies, who treated KB prior to admission and upon discharge from the rehabilitation unit.

REFERENCES

Freund, J., Hayter, C., MacDonald, S., Neary, M., & Wiseman-Hakes, C. (1999). *Cognitive communica-tion disorders following traumatic brain injury: A practical guide*. New York: Psychological Corporation.

Garrett, M. (1980). Levels of processing in sentence production. In B. Butterworth (Ed.), *Language production, Vol. 1*. New York: Academic Press.

Goodglass, H., & Kaplan, E. (1972). *The assessment of aphasia and related disorders* (2nd ed.). Philadelphia: Lea & Febiger.

Kay, J., Lesser, R., & Coltheart, M. (1992). *Psycholinguistic assessments of language processing in aphasia (PALPA)*. Hove, UK: Lawrence Erlbaum Associates Inc.

APPENDICES

APPENDIX 4.1: KB'S response to two elicitations of conversation

What have you been doing this morning?
I have been in with the physiotherapist er she has been working on my arm. . . . Er very good really. . . . Er . . . my finger in my f . . . my finger in my f . . . fingers is beginning to develop and my arm is . . . getting a nice straight position when it is holding me up . . . no . . . that's wrong isn't it? My elbow is . . . is . . . straight when it's he . . . he when it's holding my weight . . . that's what I want to say, thank you. It was a good session. I enjoyed it very much(Q) "nothing" I er had er a sleep this morning which is usually my styleer . . . (laughs) but erm I can't say I did anything this morning really er. . . . I . . . haven't no I . . . f . . . fell asleep quite a lot of the time. (Th question- What will you do this weekend?) er we'll have a nice quiet weekend er . . . go to church and go and watch some cricket that'll be about it. I think it will be/bOI/yeah . . . It will stop raining today.

Cookie Theft picture
The kitchen is in a . . . sorry. . . . The scene is pictured in a kitchen. The woman is . . . www washing cups and saucers. The water seems to be fill fill fil . . . the . . . t sorry the sink . . . filling over and water is running to the floor. Behind her back two children are . . . ch . . . stealing cookies. The little boy is on the stool and it seems to be falling over. That's it.

APPENDIX 4.2: Written stories produced by KB on a word processor

THE SUMMER

The summer of 1997 was perfect. The weather has been fine for days and days and days. People can't remember the last day it rained. Sunshine is falling from the skies.

The shortage of water is becoming a problem. The reservoirs are nearly empty. The water companies are taking severe action to the situation they face. Tankers are taking supplies from the highlands of Scotland to the empty reservoirs. It is also thought that the water companies are contemplating extraction from the sea.

Despite these problems, the countryside is beautiful and is attracting many visitors. Bob and Mary are planning a visit to the forest . . . They are aware of the danger of forest fire but think that careful preparation and execution will be sufficient.

With all the planning complete, Bob and Mary set out. Bob is a very happy man. He is thinking of the fascinating wonders of the countryside Mary has very different thoughts. Mary is in love with Bob. She is thinking of the wedding march.

They have walked in the forest for about two hours. They need a rest. Bob takes off from his shoulders, the rusack containing the picnic.

KB reported that it took him many hours to complete this. There is evidence of good sentence structuring. An occasional tense agreement across sentence problem. Sentences are, at times too simplistic where there were opportunities to combine. However, he does produce subordinated and co-ordinated clauses very well. There isn't much evidence of embedding or of relations across separate sentences, e.g., "because" or "whilst". Although one could argue that this may be a reflection of his style, I felt he would have been capable of producing a more sophisticated, cohesive text.

TWO DON'T EQUAL ONE

This is the sad story of two Scottish lads from Perth.

They are Jock Scratchy—breeder of "flies" for fisherman and his life long friend, Pee Watchett—a financier who is known for his interests in rail and bus transport.

Jock still lives in Perth. Pee is a man who lists Perth as his birthplace but could be found in London, Paris, Tokyo and New York.

Life has been tranquill for Jock. He was known at school for his woodworking ability rather than his academic skill. Jock was destined for a life of quiet moments and it was only to be interrupted by his taking the headlines once or twice in his life.

Pee was the opposite. He was always in the headlines. His school performance, he was in the top three in his class, set a target for his life.

Pee had the reputation of a leader in the financial world. He was tight-fisted: Jock was a man who knew when it was his turn to buy the drinks.

Jock saw the demand for his flies by fisherman but lacked the capital to finance his idea. Pee had lots of money but he lacked the imagination to use it well. The two men, who were schoolboy friends, were, by fate, brought together.

They were taking their "fly" business to the Stock Exchange. The fate of this business is taking much of the time of those involved in the financial world. It will fail. Jock will give his "flies" to his friends. Pee will keep his money and you will be the loser.

The above is an imaginative piece of writing with a range of verbs and tenses used. KB's sense of humour is clearly being expressed here! Occasional complex sentences were used effectively, but on other occasions I felt that he may be trying to map too many ideas into one sentence. He does have occasional word accessing difficulties which result in him expressing ideas in a complicated way.

Lexical and functionally based treatment: Effects on word retrieval and conversation

Julie Hickin, Ruth Herbert, Wendy Best, David Howard and Felicity Osborne

This study investigates whether phonological treatment for word-finding difficulties can produce long-term improvement in word finding, not only in picture naming, but also in connected speech and conversation. We present the results of therapy from two people with aphasia. We compare their response to two forms of treatment and their views of how each form of treatment impacted upon their aphasia.

Phase 1 treatment, which we will be calling lexical treatment, focused on picture naming and involved a *choice of cue*. Previous research has indicated that only semantic techniques are effective in improving word finding in the long term, and that phonological techniques produce only

short-term benefits (Howard, Patterson, Franklin, Orchard-Lisle, & Morton, 1985; Patterson, Purrell, & Morton, 1983). We hypothesised that a crucial difference between semantic and phonological treatments may be the element of choice: Only semantic tasks generally require the person with aphasia to make a choice. Here we investigate the effects of giving a choice of phonological cues, and a choice of orthographic cues, on word-finding in the long term.

In a second phase of treatment we moved away from picture naming and instead encouraged the use of targeted words in interaction related to the individual's life interests. This functionally based communication therapy differed from previous similar treatments in that it targeted specific sets of items. It involved a hierarchy of interactive tasks for developing use of the target items in conversation.

Studies analysing aphasic individuals' participation in conversations have identified word retrieval problems as a common source of breakdown (e.g., Lesser & Algar, 1995; Perkins, Crisp, & Walshaw, 1999). While cognitive rehabilitation studies have demonstrated that specific treatments for word finding can result in gains in picture naming, few attempts have been made to investigate whether there is any functional carry-over of these gains into everyday speech. Treatment studies that have adopted a purely functional approach (e.g., Green, 1982; Holland, 1991) have encountered difficulties in demonstrating the efficacy of the treatment (Holland, 1991).

Here we compare picture naming, story telling, and conversation before and after each phase of treatment. Results from the two participants described indicate that both forms of treatment lead to gains in picture naming. The carry-over to conversation is less clear-cut, with one participant showing improvement in some of the conversation measures used, and the other showing little change. The results are discussed and directions for future research are considered.

In addition to looking at quantitative assessments of performance we were also interested in how those with aphasia view their own communication and how they perceived changes resulting from treatment. This information was gathered by means of structured questionnaires.

METHOD

Design
The study is composed of three stages: an assessment stage followed by two stages of treatment. During the assessment stage a number of tests are administered to elucidate the nature of the participants' word-finding difficulties (see Table 5.2). A number of outcome measures are also administered at various points throughout the study to ascertain progress. These measures are described in Table 5.1, and the timing of them illustrated in Figure 5.1. The outcome measures are administered twice before treatment commences (assessments 1 and 2), at the end of the first phase of treatment (assessment 3), at the end of the second treatment phase (assessment 4) and finally after a period of no treatment (assessment 5). Each assessment is at least 8 weeks apart.

Informed consent was obtained prior to each of the stages, using an aphasia-friendly consent form designed by Felicity Osborne (Osborne, Hickin, Best, & Howard, 1998).

Participant details
HM is in his forties. He was married with two children, and worked as a carpenter/cabinet maker with a large shop-fitting company when he had a single left-hemisphere stroke 5 years prior to his involvement in this therapy study. Following the stroke HM and his wife separated and he was unable to see his children regularly. He lives alone now in a flat, and attends a day centre 3 days a week, where he spends his time building a model railway. HM's daughter has recently established contact with him and visits him more regularly. HM's other interests include rock music and steam trains. He has an expressive aphasia; his

FIGURE 5.1

Assessment 1

> Background Assessment

Assessment 2

> Phase 1 of Treatment

Assessment 3

> Phase 2 of Treatment

Assessment 4

> No Intervention

Assessment 5 (Follow-up)

Structure of the study.

TABLE 5.1

Assessments used during the study

Picture naming 200
The set of items used for picture naming includes matched subsets so that the influence of a range of variables on picture naming can be identified for each individual. These include imageability, frequency, familiarity, age of acquisition, operativity, and length.

Retelling the Cinderella story
Participants are asked to retell the story of Cinderella orally. The analysis of the Cinderella data involves transcription of the sample, and identification of the content words present. (We follow Bird & Franklin, 1996, in selecting nouns, verbs, adjectives, adverbs ending in -ly, and numerals as content words.) The combined spoken and written frequency of each item is computed from the Celex database (Piepenbrock & Gulikers, 1995), and mean frequency for the total content word set and the subset which are nouns is derived. In addition we look at the type–token ratio of the sets by dividing the number of different content words or nouns used respectively by the total number instances they were produced.

Word retrieval in conversation
The conversation measure analyses a transcription of 5 minutes of conversation between the person with aphasia and their chosen conversation partner (a friend or relative). As well as a qualitative overview, we used the measure to quantify success in word retrieval in conversation and compare pre- and post-treatment performance.

Communication views questionnaire
This questionnaire looks at the person's own view of their communication and is included in Appendix 5.1. Finally the treatment questionnaire (see Appendices 5.2 and 5.3) examines the person's response to the treatment.

Language control tasks
The language control tasks assess aspects of language which are not predicted to change as a result of treatment. They are: written sentence-to-picture matching (CAT); reading aloud words ($n = 52$); reading aloud non-words ($n = 26$); short-term memory (picture pointing span).

output is non-fluent, with evidence of apraxia of speech. HM's conversation partner was his key worker at the day centre.

PH is a woman in her seventies, a native of south London who has lived there all her life. She lives in sheltered accommodation in her own flat, and is involved in many of the activities available there including bingo, lunch trips, and day trips to the south coast. PH has a large and supportive family who live in the south of England, and has regular contact with some of the family members. PH sustained a single left-hemisphere stroke in 1996, 3 years prior to her involvement in the study, which resulted in aphasia. Her expressive language is fluent with frequent word-finding

problems. PH's conversation partner for the study was one of the other residents with whom she was in regular contact.

Table 5.2 shows the results of the language assessments carried out with HM and PH. It is clear from assessment items 2–5 that neither HM nor PH have marked semantic processing difficulties, yet both make semantic errors in naming, and PH's naming shows an imageability effect (item 6). HM's naming is affected by length (item 13), and he also makes phonemic naming errors (item 12). HM's difficulties with reading and repetition, combined with the length effect in naming, indicate a deficit in phonology, or a problem later in processing after phonological selection

TABLE 5.2

Language assessment in percentages prior to therapies

	HM	PH
1. Naming 200 pictures (number of correctly named items)	44	36
2. CAT Spoken word to picture matching ($n = 30$)	100	93
3. CAT Written word to picture matching ($n = 30$)	87	97
4. Pyramids and Palm Trees ($n = 52$)	94	90
5. Percentage of semantic naming errors (out of total naming errors)	52	25
6. Imageability effect in naming	N	Y
7. ADA Auditory discrimination ($n = 40$)	82	68
8. Short-term memory phonemes	1.4a[a]	2.5[a]
9. Repetition of words ($n = 152$)	73	97
10. Repetition: non-words ($n = 26$)	31	58
11. Repetition non-words: 1st phoneme correct ($n = 26$)	54	88
12. Percentage of phonemic naming errors (out of total naming errors)	20	5
13. Length effect in naming	Y	N
14. Reading words ($n = 152$)	70	97
15. Reading non-words ($n = 26$)	0	35
16. Reading non-words: 1st phoneme correct	38	85
17. Written naming ($n = 25$ for MH and 40 for HP)	16	38

[a] Number of phonemes.
The table shows participants' performance on the following: CAT—Comprehensive Aphasia Test (Swinburn, Porter, & Howard, 2004); Pyramids and Palm Trees (Howard & Patterson, 1992); ADA Auditory Discrimination from Action for Dysphasic Adults Comprehension Battery (Franklin, Turner, & Ellis, 1992). The remaining assessments are unpublished.

has been achieved. PH's superior performance in reading and repetition of words (items 14 and 9) suggests that representations in output phonology are intact, but are not always accessed. Together with her relatively intact semantic processing, this suggests that PH's difficulties lie in mapping from semantics to phonology.

The two participants differ in other important ways. Samples of conversations taken prior to the treatment show the sentence structure used in conversational speech. HM is reliant on mainly single content words to convey his meaning. He makes phonemic and semantic errors in conversation. Occasional more complex utterances are present. PH also produces some content words, and makes semantic errors, but she produces syntactically more complex sentences, often using high frequency verbs such as go, do, be, have, get, and sentences lacking in key nouns.

The following transcripts, one for each of the participants, depict the differences described (CP = conversational partner).

HM: Conversation sample

HM   yeah (1.3 seconds) and er
CP   what. Famous
HM   London /ge / dear yeah pub yeah
CP   really
HM   yeah
CP   what one was that
HM   four (2.1 seconds) four pubs
CP   you've done four pubs
HM   mmm

PH: Conversation sample

PH   mmm very nice (laughs) must 'ave been nice must have paid out what he paid. All that people (unintell.)

CP mmm
PH I mean all these
CP yeah
PH they were all out and the girls uh uh people they had were out there
CP did they
PH yeah

LEXICAL TREATMENT: WORD AND PICTURE NAMING WITH PHONOLOGICAL AND ORTHOGRAPHIC CUING, TREATMENT PHASE 1

Prior to the study reported here both participants took part in a facilitation study (Best, Herbert, Hickin, Osborne, & Howard, 2002). This study revealed that HM's and PH's word retrieval benefited from orthographic and phonological cues both in the immediate and the short term (i.e., after a delay of 10 minutes), given either a single cue or a choice of cues. This facilitation activity formed the basis of the therapy in Phase 1. The lexical approaches used in Phase 1 emphasised both phonological (word sound) and orthographic (written form) information. In this respect the therapies differed from the many treatments reported in the literature, which highlight the meaning of the word, or the meaning and the form, but rarely the form, without meaning.[1]

In the present study 100 words were treated. These were selected from the set of 200 words that had been named at pre-treatment assessments 1 and 2. (The set of 200 has naming agreement and is controlled for several variables known to affect naming in aphasia.) The set was divided into two sets of 100 matched for pre-treatment naming performance. During Phase 1 therapy, if HM or PH couldn't name a picture, or they made an error, for 50 of the pictures they were exposed to the first sound of the name with one or more distractors, and for the other 50 they were exposed to the first letter of the name with one or more distractors (see Figure 5.2). Targets and distractors were matched for syllable struc-

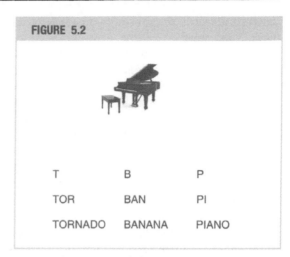

FIGURE 5.2

T	B	P
TOR	BAN	PI
TORNADO	BANANA	PIANO

Examples of exposures and distractors.

ture, but differed in terms of first letter/sound and first vowel, and were not semantically related to the target. For the first two sessions one distractor was present; this was then increased to two for the next two sessions and then three for the final four sessions.

The following outlines the procedure for the orthographic treatment.

- In attempting to name a picture, for example of a penguin, HM and PH were shown the letters P (target cue) and C (distractor cue).
- If they were still unable to name the item, they were exposed to the first letter, the first vowel and the medial consonants (if any), for example PENG or CONC.
- If still unable to name it they were exposed to the whole word for both target and distractor, for example PENGUIN or CONCRETE.
- If still unable to name the item the whole word was offered for the person to repeat, with no distractors present.
- The order of presentation of the items was randomised across sessions, as was the order of appearance of the target and distractor cues.

The procedure for the phonological condition was identical to that the orthographic treatment outlined above, but instead of seeing the written letters and words, the person was exposed to oral cues. Thus, unable to name a picture of a mermaid, the person would be told "It begins with 'duh' or 'muh' ". Additional phonological information was then given until the person could name the item, including offering the whole word in isolation for the person to repeat as the final stage of the treatment for that item.

Each of the 100 treatment items was presented once a week for 8 weeks. The treatment sessions lasted roughly 1 hour. Room was made for individualised adjustments of the treatment procedures. For example, HM had difficulty coping with additional distractors and so had three sessions with two distractors and only two sessions with three distractors.

In addition to the 100 treatment items (50 for each condition), each participant selected 20 treatment items that were personal to them and which they believed would be functionally useful to them. For example, these included words relating to home and hobbies such as gardening, shopping, and DIY. The words were presented in Phase 1 of the study in the same way as the 50 orthographic treatment items. They were also treated in Phase 2, details of which will follow.

FUNCTIONALLY BASED TREATMENT, PHASE 2

In this phase of treatment the emphasis was on the use of the 120 target words in everyday speech. To this end tasks used in the treatment sessions approximated real situations in as far as this is possible. The treatment moved gradually away from picture naming, towards the natural use of words in conversational speech. Tasks included naming to definition, and naming in a pseudo-realistic speech situation in the early sessions, making lists (shopping, inventories, aides-memoire), and then reminiscing, telling anecdotes, and conversations around chosen subjects in the later sessions. In all sessions participants had access to the pictures, and to the written cues, if they needed them. Throughout this phase a record was kept of the words produced by the participant in the sessions.

The 120 pictured items, with their written cues, were sorted into conversational categories, and made into a file, which the participants kept in their home throughout this phase.

RESULTS

Picture naming
Table 5.3 shows the results of 200- and 20-item picture naming tasks across the assessment times for each of the two participants.

Both participants made gains in picture naming for each phase of treatment, and both maintained their improved performance at follow-up two months later. For HM both treatment phases were equally effective, whereas for PH Phase 2 led to slightly greater gains in picture naming. Looking at the 20 personal items, only PH made good progress with these items in Phase 1 and maintained this at subsequent assessments. For HM it is hard to draw any firm conclusion as he could also only think of 10 words he wanted to practise and these were all quite closely semantically related (to food shopping), which may have contributed to the lack of progress (from 2 to 4 out of 10). Stability across control tasks (listed in Table 5.1) at the different assessment points suggested that improvements were due to treatment rather than to spontaneous change or possible effects of attention received during sessions.

Phase 1: Lexical treatment: Comparison of phonological and orthographic cuing
Table 5.4 demonstrates the effect of treatment for treated and untreated sets in the two conditions: treatment with phonological cues, and treatment with orthographic cues, for both participants.

As these data show, there is a very slight advantage for the orthographic technique over the phonological. PH stated that she found the orthographic technique easier as decoding the stimuli was not difficult, which may explain the slight difference between the two scores. It is somewhat surprising that HM responded to the

TABLE 5.3

Number of pictures named correctly for the 200-item and 20-item tasks across four time periods for each participant

	Pre-therapy		Following Phase 1	Following Phase 2	Follow-up
	Assessment1	Assessment2			
N = 200					
HM	90	84	110	130	115
PH	65	75	97	130	126
N = 20					
HM	not assessed	2	4	not assessed	not assessed
PH	not assessed	4	17	17	15

TABLE 5.4

The percentage of pictures named correctly by each participant following phonological and orthographic cuing in Phase 1 treatment

	Prior to Phase 1 treatment		Following Phase 1 treatment
	Assessment1	Assessment2	
HM			
Phonological (n = 50)	46	40	56
Orthographic (n = 50)	44	44	60
Untreated (n = 100)	45	42	52
PH			
Phonological (n = 50)	32	36	60
Orthographic (n = 50)	32	38	68
Untreated (n = 100)	33	38	33

orthographic cues as his reading aloud of words and particularly non-words is markedly impaired, i.e., it is difficult for him to generate phonology from visual input. It is possible that the two participants use the cues in different ways; PH sounding aloud the letters, and HM accessing a whole word representation from the combination of the picture information and the letter information. In addition, HM shows some improvement in naming untreated items (from 44% to 52%) whereas PH does not. Thus it appears that the effect of treatment generalises for HM, but is restricted to treatment items for PH.

Cinderella story telling

Table 5.5 gives the results of the analysis of the Cinderella story telling procedure. Results include the mean frequency (combined spoken and written frequency) for content words produced by the participant in retelling the story. The same measures were used for the subset of nouns. It was anticipated that an improvement in word-finding ability subsequent to therapy would lead to a reduction in the mean frequency of nouns produced, as the aphasic participant may be less reliant on retrieving high frequency items. The type–token ratio for all the content words

TABLE 5.5

Mean frequency of nouns and content words and type–token ratios (TTR) in the Cinderella story across four time periods for both PH and HM

| | Pre-treatment | | | | |
	A1	A2	Post Phase 1	Post Phase 2	Follow-up
HM					
Nouns	1.92	n/a	1.5	1.83	1.52
Content words	2.07	n/a	1.62	1.97	1.74
TTR nouns	.50	n/a	.50	.55	.58
TTR content words	.50	n/a	.57	.61	.56
PH					
Nouns	1.68	1.87	2.08	1.82	1.65
Content words	2.07	2.27	2.41	2.27	2.41
TTR nouns	.89	.56	.91	.58	.71
TTR content words	.73	.58	.88	.48	.55

Combined spoken and written frequency of each item is computed from the Celex database (Piepenbrock & Gulikers, 1995) and divided by the number of types to calculate the mean frequency. Mean frequency of nouns for normal controls: 1.75. Range: 1.64–1.87 (Bird & Franklin, 1996).

produced and for the nouns subset is also included, as it was anticipated that following therapy a wider variety of (types of) nouns may be accessible for the participants, thus producing an increase in type–token ratio.

The results of retelling Cinderella (Table 5.5) for HM showed a tendency towards a reduction in mean frequency of content words across treatments. There was no change in the type–token ratios (TTR) for either the total set of words, or the subset that are nouns. The number of types and tokens of nouns produced by HM increased from 16 (types) and 32 (tokens) (TTR = .50) to 32 (types) and 58 (tokens) (TTR = .55) after Phase 2 of therapy. They remained high at 29 (types) and 50 (tokens) at follow-up (TTR = .58).

Transcriptions of HM's narratives of Cinderella following lexical and functional treatments are given in Appendix 5.4, illustrating his improved ability to find nouns. For PH there is no change in any of the measures used. Recall that for HM the treatment effect generalised to untreated items, and for PH it did not. Thus for HM the range of words he has improved access to is potentially unlimited, whereas for PH it amounts to a relatively small number. In a connected speech task such as the Cinderella story, it is likely therefore that HM will show an improvement whereas PH will not. This is what we found. Will the same logic apply to the conversation data?

Conversation measure

A number of variables from the conversation data are available for analysis. We include here the aspects of the conversation that were thought to be sensitive to noun production in conversation. The data for those aspects of conversation that we predicted would increase as a result of treatment are given in Table 5.6. Those that we predicted would decrease after treatment are given in Table 5.7.

Looking first at aspects of the conversation in which we would expect to see improvement (Table 5.6), HM showed a steady improvement in the number of nouns used per substantive turn (i.e., per turn containing a content word). The pattern is less clear for the content words. There is improvement following Phase 1, but the low score

TABLE 5.6

Aspects of conversation predicted to increase after treatment: Nouns and content words[a] produced per substantive turn[b]

| | Pre-treatment | | | | |
	A1	A2	Post Phase 1	Post Phase 2	Follow-up
HM					
Content words/Substantive turn	1.50	1.64	1.95	1.67	2.40
Nouns/Substantive turn	0.87	0.86	1.27	1.14	1.39
PH					
Content words/Substantive turn	3.24	3.35	2.08	2.67	2.68
Nouns/Substantive turn	0.60	1.09	0.82	0.33	0.62

[a] Content words are all closed class elements: nouns, verbs, adjectives, adverbs ending in -ly and numerals.
[b] A substantive turn is any turn containing a content word.

TABLE 5.7

Aspects of conversation predicted to decrease after treatment

| | Pre-treatment | | | | |
	A1	A2	Post Phase 1	Post Phase 2	Follow-up
HM					
Total word errors[a] /speech units	0.25	0.25	0.31	0.21	0.17
Total word errors/content words	1.33	1.15	1.68	0.91	0.76
Word errors per turn	0.65	0.84	1.25	1.14	0.66
PH					
Total word errors/speech units	0.08	0.08	0.12	0.05	0.07
Total word errors/content words	0.28	0.31	0.34	0.22	0.24
Word errors per turn	0.60	0.62	0.52	0.35	0.42

[a] Word errors are semantic paraphasias, circumlocutions, phonological errors, neologisms, filled pauses and pauses.

after Phase 2 undermines this result. For PH there is no clear change as a result of treatment on any of these measures.

For aspects that we would expect to decrease after treatment (Table 5.7), HM shows a decrease in the proportion of speech units that are word errors. This is slight following Phase 2 therapy but more marked at follow-up. There is even more of a decrease following Phase 2 treatment and follow-up for the number of speech errors as a proportion of the number of content words. PH also shows this pattern of decreased number of word errors following therapy.

To summarise the conversation measures, HM, for whom the treatment effect of Phases 1 and 2[2] generalised to untreated items, and who showed some improvement in the Cinderella task, also showed improvement in noun retrieval in conversation. PH, who did not show any generalisation, improved in a more limited fashion in conversation, producing fewer speech errors after Phase 2 functionally based treatment, which directly targeted noun production in conversation.

From these data we can conclude that generalisation of treatment effects to untreated items may not only affect picture naming, but can also carry over to other speech tasks, at least for HM. If no generalisation occurs to untreated items (as for PH), carry-over to other speech activities is more limited. It is essential, therefore, that we attempt to identify which treatments lead to generalisation for which individuals.

Communication views questionnaire

Both participants completed an aphasia-friendly questionnaire about their communication with the help of the therapist at each stage of the project.

The data in Table 5.8 indicate that HM appeared to feel more comfortable with communication in general as treatment progressed (questions 1a, 1b, and 2), but that he viewed words as being harder to find in conversation at the end of treatment. He showed some tendency to view his reading and understanding as having improved (question 4a) but indicated little change in reading and understanding (question 4b).

Table 5.8 shows that PH was positive about her communication with family throughout her involvement in the research, but was less so with friends. Responses to this latter question, and to question 2, were erratic, leading one to question the validity and reliability of measures such as this. Similarly for question 3a, PH appeared to feel more and more positive about her naming abilities as the study progressed: Given the variability of her responses to other questions this must be interpreted cautiously, however.

When asked about reading, which was not

treated directly in this study, PH showed some tendency towards a more positive evaluation as the study progressed. When asked whether her reading had improved, she remained fairly stable and equivocal in her opinion.

Participants' comments about treatment

Both participants responded well to the treatment at both phases. HM enjoyed participating in therapy and appeared to become more extrovert as therapy progressed. During Phase 1, initially orthographic cues appeared to be somewhat more helpful than phonological cues, as HM tended to get the target word with less cuing information. However, this initial advantage lessened as therapy progressed. HM responded positively to being given a choice of cues and rarely chose the wrong one, although two distractors were felt to be more useful than three by the therapist and HM, possibly due to memory limitations.

During Phase 2, although HM reported finding the therapy sessions more difficult and was not able to produce many target items, he also felt that the sessions were very useful. He became more animated as therapy progressed, for example, commenting that "talking about work was good therapy".

In Phase 1 PH made good progress with the treatment and had a positive response to it, trying hard to get the words right, and concentrating well in sessions. She was aware of items that were difficult for her and was keen to get these right. PH responded well to the choice of cues used in the sessions. She reported that the element of choice was helpful, although in early sessions she found it hard to decode the set of phonological cues. This grew easier as treatment progressed. PH was able to identify which of the cues was the correct one, even if this did not cue word retrieval. In early sessions she reported that the intermediate cue (consonant vowel consonant) was effective for her, whereas the consonant + schwa was less so.

In Phase 2, PH was able to use the words in the treatment sets in natural conversations, and reported that seeing the pictures made it much easier for her to recall a word. Conversations about family, friends, health, and reminiscences

TABLE 5.8

Questionnaire results on a scale ranging from 0–12: Low numbers represent the more positive end of the scale

	Pre-therapy		Post Phase 1	Post Phase 2	Follow-up
HM					
Q1a. Communicating with family	10.1	–	–	9.5	0.3
Q1b. Communicating with friend	9.0	–	–	0.0	3.5
Q2. Communicating ideas, feelings, etc.	10.0	–	–	0.3	3.7
Q3a. Finding words in conversation	5.4	–	–	10.7	8.7
Q3b. Change in word-finding	n/a	–	–	0.7	2.8
Q4a. Reading and understanding	2.9	–	–	0.8	1.2
Q4b. Change in reading and understanding	n/a	–	–	0.8	2.4
PH					
Q1a. Communicating with family	1.1	1.3	0.0	0.5	0.0
Q1b. Communicating with friend	2.4	1.6	3.5	5.9	6.3
Q2. Communicating ideas, feelings. etc.	2.6	10.0	1.6	0.7	6.2
Q3a. Finding words in conversation	5.3	9.8	10.0	5.1	9.3
Q3b. Change in word-finding	n/a	n/a	2.4	5.1	7.4
Q4a. Reading and understanding	10.3	5.7	1.8	5.5	1.5
Q4b. Change in reading and understanding	n/a	n/a	5.4	5.0	6.6

The scales are measured from the left on lines 12 cm in length.

were most productive in terms of the number of nouns produced spontaneously. In the final session PH produced 51 nouns, 16 of which were from the treatment set. PH did not use the file of picture items in between sessions to practise the words.

SUMMARY

Two people with aphasia were presented, who showed great differences in their language profile, but little semantic impairment. HM responded well to treatment with improvements to both treated and untreated words in picture naming, and he showed generalisation to connected speech activities (telling the Cinderella story, and conversation). PH also responded well to the treatment but the effect did not generalise to untreated items, or to other speech activities except in the decrease in error production in conversation. For both participants, naming benefited from phonological and orthographic cues in a facilitation task, and this may therefore be a useful part of clinical assessment in helping to determine which people treatment may help (see Best et al., 2002, and Hickin, Best, Herbert, Howard, & Osborne, 2002 for further discussion of this issue).

NOTES

1 Note, however, that seeing a picture of each word will activate its meaning to some extent, and it may be (as suggested by Howard, 2000) that the difference between semantic and phonological therapies for word-finding difficulties has been overstated.

2 Evidence of generalisation of Phase 1 treatment is shown in Table 5.5, and that of Phase 2 treatment is provided by improvement in the set of items not treated in this phase ($n = 100$), which improved from 55% to 63% correct.

REFERENCES

Best, W., Herbert, R., Hickin, J., Osborne, F., & Howard, D. (2002). Phonological and orthographic facilitation of word-retrieval in aphasia: Immediate and delayed effects. *Aphasiology*, *16*, 151–168.

Bird, H., & Franklin, S. (1996). Cinderella revisited: A comparison of fluent and non-fluent aphasic speech. *Journal of Neurolinguistics*, *9*, 187–206.

Franklin, S., Turner, J., & Ellis, A. (1992). *Action for dysphasic adults comprehension battery*. London: Action for Dysphasic Adults.

Green, G. (1982). Assessment and treatment of the adult with severe aphasia: Aiming for functional generalisation. *Australian Journal of Human Communication Disorders*, *10*, 11–23.

Holland, A. (1991). Pragmatic aspects of intervention in aphasia. *Journal of Neurolinguistics*, *6*, 197–211.

Hickin, J., Best, W., Herbert, R., Howard, D., & Osborne, F. (2002). Phonological therapy for word-finding difficulties: A re-evaluation. *Aphasiology*, *16*, 981–999.

Howard, D. (2000). Cognitive neuropsychology and aphasia therapy: The case of word retrieval. In I. Papathanasiou (Ed.), *Acquired neurogenic communication disorders: A clinical perspective*. London: Whurr.

Howard, D., & Patterson, K. (1992). *Pyramids and palm trees*. Bury St. Edmunds, UK: Thames Valley Test Company.

Howard, D., Patterson, K., Franklin, S., Orchard-Lisle, V., & Morton, J. (1985). The treatment of word retrieval deficits in aphasia: A comparison of two therapy methods. *Brain*, *108*, 817–829.

Lesser, R., & Algar, L. (1995). Towards combining the cognitive neuropsychological and the pragmatic in aphasia therapy. *Neuropsychological Rehabilitation*, *5*, 67–92.

Osborne, F., Hickin, J., Best, W., & Howard, D. (1998). Treating word-finding difficulties—beyond picture naming. *International Journal of Language and Communication Disorders*, *33*, 208–213.

Patterson, K., Purrell, C., & Morton, J. (1983). The facilitation of naming in aphasia. In C. Code & D.J. Muller (Eds.), *Aphasia therapy* (pp. 76–87). London: Arnold.

Perkins, L., Crisp, J., & Walshaw, D. (1999). Exploring conversation analysis as an assessment tool for aphasia: The issue of reliability. *Aphasiology*, *13*, 259–281.

Piepenbrock, R., & Gulikers, L. (1995). *The CELEX lexical database* (Release 2) [CD-ROM]. Philadelphia: Linguistic Data Consortium, University of Pennsylvania.

Robson, J., Pring, T., Marshall, J., Morrison, S., & Chiat, S. (1998). Written communication in undifferentiated jargon aphasia: A therapy study. *International Journal of Language and Communication Disorders*, *33*, 305–328.

Swinburn, K., Porter, G., & Howard, D. (2004). *Comprehensive aphasia test*. Hove, UK: Psychology Press.

APPENDICES

APPENDIX 5.1: Questionnaire: Language satisfaction scale

1. How comfortable are you when communicating with a family member? (Choices: Comfortable, Uncomfortable) Or with a friend? (Choices: Comfortable, Uncomfortable)

2. How well do you let a family member/ friend know the things you most want to say? Not just your needs and wants but your thoughts, ideas, feelings or opinions? (Choices: Well, Not at all well)

3. How easy is it to find the words you want to say in conversation? (Choices: Easy, Difficult) How has this changed over the past 2 months? (Choices: Better, Same)

4. How easy is it to read and understand things now? (Choices: Easy, Difficult) How has this changed over the past two months? (Choices: Better, Same)

APPENDIX 5.2: Treatment session summary sheet: Researcher's views

1. Was today a good day or a bad day for_____?
   Good day   Average day   Bad day

   Comments:

2. How useful do you think the treatment session was?
   Very useful   Moderately useful   Not useful

3. Which type of cue appeared to be most useful? Seeing pictures again, sound cue / written cue, choosing between cues, repeating the word, saying it aloud?

4. How difficult was the treatment task?
   Easy   Moderately difficult   Very difficult

   Comments:

5. Would anything have made the session more useful?

APPENDIX 5.3: Treatment session summary sheet: Participant's views

1. Was today a good day or a bad day for in general (but especially re talking)?
   Good day   **Average day**   **Bad day**

   Comments:

2. How useful did you find the treatment session?
   Very useful   **Moderately useful**   **Not useful**

1. What was most useful—i.e., What helped you to recall a word most? Seeing pictures again, sound cue / written cue, choosing between cues, repeating the word, saying it aloud?

2. How difficult was the treatment task?
   Easy   **Moderately difficult**   **Very difficult**

   Comments:

3. Would anything have made the session more useful?

APPENDIX 5.4

Cinderella HM, After Phase 1 (T: = target)
A clock /kropin/ (T: scrubbing) and that's a pail
Mans and woman the King . . . Ber ber . . . A dog people a King . . . That's it
That's er women but old and a woman a keys and a broom pail wand but it's woman wand and it's magic that's it
Mice and pumpkin but it's massive now wedding /mat/ coaches pumpkin but /briger/ (T: bigger)
Well /tinderela/ and a man that's er people people
A clock twelve clock the slipper but cinderella
The witches No! No! A fat one /sliper/ (T: slipper)
Old people ugly /siper/ and woman but fine what's her name what's that name a slipper fine and its..
A King has er married castle that's it init? (laughs)

Cinderella HM, Following Phase 2
Now then a woman brushing bucket there's a mice a fire
A people envelope there's a King children (aunties)?? Dog as well and the King a King that's all people houses and church
Wishes two woman's wishes woman brushing and that's er water and er logs keys maybe that's it I think
That's er what's that what's that good but a bloke wishing for a star
The woman maybe logs and er clogs mice and /kumkin/ (T: pumpkin)
Dear oh dear and that's er horses and pumpkin maybe carriages gold
Kings and queens and er that er Buckingham Palace wine and song
The twelve and what's that a woman diamonds bit bigger a shoe off one shoe man as well
Wishes that's er glass shoe but wishes no no woman no
The kings and glass glass shoe and that a woman maybe nice king and clothes old clothes woman a chair / pushen/ (T: cushion)
A woman and a man castle and er maybe together and er that's it init queen.

A group approach to the long-term rehabilitation of clients with acquired brain injury within the community

Sally McVicker and Leonie Winstanley

INTRODUCTION

There is much literature documenting the extensive problems of living with a disability as experienced by clients with stroke and traumatic brain injury. The aphasia literature discusses the feelings of loss of role and reduced self-worth and productivity that result from aphasia. These difficulties can lead to avoidance, withdrawal, and isolation (Brumfitt, 1996; Parr, Byng, Gilpin, & Ireland, 1997). Hartley (1995) quotes breakdown in relationships and social isolation as some of

the devastating long-term effects of traumatic brain injury. The need for long-term follow-up in the community is discussed widely. For example, Hersh (1998) talks about "traversing the plateau" with people with chronic aphasia and Hartley (1995) discusses the long-term needs of those living with the consequences of brain injury.

This chapter discusses work carried out in the community over a period of 6 months with a group of people with acquired brain injury. Brain injury here included those with traumatic brain injury, brain tumour, and stroke either through haemorrhage (including subarachnoid haemorrhage) or infarction. While these people all experienced difficulty with executive dysfunction and communication as a result of their brain injury, the severity and characteristics of their impairment varied. The group also varied in age (between 24 and 58 years), culture and social background, and in time post-onset (6 months to 12 years). All had difficulty in coping within the community. Group members and their issues are described in Table 6.1.

The therapy described here took place as part of the service offered by the London Borough of Southwark. As part of a multidisciplinary community therapy team, we visited people living throughout the borough in their own homes, and we were struck by the stark isolation of the individual experience. Despite the diverse backgrounds and times post-onset of our clients they seemed to share a number of common issues and challenges in learning to live with their disabilities. We hoped that by bringing people together, we could enable and encourage people to "take more control of their lives" and move forwards.

The seven group members all expressed a desire to meet others and share similar experiences. The philosophy behind setting up the group drew on the social model of disability in terms of user involvement and empowerment. Group members had to decide whether to attend and to decide on the topics they wished to address (attention and memory in the first instance, and stress management in the second). Modules were run for each of these broad topics. Each one covered sessions on education, insight, identification, and implementation of strategies. Each group member gathered a personal log (referred to in the group as a portfolio).

Results of the group therapy programme suggest that awareness may be a key issue in group members' progress in the use and implementation of strategies.

Ylvisaker and Szakeres (1989) describe the difficulties manifest in executive function as deficits in problem solving, self-monitoring, directing, initiation, goal setting, inhibition, organisation, planning, and attention. These affect language and activities of daily living. In terms of communication, the group experienced such executive difficulties in the absence of or in addition to an aphasia. The measure of cognitive-linguistic abilities (MCLA, Ellmo, Graser, Krchnavek, Calabrese, & Hanck, 1995) was used for assessment in those cases where thorough assessment had not already established a clear picture of an individual's language.

Communication was characterised by poor attention and listening skills for five of the seven group members. Comprehension varied from a member who had difficulty with discourse (significantly below the standardised mean for age and education) to those who had minimal or no difficulty following conversational speech and who were able to understand complex abstract discussions. All had some memory deficits, as described by their referring therapists, their current therapist, and their own observation.

For six of the seven, their expressive language was characterised by verbosity and marked problems with planning and maintaining the focus of conversation and occasionally by some disinhibition. Some extracts of their output are given below in response to the picture description task in the MCLA.

Well it's obviously late in someone's job because they've managed to tie up their computer that there's still typing and it's half past five. I think . . . the handles are quite close to each other. Someone's obviously coming to check out how good they are at it and the person coming in is a white person and the person typing is a black person and as I say there's obviously a big fat disk of everything.

. . . the window cleaner is there . . . he she he, I think it's a man with long hair. Someone has popped into the office. He's obviously on the computer or VDU. He's late at cleaning. She looks happy. Fellow at the computer he looks happy. Man coming in the door. . . . Is it a smile of happiness on his face I can't tell? Loads of stuff in the bin. He's obviously trying to do something. It doesn't say what he's doing. There's a telephone there as well.

TABLE 6.1

Group member profiles

Group member	Cognition	Language	Social situation
SC	Marked executive problems—primarily around inhibition and lack of awareness.	Inattention and poor listening skills, compromised comprehension. Very fluent, rambling and tangential speech.	Attempting to carry on as before and failing. Angry. Everyone else to blame. Breakdown in relationships, loss of job, isolation.
JM	Mild difficulties with high level executive function (planning and organisation).	Mild receptive aphasia. Mild–moderate expressive aphasia.	Retired following stroke. Previously head of the household and earner. Now cared for by late teenage children.
JJ	Difficulty with organisation and planning, attention and memory.	Good comprehension but difficulty maintaining focus and attention. Occasionally overwhelmed and needy of clarification. Fluent, rambling, unfocused output.	Evicted from her home. Unable to work. Separated from her children (9 and 11). Dependent on Social Services. Temporarily living in an unsuitable home. Uncertain future.
ED	High level executive difficulties.	Good comprehension compromised occasionally by inattention and feeling overwhelmed. Rambling, fluent and sometimes inappropriate expressive language.	24-year-old, hip, first-class graduate interested in film and fashion. Loss of job and independence. Back with Mum.
CG	Distracted. Fair memory. Difficulty with planning, organisation, self-direction, and problem solving.	Good comprehension compromised by distractibility. Fluent, rambling, tangential speech. Often inappropriate.	Ran betting shop and focus of the family. Attempting to maintain both roles against a sea of declining health, marital tension and breakdown.
RF	Very distractible. Poor attention. Uninhibited. Lack of awareness.	Good pragmatic and basic social skills give an unrealistic impression of limited comprehension. Hindered further by poor attention skills. Fluent, rambling, unfocused chatter—humour!	Loss of job and home. Forced to move in with Mum (also dysphasic). Very difficult family situation. Social Services involvement.
SY	Limited attention and memory, impacting on executive function.	Limited comprehension (< paragraph level). Fluent but disordered and unfocused content of speech.	Previous owner of a chain of restaurants and head of a family of six. Marked changes in roles and economic status.

Three group members also had more specific difficulties with language in addition to the cognitive deficits affecting expression. These included semantic errors, overuse of non-specific terms such as "obviously", "still", and "together", repetition, and some word-finding difficulties.

There was one member whose expressive language was markedly different from the rest of the group. In his case his moderate expressive dysphasia overshadowed his mild cognitive communication difficulties. He had difficulty with word finding and his speech was slow and hesitant, due in the main to difficulties of planning his sentences. It took him time to complete simple sentences, although they were usually concise and well focused.

> . . . It's . . . a . . . um . . . taking long to the doctors . . . an . . . em . . . I take L with me because er she understand my situation . . . and can enhance my situation . . . Be clarified . . . She can explain it better . . .

He also had mild receptive aphasia. His excellent pragmatic, attention, and listening skills contrasted with his colleagues' weaknesses in these areas. In spite of these differences he was adamant that he should join the group. He perceived his "speech" as being a major barrier to his progress and ability to partake in wider activities. He was determined to maximise therapy input and joined the group in addition to other groups running locally and elsewhere.

Despite their marked differences linguistically, socially, in age, and in time post-onset, the one common and uniting factor experienced by all was their difficulty in coping within the community and in learning to live with their disabilities. The people who met were profoundly affected by loss of role and lack of confidence, resulting in avoidance and isolation. All faced loss of their occupational role either permanently or in the immediate future. For all the clients, their social role within the family and community was changed. For example, one was a first-class graduate with a promising career; another was evicted from his flat and lost his former bachelor lifestyle, returning to live with his mother in a very turbulent family situation. Advocacy and Social Services were involved for many of these people.

PROCEDURES: RATIONALES FOR THE GROUP THERAPY

The rationale for group intervention stemmed from the premise that this group of individuals all expressed a clear desire to meet with others who had similar experiences. In response to this desire, and with no alternative peer group support locally, the therapists decided to see them together in a group setting to encourage peer interaction and discussion about common experiences.

From previous experiences with facilitating groups, it was felt that being in a group offered an extra dimension to the therapeutic process that is not available from individual therapy. The main advantages of group work were:

- providing peer support (Brumfitt, 1995; Fawcus, 1989; Pound, Parr, Lindsay, & Woolf, 2000)
- providing constructive feedback from peers (Brumfitt, 1995; Elman & Bernstein-Ellis, 1999; Pound et al., 2000)
- facilitating increased levels of awareness of difficulties and strengths (Malia, 1997; Malia & Brannagan, 1998; Sohlberg, Mateer, & Stuss, 1993)
- learning/sharing strategies with peers (Pound et al., 2000)
- learning through modelling from peers/ therapists (Bandura, 1997; Pound et al., 2000)
- practising social skills and developing identity in a safe group environment (Pound et al., 2000), and to extend this into their community (Margie, Saunders, & Dickson, 1987)
- reducing isolation (Parr et al., 1997; Sarno, 1981).

From the caseloads held by the therapists at the time, a number of criteria were considered when offering group intervention to individuals with a brain injury.

These included:

- an expressed interest in meeting others
- a level of attention and memory skills sufficient to enable them to meet the requirements of weekly attendance at the group
- enough understanding of language to follow single concepts when framed concretely
- the ability to communicate ideas effectively either via speech or total communication
- a level of activity tolerance sufficient for them to cope with travel to and from the group and participate in a 2-hour session
- the ability to travel to the group independently of therapists (a level of travel training was included to facilitate this—including training to use bus services).

From the 12 potential candidates identified and interviewed as possible group members by therapists, 7 elected to attend. From those 7, 2 individuals had issues that were best addressed in individual therapy and this separate input continued alongside the group-based intervention. Examples of individual work included personalised anger-management and wider liaison and planning with statutory and non-statutory services.

METHODS

In keeping with the social model of disability (Beresford & Croft, 1993; Oliver, 1990) the aim was to facilitate the group to be self-directed and member-focused rather than therapist-led and dependent. It was hoped that this philosophy would assist group members to feel more confident in defining their own identities and destiny.

Accordingly, we looked to draw the specific aims of therapy from discussion and the concerns raised by the group as a whole. The role of the therapist in these discussions was to act as a facilitator, probing issues if required and drawing

discussion points together in a format that allowed the group members to reflect on their discussion and prioritise the issues they had raised.

There were three modules to the group programme. In the first module, lasting for 6 weeks, group members became acquainted, initiated ideas, and set the baseline for the following two modules. The second and third modules were each run for 8 to 10 weeks. Each one was structured into a triad and covered aspects of education, awareness, and implementation of strategies

No standardised outcome measures were used as they were not considered to be sensitive enough to pick up on the complexity or nature of change. We aimed to use an eclectic mixture of outcome measures.

1. SMART goals. Goals were set that were Specific, Measurable, Agreed, Realistic, and Timed (SMART: Whitmore, 1996). These goals were set and re-evaluated with the group members as part of the therapeutic group process.
2. Checklist of listening behaviours adapted from Hartley (1990) (Appendix 6.1).
3. Assessment of client behaviours in group activities (Tipton & Einbinder Kaye, 1992). This measure was ongoing within the group.
4. Self-rating questionnaire focusing on memory, attention, and communication written for the group (Appendix 6.2).
5. Dartmouth COOP function and health status measure for adults. This was used to measure quality of life (Johnson, 1989).
6. The "blobby men" rating (Figure 6.2) complemented the outcome tools used.

THERAPY

Module one: Six group meetings
The first module focused on getting to know one another. Group-gelling was facilitated through a variety of fun warm-up exercises, group discussions, and explorations as to why each group member had decided to attend.

In the first meeting with the group, four goals were set:

- Goal 1: that the group will establish a working rapport
- Goal 2: jointly to establish group ground rules
- Goal 3: to identify the issues that the group wished to address and identification of future goals for the group
- Goal 4: to decide if they wished to join the group.

Sessions were initiated by introducing the use of a gym ball passed amongst the group, with a memory or descriptive task associated with receiving or passing the ball. Further warm-up tasks attempted to strike a balance between conversational discussions and non-verbal tasks. These tasks aimed to focus on the wider aspects of communication, for example, gesturing opening a present and guessing the contents, or a more physical task of moving to corners of the room depending on the person's responses to closed questions.

Given the cultural and social diversity of the group it was essential to establish ground rules for the group early on to ensure that issues of equal opportunity were addressed.

Members were asked to complete two grids: one of activities undertaken pre-morbidly, and one of activities currently involved in. This was used to stimulate discussion around the changes experienced in a variety of spheres. It prompted much comment on both negative and positive aspects of living with brain injury and became the foundation for future discussion. Brainstorming sessions were employed to encourage the group to think of all the issues facing them. The group prioritised these issues and identified areas to focus on in future modules.

Module two

The following personal goals were agreed upon with the group at the beginning of the second module.

- Goal 5: to be able to express what is meant by the term attention/memory

- Goal 6: to identify strengths and weaknesses with regard to attention/memory
- Goal 7: to identify one strategy to help promote better attention/memory
- Goal 8: to keep a log of the above.

The areas to be covered in this module included:

- orientation
- visual inattention
- auditory inattention
- external/internal distractors
- storage and retention of information (memory).

Each of the group members had a level of attention and or memory deficit as shown through formal assessment, observation, and interview. The first part of the module was designed to educate and provide the group with accessible verbal and written information about the basic concepts and terminology for attention and memory. This was done through discussion of simple illustrated handouts and listening games (What can you hear in the room? What's on your mind?). Video feedback, self-rating scales, and peer evaluation were utilised to promote individual recognition and acceptance of strengths and weaknesses. The rating scale used for this is given in Appendix 6.2. These were self-evaluated through the use of personal logs. Appropriate strategies for use in daily life were identified and members selected handouts of their chosen strategies. Strategies varied from the use of simple cues (alarm clocks, diaries) to the use of discussed and practised strategies; for example, the "feedback loop", which aimed to focus the group to listen, monitor, and indicate comprehension. The handouts varied from a simple cartoon to convey a single idea, such as the use of a diary, to a much fuller and more comprehensive account of the strategies used (to "help remember something you have to do", for instance.) This variety in the complexity of information provided was intended to make the information accessible to all at whatever level of comprehension they felt comfortable with. "Homework" tasks were given to practise outside the group and as a way of bringing feedback to the next session based on the degree of success.

For example, group members were asked to bring a snack for all to share in the next week. Only SY managed to remember this, and he triumphantly produced a tin of tuna! Discussion on strategies for remembering ensued, including some thoughts on making links by association. It was essential to encourage practice outside of the group in a real-life situation to measure if individuals in the group were able to generalise the skills and strategies learnt in therapy.

Module three

The third and final module in the programme dealt with stress management. The programme used was adapted from an Open University manual on handling stress (Bailey & Lorna, 1992). The goals for this module were:

- Goal 9: to identify the positive and negative aspects of stress in their life
- Goal 10: to identify a relaxation strategy that they would feel comfortable using
- Goal 11: to identify a strategy for coping with negative stress
- Goal 12: to identify what is unhelpful in dealing with stress.

As part of the initial stress education, the group identified what stress is and identified positive and negative aspects through a brainstorming session. The first session ended with a short talk by each group member on what a stress-free lifestyle might be for them. This provoked further discussion on the more positive aspects of stress and that life would be dull without some level of stress.

The group was given a set of tasks to complete that would provoke an amount of stress (refer to Appendix 6.3 for sample session plan). This exercise was used to facilitate group members' insight into their own stress symptoms and to increase body awareness. Each group member completed their own stress-rating scale (Powell, 1992).

The group was asked to feed back on each other's posture and body language and their perception of the degree of stress present. Body diagrams were then used to illustrate the short-term effects of stress (fight or flight reaction) and the long-term effects of negative stress on the body (ulcers, raised blood pressure, and muscle pain).

The group identified the effects to include physical, behavioural, social, and emotional aspects but they focused more on the social and behavioural effects of stress, citing examples including difficulties sleeping, avoidance of situations, increased confusion, and increased difficulty in listening or in finding the right words.

The group then identified lifestyle and life events as contributory aspects to stress. This led to an emotional and revealing discussion from individuals about their brain injury in terms of its impact as a major life event.

Adaptive and maladaptive mechanisms for coping were identified. Therapists role-playing a scenario with different outcomes facilitated discussion. The group members were then asked to identify the most appropriate solution and give reasons for their choice. From this the group identified passive, aggressive, and assertive behaviours and was not only able to see the positive and negative aspects of each one on an empirical level, but was also quick to explain their habitual behavioural patterns.

Adaptive strategies such as goal planning, time management, assertiveness, relaxation, humour, and breaking the cycle of negative self-talk were introduced and discussed.

A relaxation exercise was included at the end of each session. This attempted to introduce the group to a variety of relaxation techniques. These included breathing, progressive muscular relaxation, visual imagery, and elements of yoga and the Alexander technique (Barlow, 1990). The physiotherapist (from the therapy team) was brought in to lead some of these exercises.

Finally the group was introduced to local community resources. Therapists hoped this would extend the generalisation of the skills gained by establishing ongoing routines. Each member of the group completed a stress action plan, which identified adaptive strategies and when and for how long to employ them.

At the end of this module each group member was given assistance in writing an individual goal for the use of their identified strategy in a real-life situation, which would then be reviewed at the end of the module. Therapists observed and reinforced the practice of these strategies throughout the third module.

Goals were also rated at the end of this third module. This included self-evaluation of the success of their strategy for improving attention and memory that had been identified for further development in the second module.

RESULTS

Outcome measure 1—SMART goals

SMART goals 1–4 were achieved by all group members. However, one group member elected to withdraw from the group (group goal 4), saying that she felt that she did not have any difficulties and wanted to resume her previous lifestyle and return to work immediately. Consequently there are no other sets of results for this group member.

SMART goals 6 and 9 were the goals that required the identification of strengths and were achieved by all. However, two group members were only able to articulate these verbally and they were not able to make the significant leap of applying the consequence of these issues to their daily lives. This was not rated by the goals set.

SMART goals 7, 10, and 11, which focused on the identification and use of strategies, were again achieved at re-rating but have not been rated since. From continued contact with individual group members, however, we would suggest that four of the six have maintained regular daily use of strategies.

Outcome measure 2—checklist of listening behaviours

The results from the checklist of listening behaviours are summarised in Table 6.2.

Three of the six group members showed a consistent and significant improvement. One (CG) stayed the same, and on closer analysis this was due to increased distractibility counteracting the gains in her actual listening and comprehension skills. This was due to internal distraction caused by much personal anxiety and change. Two members had a slight decrease (SY and RF). As their

TABLE 6.2

Listening behaviours rating scale summary

Group member	Rating	
	Pre-course (Max. score = 80)	*Post-course (Max. score = 80)*
SY	30	25
ED	53	66
RF	33	32
CG	51	51
JM	60	65
JJ	48	60

familiarity in the group increased they became less inhibited and more distracted. This was perhaps a more accurate reflection of their natural communication amongst family and friends.

Outcome measure 3—assessment of client behaviours in group activities

The ongoing assessment of client behaviours through group activities is divided into three sections: functioning within the group, communication, and cognition (Figure 6.1).

The pattern of results in all three is similar. Four of the group members improved in all areas. Once more SY and RF did not show improvement; they were consistent on communication and cognition but decreased for functioning within the group. As discussed above, their decreased inhibition influenced their ability to work effectively within the group.

Outcome measure 4—self-rating questionnaire

Results on the self-rating questionnaire are summarised in Table 6.3. It was hoped that this measure would reflect the group members' insight into the progress in managing their memory, attention and communication skills. From the table it is possible to see that three of the group members, ED, JJ, and JM, perceived a change and improvement in their attention, memory, and listening skills. This improvement is echoed

FIGURE 6.1

a. Ongoing assessment of client behaviours in group activities: Functioning within a group

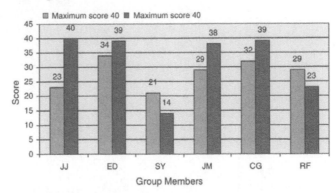

b. Communication

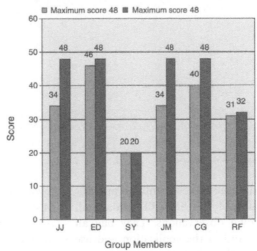

c. Cognition

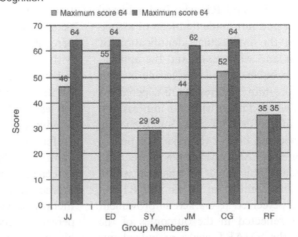

Ongoing assessment of client behaviours in group activities.

TABLE 6.3

Self-rating questionnaire (Always = 4, Sometimes = X, Never = 0)

	ED		RF		SY		JJ		JM	
Question	Initial	End	Initial	End	Initial	End	Initial	End	Initial	End
1	X	4	X	X	X	X	X	4	4	X
2	X	4	X	X	4	4	X	X	4	X
3	X	4	X	X	X	X	X	4	X	X
4	4	4	X	X	X	4	X	4	4	4
5	X	4	4	4	4	4	X	4	X	4
6	X	X	4	X	X	X	X	X	X	4
7	4	4	4	X	4	4	X	4	4	4
8	X	X	X	4	4	4	4	4	4	4
9	4	4	X	4	4	4	X	4	4	4
10	4	4	X	X	X	X	X	4	4	4
11	4	4	X	4	X	X	0	4	4	4
12	X	X	X	X	X	X	X	X	4	4
13	X	4	4	4	X	X	X	4	4	4
14	4	4	4	X	4	4	X	X	4	4
15	X	4	X	X	X	X	X	X	X	X
16	X	X	X	4	0	0	X	X	0	0
17	0	X	X	X	X	X	X	X	X	X
18	X	4	4	4	X	X	X	4	4	4
19	4	4	4	4	X	X	X	4	X	X
20	X	X	X	X	X	X	X	4	X	0

in the rating scales, the achievement and application of the results of the SMART goals, and, of course, our own observations. They had all grown in insight and in the application and use of strategies within their daily lives.

The results of SY and RF, who had achieved their goals but had not made that leap of association between the intellectual identification of their strengths and weaknesses and the application of the consequence to issues arising in their daily lives, were more interesting. SY perceived little change, which tallied with our impressions, the outcome of the SMART goals, and the rating scales. He appeared unable to make that link in applying strategies. At 12 years post-onset, had he already adapted as far as he was able within the support and comfort of his family? RF, on the contrary, perceived a marked improvement that was not reflected in the outcomes of the rating scales, the SMART goals, or indeed our

own impressions. He perhaps lacked a degree of insight.

The "blobby men" rating was also an attempt to seek the perceptions of the group into their own progress (see Figure 6.2). Whilst similar trends prevail, at some level individual difficulties persist and we suggest that this may dampen their perceptions of their achievements. For example, with reference to ED and JJ this is true.

ED moved sidewards. To her this reflected a greater security and a better ability to cope; she felt less "out on a limb", less precarious. JJ moved notably up the tree, but only so far. She too felt "safer" and that she had progressed, but was not finally out there and confident on the top. JM perceived himself as being well supported (as indeed he was by family and the considerable therapy backup he was receiving at the time). RF perceived success but his limited application of his goals and his limited awareness make his

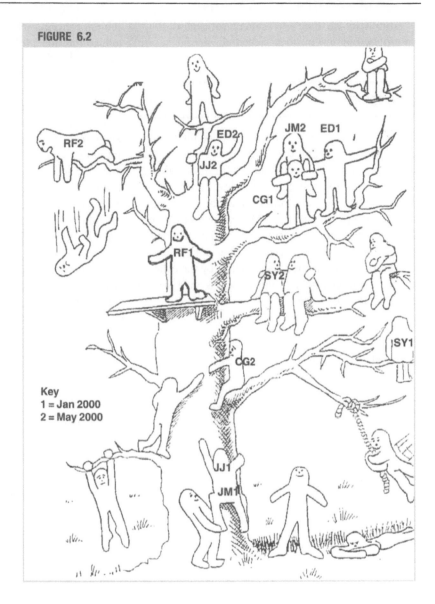

FIGURE 6.2

Key
1 = Jan 2000
2 = May 2000

Blobby men rating
pre- and post-group.
Adapted from *Games
without frontiers: Fun,
growth & development
games for group workers*
(Wilson, 1992).

achievements more precarious. He felt he was doing "fine" on the one hand but, on the other, it is clear that he had some inkling of the fragility of his situation. SY, alongside our perceptions, moved only sidewards. However, it is of note that he placed himself out on his own and alone, to begin with, but felt supported and befriended by the end. CG's drop down the tree is interesting: She felt extremely anxious because of her uncertain medical situation, and perceived herself to be "hanging on for dear life" in spite of her strong cognitive and linguistic strengths.

Anxiety clearly impeded her progress and her self-perceptions.

Outcome measure 5—Dartmouth COOP function and health status measure for adults

Reassessment on the Dartmouth COOP was not carried out. On initial assessment it was felt that this measure was not sensitive enough to detect the subtleties of change experienced and reflected in the intricate analysis of the specific individual behaviours looked at in the above checklists.

An overall summary of changes for each of the group members is given in Table 6.4.

DISCUSSION

Our clients' common need to learn about brain injury and to share this with others who had experienced similar circumstances far outweighed their differences in symptoms or levels of ability. The member who had more pronounced expressive language difficulties (JM) learned to value and recognise his own strengths as an excellent listener, which he had previously overlooked. This recognition was also fed back to him by the other group members, which appeared to give him additional confidence.

New concepts were presented in the group in concrete terms, with pointers given for further study and reflection for any of those members who felt able and motivated to do this. Indeed, this happened with one group member, who offered to bring her research findings back to the group. This member also opted to continue to participate in the group in spite of being given the option to attend a smaller, more focused discussion and research-based group at the end of module two. She fed back that from the group she greatly valued the opportunity to meet, share, and understand others' similar experiences and that she felt comfortable with the pitching of group activities.

This group aimed to be therapeutic and to give members the insight and strategies to enable them to make the changes needed to manage their daily

TABLE 6.4

Summary of results

Group member	Listening rating scale	Rating scale 'Function within the group'	Communication	Cognition	Self-rating questionnaire	Blobby rating
SY	Declined	Declined—disinhibition?	No change	No change	Minimal change	More support?
CG	No change	Improvement	Improvement	Improvement	No rating (ill at time of rating)	"Hanging on"
ED	Improvement	Improvement	Mild improvement	Improvement	Perceived improvement	"Safe holding on, but doing well"
JJ	Improvement	Improvement	Improvement	Improvement	Perceived improvement	"Safe holding on, but doing well"
JM	Improvement	Improvement	Improvement	Improvement	Perceived improvement	"Well supported and doing well"
RF	Minimal decline	Declined—disinhibition?	Minimal improvement	No change	Perceived improvement	"Soaring but precarious"

lives more effectively; for example, "feeding back when you haven't understood", or the use of a diary to record important information. We wondered whether timeliness of intervention is a critical factor. Four members were between 1 and 2 years post-onset. One, however (SY), had received his injury 12 years before and the remaining two attended within 6 months of their insult following discharge from the acute sector. Six months may be too early in the bereavement process for most to be able to address the gritty issue of adaptation and strategy use—often people are more focused on recovery and getting back to "normal". Also, at 6 months post-onset, individuals have not actually experienced living in the community with their disabilities, nor grasped the full impact and implications of their insult. For the woman who withdrew from therapy this was certainly true. Another woman, CG, at 6 months post-onset, had insight but was still in shock and trying to continue her life to meet others' expectations in fulfilling her role as wife, mother, and earner. In addition she had continuing medical problems, which caused extreme anxiety and uncertainty. For SY, in the 12 years since his injury, life had changed dramatically and the family had routines in place. For this person the group offered the opportunity for support, socialisation, and an educative update.

For the four members between 1 and 2 years post-onset, the timing and focus of the group appeared to be good. They had all received much previous therapy in the acute and rehabilitative settings as in-patients. On discharge, the reality of an unstructured, non-institutional day was a shock. The isolation, scope of change, and the exhausting demands placed on both physical and mental stamina by attempting to live a normal daily routine resulted in low mood and an inability to cope. For some this meant spending days in bed, for others a fostered dependency on carers, or Social Services exceeding their needs and causing additional stress and breakdown of family relationships. None were able to fulfil the full expectations of their previous roles and they mourned this loss. Their executive difficulties made it problematic for them to initiate, organise,

plan, and direct their days. Communicating with family, friends, and the public was challenging and draining, particularly as these difficulties are often subtle and go unnoticed. All articulated a sense of isolation and bewilderment and a desire to meet with those who had some understanding of their situation.

Meeting each other in a group was evaluated as providing the peer support, feedback, and structured approach to learning that group members sought. It also provided a safe environment within the community to discuss, experiment, and evaluate their progress and strategies away from the stress of their social situation. The problem-solving style of the group aimed to equip individuals to use this approach directly in daily living in the long-term. Being based within the community setting, in a healthy-living centre, gave the advantage of direct application of the approach to the practical and relevant challenges of life. The group meetings built and expanded on some of the work achieved in previous rehabilitation settings. It encouraged generalisation and carry-over of skills that may not have been achieved without this additional reinforcement.

Awareness appeared to play a major role in the relative ongoing success achieved by the group members, as rated by the therapists and through self-evaluation. The woman who felt she had no difficulties withdrew from therapy completely. Subsequent follow-up has identified failed employment, alienated family and friends, anger, and a continuing pattern of blaming others for her situation. It is extremely difficult to know how to help her other than by "leaving the door open".

A model of awareness has been discussed by Stuss (1991) and Malia and Brannagan (1998) (Figure 6.3). They describe intellectual awareness as an ability to indicate (verbally or non-verbally at some level) a cognitive knowledge of a change in function. They then describe two other levels of awareness: emergent and anticipatory awareness. Emergent awareness is when the person can recognise this difficulty at the time it is occurring and know why it is happening without the need for feedback. At the top of the awareness

FIGURE 6.3

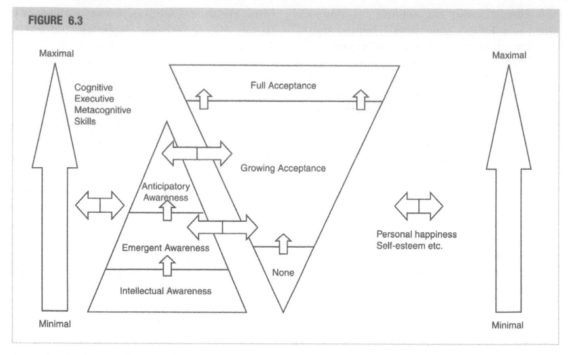

Model of awareness after Stuss (1991) and Malia and Brannagan (1998).

hierarchy, anticipatory awareness describes the ability to predict likely problems arising from their particular disabilities. Acceptance dovetails the level of awareness and develops alongside it. The authors also point out that awareness is not an all-or-nothing phenomenon, but that levels of awareness vary across different domains of functioning. For example, a person may be aware of his physical difficulties at the anticipatory stage, independently using an adaptive walking aid. He may also be aware at the intellectual stage that he has memory problems but be unable to connect this with a tendency to forget appointments or the need for a diary. The model also indicates that the level of individual personal happiness and cognitive skills has an influence on the individual's ability to progress through the hierarchy of awareness and acceptance. Denial and awareness deficits due to brain injury often coexist and can present with similar behavioural manifestations, so can be clinically difficult to distinguish. However, at some level (consciously or subconsciously), denial indicates a degree of awareness and may be part

of a natural psychological defence mechanism. Past experiences and values influence denial. The meaning of illness varies from person to person and is linked to personality, life experience, and culture (Malia & Brannagan, 1998).

Applying this model to the group, a summary of the relationship between time post-onset, "recovery", and awareness is drawn up in Table 6.5.

Table 6.5 relates to the results given in Table 6.4. The two members whose rating scale scores declined, SY and RF, achieved their goals but were unable to apply their knowledge to daily living. The authors suggest that they had an intellectual level of awareness and were therefore able to articulate their strengths and weaknesses and the strategies they felt may be helpful (with regard to cognition and communication), but in reality had great difficulty in applying this knowledge. This might explain their decline in rating scales and perhaps their limited progress. Additionally they had limited attention, and according to the model, attention is a prerequisite for working

TABLE 6.5

A summary of the relationship between time post-onset, "recovery", and awareness as defined by Stuss (1991) and Malia (1997)

Time post-onset	Recovery	Awareness
One at 12 years	Limited progress	Intellectual awareness
One at 6 months	Stable, progress hampered by external factors	Elements of anticipatory awareness
Four at 1–2 years	Three out of the four members at this stage made good progress	Elements of anticipatory awareness
	One out of the 4 members at this stage, made limited progress	Intellectual awareness
(One opted out: 6 months)	Opted out	No intellectual awareness or denial?

through the hierarchy. For one of these two members, being 12 years post-onset, timeliness may also have been significant. The other, however, fell within the 2-year bracket.

The other group members all progressed and, by the end of module three, would appear to show elements of anticipatory awareness. This is evidenced through their independent use of strategies and their growing ability to generalise. The one woman who did not make such notable progress and whose scores remained similar, suffered during this period from extreme anxiety and emotional turmoil due to difficult home and medical circumstances. Timeliness may also have been a factor for her at 6 months post-onset.

We have discussed the results from our perspectives as clinicians, using the eclectic range of outcome tools we had selected. These undoubtedly looked to assess "change" and to pick up on "improvements" as a result of intervention. We thought to ask the group members for their perspectives: What is recovery? Is it synonymous with "change" and "improvement"? What, then, is therapy all about? As you will see from Figure 6.4, their interpretation was much broader. Recovery, it seemed, was reached through dialogue (both internal and external): the grappling with emotions of loss and grief, the hopes and aspirations of what might be, the broader understanding, knowledge, and perceptions reached

through experience and, in their case, through mutual discussion and sharing.

Therapy here had served to provide a structure and a facilitative forum for considering recovery. On the one hand, we attempted to maintain a client-centred approach throughout, consistent with the social model. We achieved this by seeking the group's views about the issues to be addressed and by joint goal setting. On the other hand, the group required some input from the therapists; for example, group ground rules were essential. The therapist facilitated the group in the initiation, planning, and implementing of activities. With respect to communication, the therapist sometimes pointed out reasons why conversation or speech was problematic. It is our view that at this stage of recovery in the community, a significant role of the therapist is to act as a facilitator, advocate, and educator.

Group members' views highlight the importance of long-term support. The need for long-term follow-up is further emphasised by the premise that awareness and psychological adjustment are not static but develop over months and years. It could therefore be argued that specialist community follow-up is one of the most appropriate ways of ensuring that people with a brain injury continue to receive appropriate support months or years post-insult to enable them, as they say, "to live their lives".

FIGURE 6.4

Recovery

- knowledge and understanding of injury
- acceptance of life—can take a long time
- awareness of situation
- how long?
- going home so I will be ok
- recovery = back to "normal"
- unsure how far I will recover
- not possible to be the same
- disabled—other people's attitudes
- communication–re what has happened and how you feel; need to discuss with others—people who understand (professionals; friends; family; colleagues; and people who have similar problems)
- support in the long-term
- fatigue—body doesn't recharge in the same way as before injury

Therapy

- helping people to understand—working towards acceptance
- possible changes to help with coping
- joint discussion
- increased confidence to attempt things and live your life
- good to have back-up support

Group member's views on what is meant by "recovery" and "therapy".

REFERENCES

Bailey, N., & Lorna, S. (1992). *Handling stress. A pack for group work. Teaching pack*. Oxford: Oxford University Press. Open University in association with the Health Promotion Authority for Wales and the Health Education Authority Buckingham.

Bandura, A. (1977). *Social learning theory*. New York: Prentice Hall.

Barlow, W. (1990). *The Alexander principle*. London: Gollancz Paperback.

Beresford, P., & Croft, S. (1993). *Citizen involvement: A practical guide for change*. Basingstoke, UK: Macmillan.

Brumfitt, S. (1995). Psychotherapy in aphasia. In C. Code & D. Muller (Eds.), *Treatment of aphasia: From theory to practice*. London: Whurr.

Brumfitt, S. (1996). Losing your sense of self: What aphasia can do. In C. Code & D. Muller (Eds.), *Forums in clinical aphasiology* (pp. 349–354). London: Whurr.

Ellmo, W.J., Graser, J.M., Krchnavek, E.A., Calabrese, D.B., & Hanck, R. (1995). *Measure of cognitive-linguistic abilities*. Vero Beach, FL: The Speech Bin.

Elman, R.J., & Bernstein-Ellis, E. (1999). Aphasia group communication treatment: The Aphasia Centre of California approach. In R.J. Elman (Ed.), *Group treatment of neurogenic communication disorders: The expert clinician's approach*. Boston: Butterworth-Heinmann.

Fawcus, M. (1989). Group therapy: A learning situation. In C. Code & D. Muller (Eds.), *Aphasia therapy* (pp. 113–120). London: Cole & Whurr.

Hartley, L.L. (1990). Assessment of functional communication. In D.E. Tupper & K.D. Cicerone (Eds.), *The neuropsychology of everyday life. Volume 1: Assessment and basic competencies*. (pp. 125–167). Boston: Kluwer Academic.

Hartley, L.L. (1995). *Cognitive-communication abilities following brain injury: A functional approach*. London: Singular Publishing Group.

Hersh, D. (1998). Beyond the "plateau": Discharge dilemmas in chronic aphasia. *Aphasiology, 12*, 207–243.

Johnson, D. (1989). *The Dartmouth COOP function and health status measures for adults*. Hanover, NH: Trustees of Dartmouth College, Dartmouth Medical School.

Malia, K.B. (1997). Insight after brain injury: What does it mean? *Journal of Cognitive Rehabilitation, 15*, 10–12.

Malia, K.B., & Brannagan, A. (1998). *Insight workshop*. York, UK: Brain Tree Training.

Margie, O., Saunders, C., & Dickson, D. (1987). *Social skills in interpersonal communication*. London: Croom Helm.

Oliver, M. (1990). *The politics of disablement*. London: Macmillan.

Parr, S., Byng, S., Gilpin, S., & Ireland, C. (1997). *Talking about aphasia*. Buckingham, UK: Open University Press.

Pound, C., Parr, S., Lindsay, J., & Woolf, C. (2000).

Beyond aphasia. Therapies for living with communication disability. Oxford: Winslow Press.

Powell, T. (1992). *Stress inventory—effects of stress.* (*Adapted from Work Stress Inventory.*) Buckingham, UK: Open University Press.

Sarno, J. (1981). Emotional aspects of aphasia. In M.T. Sarno (Ed.), *Acquired aphasia.* New York: Academic Press.

Sohlberg, M.H., Mateer, C.A., & Stuss, D.T. (1993). Contemporary approaches to the management of executive control dysfunction. *Journal of Head Trauma Rehabilitation, 8*, 45–85.

Stuss, D.T. (1991). Disturbances of self-awareness after frontal system damage. In G.P. Prigatano & D.L. Schacter (Eds.), *Awareness of deficit after brain injury.* Oxford: Oxford University Press.

Tipton, A., & Einbinder Kaye, M. (1992). *Ongoing assessment of client behaviours in group activities.* Tucson, AZ: Therapy Skill Builders.

Toglia, J. (1991). Generalization of treatment: A multicontext approach to cognitive perceptual impairment in adults with brain injury. *American Journal of Occupational Therapy, 45*, 505–516.

Whitmore, J. (1996). *Coaching for performance.* London: Nicholas Brealey.

Ylvisaker, M., & Szakeres, S.E. (1989). Metacognition and executive impairments in head injured children and adults, *Topics in Language Disorders, 9*, 34–49.

Ylvisaker, M. (1992). Communication outcome following traumatic brain injury. *Seminars in Speech and Language, 13*, 239–251.

APPENDICES

APPENDIX 6.1: Cognitive-communication abilities following brain injury

Checklist of listening behaviours

1. Easily distracted by irrelevant noises or movement.
2. Inhibits internal thoughts (facial expression consistent with speaker's message, listening rather than planning what to say).
3. Not easily overwhelmed (copes well with multiple stimuli, e.g., visual and verbal information or many people present).
4. Refrains from doing other tasks that might distract speaker.
5. Refrains from interrupting the speaker.
6. Shifts attention in group as speaker changes.
7. Waits until directions/information is completed before starts.
8. Maintains eye gaze towards speaker.
9. Comprehends paralinguistic aspects of communication (vocal tone, loudness and fluency).
10. Picks up well on non-verbal cues (e.g., gestures, drawing) to interpret the situation and assist comprehension.
11. Is able to follow conversation well irrespective of the complexity, rate, or length of the message.
12. Asks for clarification or repetition when unsure of message.
13. Comments indicate a thorough understanding of speaker's intent.
14. Initiates questions/comments relevant to topic of discussion.
15. Indicates level of understanding through verbal or non-verbal means.

(Adapted from Hartley, 1995.)

APPENDIX 6.2: Self-rating questionnaire

The group member is asked to rate him or herself on each of the items below: The choices are *Always, Sometimes, Never*

Do you remember the names of the people in the group?
1. Do you remember the instructions in the group?
2. Do you remember what was talked about last week in the group?
3. Do you use anything to help you with your memory for the group, e.g., a diary, a calendar, notebook, post-it notes?

Attention
4. Do you pay attention when a person is talking to you?
5. Are you easily distracted in the group?
6. Do you keep track of what is happening in the group?

Communication/Conversation
7. Do you look at the person who is speaking?
8. Do you keep your concentration in group discussions?
9. Do you understand what is being said in the group?
10. Do you ask for help and explanation if you don't?
11. Are you a good listener?
12. Do you give yourself and others time to communicate?
13. Do you keep track of what you are saying?
14. Do you start new topics of conversation?
15. Do you talk when others are talking?
16. Do you tell stories and jokes?
17. Do people understand you when you talk or give information?
18. Do you ask questions/make comments relevant to the discussion?
19. Do you do a lot of talking?

APPENDIX 6.3: Sample of stress management session

- Introduction and warm-up
  (What I feel good about and one thing that stresses me out)
- Recap on what is understood by stress
- Fill out stress questionnaire
- Recap goals
- Exercise to monitor what it feels like to experience a level of stress
  (Two group members to take everybody's orders for coffee, make a note of it and work out the pricing and change required)
- Brainstorm (how did it feel?)
- Identify the mental, physical, social and emotional reactions experienced by the group
- Clarification of these headings and link to the stress chain
- Add an extra example from experience
- Relaxation exercise (yoga, exercise: tense—relax—and imagine)

"What's in a name?" Improving proper name retrieval through therapy

Ann Montagu and Jane Marshall[1]

Outlined here is a therapy study with a 61-year-old woman (SH) with aphasia. SH underwent a heart bypass operation in 1993 and right carotid endarteroectomy in October 1995. On 1 December 1995, she had a left-hemisphere infarct stroke in the left parietal region with involvement of the left Sylvian fissure. This led to mild–moderate oropharyngeal dysphagia, right-sided weakness, mild receptive and expressive dysphasia, and dyspraxia. SH walked with great effort and often relied on a wheelchair when going out. She had normal hearing. She wore glasses and had no vision in her left eye. Following her stroke, she regularly took Prozac for depression. SH steadfastly asserted her independence and lived alone. Her three children and five grandchildren visited regularly, but apart from this she had few opportunities to mix with others.

SH initially received 9 months of domiciliary speech and language therapy once or twice a week, followed by some group therapy locally. She then began attending a university-based aphasia group but had not gone consistently due to transport and mobility difficulties.

SH communicated quite well but she demonstrated some clear word-finding difficulties that affected and frustrated her in conversations. Whilst she displayed some general anomia, it was her difficulty with proper names, i.e., names of people and places, that seemed to cause her particular distress. In instances of proper noun anomia, SH was often quite dependent on her communication partner to help repair the conversation. The following extract from a conversation with SH about her grandchildren illustrates this:

AM: And he's (your son) got twins?

SH: No two young girls

AM: Not twins, very similar in ages. Who's the eldest?

SH: Erm oh Anne er Anne er Nelly, Nelly

AM: So Nelly's the eldest and then there's. . . .

SH: there arem (Scratching head) Nelly and (gestures to photos behind her)
Oh (looking frustrated)

AM: Is it Chloe?

SH: Yeah

AM: I thought they were twins

SH: No no

AM: I think it's because that photo you showed me

SH: They're together

AM: They look identical as well, . . . they're close in age

SH: Yes, one year something . . . but erm I can't remember names at all, bit hard . . .

The practical importance of proper nouns for SH was clear. For example, proper nouns were vital for her to impart autobiographical information to others and carried emotional weight. More widely, we could imagine the difficulty she might have in introducing herself or greeting others without using proper names. Furthermore, she could not use a synonym in place of a proper noun as is often possible with common nouns. The purpose of this study, therefore, was to discover if therapeutic interventions could facilitate her retrieval of proper nouns.

COMMUNICATION PROFILE

Formal assessment results for SH are listed in Table 7.1.[2]

SH's comprehension had not been formally tested in the recent past. Previous SLT reports pointed to high-level comprehension difficulties at a complex sequential ideational level. Her score on the auditory synonym judgement test, although very good, supported this (see Table 7.1). Additionally, SH reported difficulties with increased auditory load, e.g., when listening to the TV news, and found greater difficulty when communicating with more than one person. However, in normal conversation, she coped well with little or no facilitation. She also picked up on humour well, as the following post-therapy extract, where she was talking about the comedian Ali G, illustrates:

SH: Oh my man

AM: Who's your man?

SH: Ali G

AM: Cos you can laugh at the TV

SH: Oh no no not only that, I like him

AM: Oh do you think he looks good as well?

SH: Oh /g/ gorgeous. No I think he's gorgeous (laughing). You know because you know so funny and erm I just like him very much oh yeah I like him

Formal and informal testing indicated that SH read single words and short sentences aloud well. Informal testing showed she could capture the general meaning of short newspaper articles. However, she did not feel confident in this medium and repeatedly said "I can't read" and typically only read TV listings in newspapers.

Anomic difficulties were evidenced by phonological errors that resulted in real and non-word substitutions, e.g., /konifə/ → /koribə/, conduit d'approche, circumlocution, hesitancy, and verbal groping. Additionally, she often produced pronoun reversals and made occasional morphemic errors. Formal testing suggested that her single word repetition was quite good, but she had greater difficulty with words containing three or more syllables. SH wrote her name, copied words, and wrote some three- to five-letter words accurately. However, she was not confident about writing and found it effortful. Although she sometimes finger-wrote as a self-cuing mechanism, she did not spontaneously write in her everyday communication.

TABLE 7.1

Formal assessment results (SH)

Assessment name	Date administered	Score
PALPA Minimal Pair Discrimination	01/99	35/36 same 31/36 different
PALPA Syllable Length Repetition	01/99	6/8 one syllable 6/8 two syllables 4/8 three syllables
PALPA Auditory Synonym Judgement	01/99	29/30 high imagability 25/30 low imagability
PALPA Reading Aloud Picture Names	03/99	16/20
PALPA Written Picture Naming	03/99	7/20
PALPA Picture Name Repetition	06/99	13/20
PALPA Spoken Picture Naming	06/99	14/20
PALPA Written Picture Names to Dictation	06/99	7/20

SH was a very communicative person, using intonation, humour, sarcasm, gesture, and facial expression well to convey meaning during her conversations. She was very aware of her difficulties, which she approached with some humour but also, at times, with considerable frustration.

PROPER AND COMMON NOUNS

Various assessments were carried out to further investigate SH's comprehension and production of proper and common nouns.[3]

Face recognition

This test used 40 pictures of famous people, each of which was paired with a non-famous distracter similar in appearance to the target. The pictures were randomly mixed and SH asked to provide a yes/no answer in reply to the question "have you seen this person before?". SH scored 91% on this task, demonstrating intact face recognition.

Name comprehension

The 40 pictures used in the previous task were combined with 20 pictures of famous places, 20 high-familiarity common nouns, 20 low-familiarity common nouns, and 15 pictures of personal significance to SH, e.g., pets and family members. Her ability to recognise the spoken name of each picture was tested using the format "is this . . . ?", randomly alternating between targets and distracters. For example, when shown a picture of Roger Moore, she might be asked "is this Harrison Ford?". SH scored 100% on this task, showing no difference between proper and common nouns.

Name production

SH was asked to name all five groups of pictures used in the comprehension task (Table 7.2). Where she was unable to name the target, she was provided alternately with either a semantic or a phonemic cue. For example, the semantic cue for the picture of London was "it's our capital city".

A comparison of proper name production with common noun naming revealed no significant difference for SH ($\chi^2 = 0.36$). Interestingly, when we

TABLE 7.2

Raw scores and percentage correct of SH's proper noun and common noun naming

SH	Famous people	Famous places	Personally familiar	Common nouns	
				High fam	Low fam
Uncued response	13/40 (33%)	11/20 (55%)	11/15 (73%)	12/20 (60%)	9/20 (45%)
Phonemic cues	11 correct	1 correct	3 correct	2 correct	
Semantic cues	1 correct	1 correct			

analysed common and proper nouns removing the personally familiar scores from the latter group, we found that again there was no difference between the two groups ($\chi^2 = 1.5$)

The second analysis examined differences within the proper nouns group, comparing famous people and famous places. For SH this was not quite significant ($\chi^2 = 3.28$, $p < .10$). Arguably, had there been equal numbers of stimuli in both groups, we might have seen a significant difference between the two groups for SH.

Third, naming scores for famous people and personally familiar names were compared to test for an effect of familiarity. For SH, production of personally familiar names was significantly better ($\chi^2 = 7.40$, $p < .01$). The stimuli chosen by her were all family names as opposed to a mixture of personally familiar place names and family names. Hence, this effect was a pure familiarity effect as opposed to a combined effect of familiarity and place name preference.

The fourth analysis tested for a familiarity effect within the common noun group. Whilst there was no significant familiarity effect ($\chi^2 = 0.9$), she scored marginally better with the high-familiarity group.

Overall, SH benefited more from phonemic than semantic cuing when naming, correcting 11 famous people's names when given a phonemic cue. She also produced some particularly rich circumlocutions, indicating good semantic knowledge of the targets. For example, for Bill Clinton and Nelson Mandela, her responses were "American . . . naughty boy him" (this was at the time of the Monica Lewinski affair) and "Africa

. . . in prison for years . . . his wife wasn't nice either" respectively. Circumlocuting was a successful strategy for her, on five occasions precipitating the correct naming of a famous person. Perhaps this explained why semantic cues weren't effective. If she could provide her own cues, additional information from the therapist might not be helpful. Moreover, her circumlocutions often included place names, thereby supporting the previous analysis that place names were slightly easier (though not significantly) to produce than famous people's names.

THERAPY RATIONALE

Proper nouns

Whilst the results from the above assessments suggested that proper nouns did not represent a distinct deficit for SH, since comprehension or naming of proper nouns was no worse than common nouns, it became clear that SH's proper noun anomia had a potentially profound impact on her ability to interact in conversation. For example, her difficulty recalling the names of her grandchildren was distressing for her and her family/friends alike, critically compromising her ability to take part in conversations. With this in mind, it became important to discover if word-finding therapy could facilitate her retrieval of proper nouns and if treatment effects would generalise to improve access to proper nouns at sentence level. Perhaps therapy could also affect other areas of communication and word production skills?

In addressing these issues for SH, we were also tackling some interesting questions about word-finding therapy. Whilst such therapy is known to be effective with common nouns (e.g., Howard, Patterson, Franklin, Orchard-Lisle, & Morton, 1985; Marshall, Pound, White-Thomson, & Pring, 1990; Nickels & Best, 1996a,b), there are few studies looking at treatments for proper noun anomia. Would proper nouns respond to therapy as effectively as common nouns and, if so, would the therapy be similar to that used for commons? Moreover, would therapy affect naming tasks (e.g., naming from description) other than picture naming?

Linking semantics and phonology

SH's excellent results on comprehension tasks and the richness of her circumlocutions indicated that her impairment lay at a level below semantics. Her ability to read aloud regular and irregular single words showed she could access the phonological output lexicon. This suggested that her naming difficulties probably resulted from an impairment in the route connecting semantics with the phonological output lexicon.

This hypothesis influenced the design of therapy. First, we wanted to include some element of picture–word matching. Semantic tasks may aid word production (Howard et al., 1985), even in cases such as SH where a limited or no semantic deficit has been shown (Marshall et al., 1990). If, as well as accessing semantics, the task involved an element of reading the words aloud, SH would also be accessing the phonology of each word. She might therefore learn through this task to make links between semantics and phonology.

Errorless technique

SH was prone to depression and she seemed to benefit from a high level of success and encouragement. For this reason we felt that an errorless therapy technique would be successful. Errorless techniques work on the premise that the prevention of error in therapy can be beneficial. This approach differs from traditional anomia therapy, where the subject is consistently presented with initial failure in naming attempts before any remedial action is taken. This errorless technique has its origins in memory rehabilitation (e.g., Parkin, Hunkin, & Squires, 1998; Wilson, Baddeley, & Evans, 1994) but has rarely been applied in aphasia (though see Dare & Franklin, 1999). It has, however, been applied to the treatment of proper names, although not with aphasic people (Parkin et al., 1998). The therapy is typically "user-friendly" in nature and this, combined with some positive outcomes in recent research, made it a good option for SH.

Writing

Finally, it was important to involve some element of writing in therapy as SH had expressed a desire to work on her written skills.

THE THERAPY STUDY

Initial assessment

SH chose 60 pictures: 20 famous people, 20 famous places in London, and 20 personally familiar people/pet names. She selected words that were particularly important or familiar to her. All 60 words were initially assessed, as follows, in three conditions over four sessions lasting approximately 1 hour each. Again, to be judged correct, responses had to be no more than one phoneme different from the target.

Single items

- Spoken picture naming assessment, with each picture presented to SH on a blank piece of paper.
- "Quiz"—SH was asked to give spoken responses to a quiz. The question might, for example, be "Who sang *Like a Virgin*?" (Madonna) or "Where did Charles and Diana get married?" (St. Paul's Cathedral).

Conversations

SH took part in three conversation tasks, one for each proper name category being investigated, each lasting approximately 10 minutes. The aim was for SH to discuss with the therapist a topic that would require her to access some proper names within the category being tested. When considering famous people, for example, the conversation centred on television comedians and singers that she liked and why she liked them. Similarly, when discussing her personally familiar names, she was asked to talk more about her family, their characters, and their interests.

Therapy

Following initial assessment, the words were divided into a treated and an untreated set, each containing 30 words (10 from each proper name category). Responses on the picture naming assessment for each category were collated and equal numbers of correct and incorrect answers assigned randomly to both sets. Five sessions of therapy took place over a 6-week period, involving one 60-minute session each week and four sets of homework completed by SH between the first and last session.

Therapy in each session was divided into two parts with a third homework task.

Part 1: Cued naming

In week 1, each picture was presented individually together with the target name; e.g., with "Ali G", SH was told "This person begins with 'A' and his name is 'Ali G' ". SH was simultaneously shown a card with "Ali G" written on it. She was asked to repeat and then copy the name. Each week the complexity of the task increased by adding distracter names to the card on which the target was written. SH had to read the names and pick the correct one before repeating it and copying it down. Informal assessment had shown that SH could repeat and copy single words and her semantic knowledge was sufficient for the distracters not to put her off. This helped maintain interest each week but did not affect SH's success in performing the task, thereby retaining the errorless aspect of the therapy.

Week 2: Two distracters belonging to broadly the same category were chosen. For example, for the target "The London Eye", the distracters were The Louvre and The Spanish Steps.

Week 3: Two distracters more closely belonging

to the same category were chosen. For the aforementioned target, the distracters were The Planetarium and The London Aquarium.

Week 4: Two distracters visually and/or phonologically related to the target were used. For example, for the target "The London Eye", the distracters were The London Fly and The London Pie.

Week 5: The same distracters were used as the previous week but, before being shown the card, SH was asked to write the first letter of the target herself without being given a cue.

Part 2: Naming pictures without cues

This part involved spoken naming of all 30 pictures without cues. In cases where SH was unable to name the picture, SH elected to look at her own written version of the name and read this aloud.

As the therapy sessions evolved, SH automatically repeated the name after she had copied it, so that in each therapy session she made three attempts at each of the treated items. Previous research shows that this level of repetition can be effective in the treatment of anomia (Miceli et al., 1996).

Part 3: Homework

The treated set was split into two smaller sets of 15 words each. SH was given each set alternately each week at the end of the session, so that between weeks 1 to 6 she worked on each set twice. Each picture was presented with four written words that SH was instructed to read aloud. These were the correct name (e.g., Jerry Springer), a close semantic distracter (e.g., Robert Kilroy-Silk), a more distant semantic distracter within the same category (e.g., Jude Law), and a distracter belonging to another proper name category (e.g., Lake District). Distracters were not drawn from the treated or control sets. SH was required to select the correct name from the distracters and record her choice (✔) on a chart. There was room for SH to have five attempts at each picture during the week.

During therapy, SH was given regular feedback and encouragement. There was some discussion about the nature of the proper names being targeted, particularly, for example, names that were longer, which SH found more difficult. Some conversation also naturally arose during sessions, especially about some of the targeted famous people who were particularly topical. As therapy progressed, the homework record charts were enlarged at SH's request, allowing her to copy the target name onto the chart so she could work more on her writing skills. Moreover, she spontaneously tried to self-cue her spoken output by finger-writing names.

POST-THERAPY ASSESSMENT

Post-therapy assessment took place over four sessions during the 2 weeks immediately following the final therapy session. All assessments carried out initially were repeated. In addition, for the treated set of words, SH was asked to complete a written picture naming test. Whilst she had refused in the pre-therapy stage as she felt she "could not write at all", SH agreed to do the test after therapy.

FOLLOW-UP MAINTENANCE ASSESSMENT

All assessments carried out immediately post-therapy were repeated during a 2-week period 2 months after the end of therapy. Additionally, we were interested to explore SH's thoughts about the changes she had noticed in her communication during therapy. We considered either having a general discussion with her or asking her to complete a questionnaire. In the event, we decided upon a discussion structured by a questionnaire, because we felt that a questionnaire would provide more specific information and would be less "leading" for SH than a general discussion alone.

Fifteen questions were divided into four sections—talking, writing, reading, general. Each question was presented in a yes/no format and the questionnaire was balanced such that there were almost as many expected no answers (7) as there

were expected yes responses (8). For example, for the question "I can name all the people worked on more easily" we expected an affirmative response, whereas for the question "I can write a letter more easily", we expected a negative response. We felt it important to have a mixture of yes/no replies and purposefully try to elicit some no answers due to issues of compliance.

RESULTS

Naming and quiz assessments
Tables 7.3 and 7.4 summarize the raw data from these assessments. McNemar and chi square tests were used to analyse this data.

Spoken picture naming improved over the course of the study for treated and untreated sets, with the former reaching near ceiling post-therapy and after the maintenance period. McNemar tests showed that, for the treated set, improvement was significant post-therapy ($\chi^2 = 13.06$, $p < .001$) and again at follow-up ($\chi^2 = 11.07$, $p < .001$) when compared with the pre-therapy scores. The untreated set improved slightly post-therapy but this was not significant ($\chi^2 = 0.57$) when compared with the pre-therapy scores. However, interestingly, the control set significantly changed at follow-up from the pre-therapy score ($\chi^2 = 6.125$, $p < .02$) and between the post-therapy and follow-up assessments ($\chi^2 = 7.7$, $p < .01$).

Likewise, in the quiz condition—an alternative naming assessment—SH scored almost 100% with the treated set at both assessments following therapy. When contrasted with pre-therapy scores using the McNemar test, this gain was significant both post-therapy ($\chi^2 = 9.6$, $p < .01$) and at follow-up ($\chi^2 = 12.07$, $p < .001$). As with the naming assessment, the gains in the famous people and personally familiar categories of the treated set are particularly striking, and for both assessments the famous places lagged slightly behind. Turning to the control set, however, all categories displayed gradual improvement in the quiz condition. Using the McNemar test to compare pre-therapy scores with scores post-therapy and at

TABLE 7.3

Naming assessment (raw data)

Time of assessment	Famous people	Famous places	Personally familiar	Totals
	Proper name category			
Pre-therapy				
Treated	3/10	4/10	6/10	13/30
Untreated	3/10	4/10	6/10	13/30
Post-therapy				
Treated	9/10	9/10	10/10	28/30
Untreated	4/10	5/10	7/10	16/30
Follow-up				
Treated	10/10	7/10	9/10	26/30
Untreated	7/10	8/10	9/10	24/30

TABLE 7.4

Quiz (raw data)

Time of assessment	Famous people	Famous places	Personally familiar	Totals
	Proper name category			
Pre-therapy				
Treated	5/10	5/10	5/10	15/30
Untreated	3/10	3/10	7/10	13/30
Post-therapy				
Treated	10/10	8/10	10/10	28/30
Untreated	5/10	7/10	8/10	20/30
Follow-up				
Treated	10/10	9/10	10/10	29/30
Untreated	9/10	7/10	8/10	24/30

follow-up, this change was significant post-therapy ($\chi^2 = 5.14$, $p < .05$) and following the maintenance period ($\chi^2 = 7.69$, $p < .01$). Possible reasons for the gains in the control set are considered later.

Chi square analyses were used to examine the differences between the treated and control sets at the post-treatment and follow-up stages. Crucially, these showed that in the quiz condition post-therapy ($\chi^2 = 6.67$, $p < .01$) and at follow-up ($\chi^2 = 4.04$, $p < .05$), the treated group performed significantly better than the untreated group, pointing to an effect of therapy rather than generalised spontaneous improvement. In the naming condition, the chi square result was also significant post-therapy ($\chi^2 = 12.27$, $p < .001$) but not at follow-up ($\chi^2 = 0.48$). However, the differences between the two assessment conditions should be interpreted with caution as the actual differences in the raw scores were minimal.

Writing assessment

This assessment used the treated set only as stimuli (Table 7.5). SH achieved most success with the personally familiar names, a functionally positive result that was further corroborated by the qualitative assessment measures (see below). Moreover, at the follow-up assessment, SH was also able to spell four personally familiar names correctly from the untreated set. Place names and famous people names showed poorer performances but their scores were on a par with the written

naming scores, cited in the *Communication Profile* section earlier, where SH scored approximately 35%.

Assessing conversations

Table 7.6 conflates the results from the conversations from all assessments. A 5-minute window of each conversation was chosen for informal analysis. Sections were chosen from the first 5 minutes of the conversation in the first two categories and from the second 5 minutes in the personally familiar topic. This was because in the latter category, the subject matter was initially slightly tangential.

The analysis aimed to identify how many proper nouns SH accessed and the strategies/coping techniques she adopted in instances of proper name anomia. Also, if repair was necessary, identifying who initiated it and how the repair was achieved. Three categories of repair were recorded:

- self-initiated, self-repair (SISR), e.g.,

    SH: do, dom, D O, Dome

TABLE 7.5

Written picture naming—% correct

	Post-therapy	*Follow-up*
Famous people names	40%	30%
Famous place names	40%	10%
Personally familiar names	70%	90%

TABLE 7.6

Analysis of conversations

	Pre-therapy	*Post-therapy*	*Follow-up*
Number of proper names	7 given correctly 9 others attempted	18 given correctly 4 others attempted	12 given correctly 2 others attempted
Strategies/Coping techniques	• Circumlocution • Finger writing • Verbal groping • Verbal spelling • Gesture • Environmental props • Frustration	• Verbal groping • Finger writing • Circumlocution • Gesture • Frustration	• Circumlocution • Verbal groping • Finger writing • Gesture • Frustration
Types of repair	3 SISR 7 SIOR—repair often very long	3 SISR 3 SIOR	2 SISR 1 SIOR 1 SIOUR

SISR: self-initiated, self-repair. SIOR: self-initiated, other repair: SIOUR: self-initiated, other unable to repair.

- self-initiated, other repair (SIOR), e.g.,

  SH: Erm the um, /kor/ /kori/ /kori kaet/. Excuse me (finger writing) C Wharf.
  AM: Canary Wharf

- self-initiated, other unable to repair (SIOUR), e.g. (topic—famous places)

  SH: Yes and three two where the fire started here up there near (unintelligible) fire was near St Pauls
  AM: The great fire years and years ago
  SH: Oh yeah. When they come everything off . . . erm . . . erm then place there there in the city there where the that man sit on a /hɔ/ horse horse. When the thing out of him (points to shoes) the things on. When this man siting on the horse . . . the man who did it got the things off. Yes a big statue (5 turns later)
  AM: I can't think what he's called.

SISR was recorded even where SH eventually accessed the proper name through self-cuing. Hence, the total number of repairs noted in the table may exceed instances of proper names that were unsuccessfully attempted. For example, at the pre-therapy stage, there were 10 repairs but only 9 proper names were unsuccessfully attempted— this was because 3 instances of SISR resulted in SH achieving the proper name correctly.

Comparing the number of successfully attempted proper names with unsuccessful ones showed that SH's access to proper names in a conversational context improved during therapy. Pre-therapy, those names attempted unsuccessfully outweighed those given correctly. This improved dramatically to a ratio of about 4:1 and then 6:1 (successful:unsuccessful) in the maintenance period. In other words, at follow-up, for every six proper names accessed correctly, there was only one that she was unable to achieve. Crucially, the names accessed weren't just those from the therapy set. They included some that didn't appear in the study (e.g., Regent Street, Soho), as well as some from the control group (e.g., David, Billie).

Alongside this, the need for repair within a conversation decreased post-therapy and further at follow-up. Moreover, the balance within the conversation altered post-therapy. Pre-therapy, the repairs were often quite long and drawn out, typically involving SIOR.

Example: Conversation topic—famous people—pre-therapy

SH: I love that girl, fat one er two, two girls
AM: What channel are they on
SH: Two er one Oh not on now
AM: What sort of shows do they do?
SH: They take two girls, one older than the other and one big girl
AM: One big one. What colour hair has she got?
SH: Black
AM: Is she married to
SH: Yes a black one, I can't remember the name
AM: Do you mean Lenny Henry? So you're talking about French and Saunders
SH: Yes yes

As instances of repair decreased, the overall ratio of SIOR to SISR became more equal, although the strategies SH adopted to manage any difficulties remained similar. In turn the repairs became generally shorter, as exemplified below.

Example: Conversation topic—famous people—post-therapy

AM: Fantastic so we've got Ali G
SH: (laughs) And erm Cliff Cliff /kilver kilv kri kris/ no Cliff Richards

Example: Conversation topic—family— post-therapy

AM: So she's taking after you isn't she with your animals
SH: Yes . . . There's Nicky no sorry oh well oh erm /daenel daenel/ Chloe

Questionnaire

SH's questionnaire (Table 7.7) was completed at follow-up. This used a yes/no format and was administered before SH knew the results of the follow-up assessments. We expected SH would give eight yes and seven no responses. Eight of the areas were ones we hoped would be affected

TABLE 7.7

SH's questionnaire

Section	Question	Expected response	Actual response
Talking	I can name all the people worked on more easily	Yes	Yes
	I can name all the places worked on more easily	Yes	A lot, not all
	I can speak to my grandchildren more easily using their names	Yes	Yes
	I can name all people and places better	Yes	No
	I can talk more easily about a TV programme I have enjoyed	No	Not sure
Writing	I can write the words worked on more easily using pen and paper	Yes	Yes
	I can write the words worked on more easily on the computer	Yes	Yes
	I can write a letter more easily	No	No, letter too long
Reading	I can read people's names and place names more easily	Yes	Yes, individual ones
	I can read my computer magazine more easily	No	Yes, little bits
	I can read the newspaper more easily	No	No
General	I am more confident talking to my family	Yes	Yes
	I am more confident talking to strangers	No	Yes
	I can talk more easily in a difficult or new situation	No	No
	I am more confident talking on the phone	No	Yes

by therapy but seven were considered beyond the scope of treatment. Whilst our predictions were generally correct, in the event, SH gave nine yes responses, four no responses, and two other responses. Overall, as her answers to question 2 in the "talking" and "reading" section demonstrated, she was more able to give differential and qualified answers than we had expected.

SH's responses to the questionnaire suggested she perceived positive effects of therapy. For example, she noticed an improved ability to access people's names such as those of her grandchildren. This corroborated what was said earlier regarding the increased numbers of proper names she was able to access in conversation post-therapy.

Moreover, SH remarked on an improved level of self-confidence when talking to her family, to

strangers, and on the phone. Alongside this, an overall reduction in her frustration was noted in conversation. Indeed, pre-therapy, her frustration was particularly noticeable when discussing her family. For example, at one point she sighed saying ". . . (I) can never say it their names".

SH's responses also indicated encouraging effects to aspects of communication and word production skills aside from speech. She reported improved writing of proper names, particularly family names, when using conventional writing and when writing on the computer. Indeed, she wrote family Christmas cards and produced a small friends/family telephone directory on the computer. Interestingly, SH also informally commented that, when a word-finding difficulty arose, she now knew the first letter of the word more often and spelling this on her hand or saying it helped her access the word. Whilst this was a strategy SH sometimes used prior to therapy, her spontaneous comments suggested it was a technique of which she was more aware and one she now used more frequently and successfully. This also substantiated what we said earlier; that repair was now more equally shared between SH and her communication partner.

Finally, SH remarked on improved reading ability. Specifically, she found individual names easier to read and parts of her computer book more accessible. Whilst we might have predicted the former observation, the latter was a less anticipated response.

DISCUSSION

This single case study investigated whether proper nouns could be facilitated through treatment. We were also interested in whether therapy could affect a range of spoken naming tasks as well as other communication skills.

Therapy effects

The quantitative results showed that SH's spoken proper noun retrieval significantly improved following therapy. Positive changes were seen in a range of naming tasks including picture naming and naming from definition ("quiz"). The difference between the treated and untreated sets was significant post-therapy in the naming and "quiz" conditions, suggesting that gains were attributable to therapy rather than to generalised spontaneous improvement. Overall, these results showed that retrieval difficulties with proper nouns are remediable to some degree.

Was there any generalisation?

Despite the fact that the therapy tasks were very remote from normal communication, the results suggested some generalisation to tasks that at least approximated to natural conversation. SH's access to proper nouns in a conversational context improved over the course of the study and

the gains were well maintained. She acknowledged her ability to finger-write when a word-finding difficulty arose, arguably indicating an enhanced ability to self-cue. Moreover, the balance within a conversation became more equally shared between SH and her conversation partner. Alongside this, and in part unexpectedly, SH felt her overall confidence in conversations with her family, strangers, and on the telephone had increased. Such results indicated a positive change in SH's sense of communicative "competence" (Kagan, 1998) and her ability to access the conversational floor.

As yet, most research has looked specifically at the effects of treatment on naming (e.g., Nickels & Best, 1996a,b). Few studies have considered the relationship between the treatment effects on confrontation picture naming and word retrieval at the sentence level (though see Hickin, Herbert, Best, Howard, & Osborne, 2006; chapter 5 of this volume). As such, this study represents an important area for further investigations. This study suggested that anomia therapy as specific as this might have more far-reaching effects on word production in conversation and on self-confidence than has been thus far recognised. How, though, was this achieved without "transfer" tasks being included in therapy? Perhaps SH's previous therapy experiences enabled her to make use of newly acquired skills, without them having to be explicitly "transferred"? Perhaps also the personal relevance of the stimuli for SH meant that therapy boosted her ability to retrieve these words that she already regularly attempted, such that specific "transfer" tasks were not required? It is probably also important that some improvement occurred in the naming of untreated items. Without such generalisation it may be difficult to achieve positive effects in tasks other than pure naming.

Evaluating generalisation and the reasons for it in aphasia therapy is notably difficult (Worrall, 1998). Standardised formal tests are generally impairment-based and don't reflect more functional progress. In the absence of an assessment tool sensitive enough to measure subtle functional change, clinicians typically devise specific measures (questionnaires, etc.) for unique situations. But, as previously mentioned, controlling against patient responses aimed at "pleasing" the therapist is difficult. As regards our qualitative measures, future adaptations would involve a pre- as well as a post-therapy questionnaire with SH to more accurately measure change. SH's questionnaire was also limited in terms of the responses expected from her and greater scope for differentiated responses would have been useful. Crucially, such a measure should also be administered by a "blind assessor" or someone not otherwise involved in the study. Finally, our measures could have been supplemented by pre- and post-therapy observations of SH discussing specific topics with a relative, for more "natural" conversation data. Further work in this area and the development of a subtle and holistic assessment tool to measure functional change/outcomes is crucial to proving the practical relevance and efficacy of impairment-based aphasia therapy to daily life.

We also considered therapy effects on SH's reading and writing. The greatest success was seen in her writing of family names, both in her written naming score and in her questionnaire responses. The absence of any recent pre-therapy data meant that we were unable to quantify the degree of change in her written skills. Whilst we might have expected some improvement in her writing of treated words, SH's generalisation of her written skills (e.g., to writing Christmas cards) was not predicted. Perhaps regular copying of proper names and improving SH's spoken retrieval of proper nouns generalised, at least for personally familiar names, to her written output. Perhaps also much of this change can be attributed to SH's high level of motivation. Indeed, she was particularly motivated to work on her written skills, even requesting an adaptation to the homework to give her extra practice. Moreover, one of her main hobbies was working on her computer and she was certainly getting general writing practice through its use (e.g., writing the telephone directory).

Apart from improved reading of people and place names, we did not expect to see any change in SH's reading. In fact, SH reported improvements in this area as well as finding "little bits" of her computer magazine easier to read. SH's reading ability was not recently formally tested. As with the writing skills, this outcome must be treated with caution. In particular, the problem of compliance may encourage SH to inflate the positive effects of therapy (although this was not observed on all questions). Alternatively, the process of therapy might have had unpredicted and far-reaching effects, increasing SH's confidence in all her communication skills, including those that were not the focus of therapy. Evidently, although our questions remain unanswered, it would have been useful to explore more fully the changes SH felt she had made in her communication skills. Moreover, we see the importance of unpacking how therapy works, of which more is said below.

Why did the controls improve?

In both the naming and quiz condition there was a gradual change in response to the control items. In the former, this reached significance at the follow-up assessment and, in the latter, we saw significant change post-therapy and at follow-up when compared to the pre-therapy scores. We can speculate as to the reasons for this. Given the relatively small corpus of words, there may have been an effect of repeated testing, or maybe SH's naming ability displayed day-to-day variability. Whilst we know that naming ability in aphasia varies according to factors such as fatigue and stress, this explanation accounts neither for the striking and well-maintained gains in the treated set post-therapy, nor the gradual change in the control set. Were these results a sign of ongoing spontaneous change, or did they reflect the generalisation of therapy effects?

In an attempt to answer these questions, we re-tested SH on the famous people and common noun naming assessments used in the initial assessment stage, following the end of the therapy study. She showed improvements on both, scoring 18/40 and 30/40 respectively. Functionally, this was an excellent result. It also suggested that SH was not simply improving on items that had been repeatedly tested. What is less clear, however, is whether gains reflected generalisation of therapy or some ongoing spontaneous improvement.

Repeated baseline assessments could help resolve this, as could the pre- and post-therapy assessment of untreated functions.

Therapy content

We were interested in the type of therapy to which proper nouns would respond. Would tasks known to facilitate common nouns be effective with proper nouns or would proper nouns require a special technique more reflective of their characteristics? Since proper nouns were not a distinct category for SH, we predicted that she might respond to techniques traditionally used to facilitate common noun retrieval in aphasia (e.g., word to picture matching, repetition). This proved to be the case, indicating that proper and common nouns do respond to similar therapeutic methods.

Where our study differed, however, was in its use of an errorless technique, which works on the premise that the prevention of error in therapy can be beneficial. Positively, it represented a relatively straightforward and uncomplicated technique. Against this, though, we were initially concerned that the repetitive nature of the therapy might seem monotonous to SH. However, SH routinely completed the homework tasks each week and never complained of boredom during the therapy sessions. On the contrary, she seemed highly motivated and particularly amused by the famous people and personally familiar stimuli, which often stimulated discussions around the subjects concerned. Such results indicated that errorless therapy may be beneficial for some anomic patients and particularly those who respond to a high level of success. This technique therefore deserves more clinical attention.

One final point about the content of therapy relates to the number of assessment sessions compared to therapy sessions. Our reason for doing such extensive assessment was that we wanted to look at more than just the effect of therapy on naming; we also wanted to measure more conversational tasks and SH's perception of change. In the event, SH did not seem concerned about the number of assessments, but viewed them positively as more opportunities to use her speech.

CONCLUSIONS

In showing that proper noun retrieval was improved by therapy, we have highlighted the value of routinely including proper nouns in therapy programmes. The communicative importance of proper nouns in daily interactions makes such inclusion especially necessary.

The therapy programme in our study used simple techniques and was relatively economical in terms of clinical time, making such an approach relevant and readily applicable in a typical outpatient or domiciliary setting. Equally encouraging were the indications of more widespread and generalised effects of therapy. Not least, SH developed greater insight into her aphasia and an increased capacity to self-cue in instances of proper noun anomia. Finally, her increase in confidence in conversations indicated an enhanced sense of communicative "competence" (Kagan, 1998) and a positive impact on her perceived level of participation.

ACKNOWLEDGMENTS

The Stroke Association's Grant number 16/98 awarded to: Jane Marshall, Jo Robson, Tim Pring and Shula Chiat for the study entitled "The production and comprehension of proper names in aphasia: A therapy study".

We are grateful for the advice of Jo Robson in the early stages of this study. Our final thanks are to SH, who participated with such enthusiasm and good humour.

NOTES

1 This study formed part of an MSc project supervised by Jane Marshall.
2 Please note that this section has been compiled mainly from data from informal assessments

and observations. Formal assessment data for SH is scant but is used to support the former. Such formal tests were not administered by the authors.

3 The tasks described in this section were based on those used in Robson, Pring, Chiat, Marshall, & Montagu (2004).

REFERENCES

Byng, S. (1998). What is aphasia therapy? In C. Code & D. Muller (Eds.), *The treatment of aphasia: From theory to practice*. London: Whurr.

Dare, M., & Franklin, S. (1999). *Errorless learning in anomia therapy*. Paper presented at the British Aphasiology Society Biennial International Conference, London, 1999.

Hickin, J., Herbert, R., Best, W., Howard, D., & Osborne, F. (2006). Lexical and functionally based treatment: Effects on word retrieval and conversation. In S. Byng, J. Duchan, & C. Pound (eds), *Aphasia therapy file, Vol. 2*. Hove, UK: Psychology Press.

Howard, D., Patterson, K.E., Franklin, S., Orchard-Lisle, V., & Morton, J. (1985). The treatment of word retrieval deficits in aphasia: A comparison of two therapy methods. *Brain, 108*, 817–829.

Kagan, A. (1998). Supported conversation for adults with aphasia: Methods and resources for training conversation partners. *Aphasiology, 12*, 816–831.

Lesser, R., & Milroy, L. (1996). *Linguistics and aphasia: Psycholinguistic and pragmatic aspects of intervention*. London: Longman.

Marshall, J., Pound, C., White-Thomson, M., & Pring, T. (1990). The use of picture/word matching tasks to assist word retrieval in aphasic patients. *Aphasiology, 4*, 167–184.

Miceli, G., Amitrano, A., Capasso, R., & Caramazza, A. (1996). The treatment of anomia resulting from output lexical damage: Analysis of two cases. *Brain and Language, 52*, 150–174.

Nickels, L., & Best, W. (1996a). Therapy for naming disorders (Part I): Principles, puzzles and progress. *Aphasiology, 10*, 21–47.

Nickels, L., & Best, W. (1996b). Therapy for naming disorders (Part II): Specifics, surprises and suggestions. *Aphasiology, 10*, 109–136.

Parkin, A.J., Hunkin, N.M., & Squires, E.J. (1998). Unlearning John Major: The use of errorless learning in the reacquisition of proper names following Herpes Simplex Encephalitis. *Cognitive Neuropsychology, 15*, 361–375.

Robson, J., Pring, T., Chiat, S., Marshall, J., & Montagu, A. (2004). Processing proper nouns in aphasia: Evidence from assessment and therapy. *Aphasiology, 18*, 917–935.

Wilson, B.A., Baddeley, A., & Evans, J. (1994). Errorless learning in the rehabilitation of memory impaired people. *Neuropsychological Rehabilitation, 4*, 307–326.

Worrall, L. (1998). The functional communication perspective. In C. Code & D. Muller (Eds.), *The treatment of aphasia: From theory to practice*. London: Whurr.

8

Symptom-based versus theoretically motivated therapy for anomia: A case study

Lisa Perkins and Fiona Hinshelwood

BACKGROUND

The therapy study described in this chapter arose in response to a conflict that therapists frequently experience in clinical work. This is the time pressure created by large caseloads and the need to provide effective therapy. Therapists often respond to large caseloads by seeing as many clients as possible. In doing this, however, there is a danger of failing to provide anyone with an effective service.

This project involved a case study to compare the outcome of symptom-based therapy, delivered in the context of an existing large caseload with little attention to assessment, with a period of theoretically motivated therapy in which more time was devoted to the assessment and planning and less to the delivery of intervention.

THE CLIENT AND INITIAL SYMPTOM-BASED THERAPY

FR was a retired factory worker who lived with his wife. Their two daughters lived nearby with their families. At the age of 68, FR suffered a left-hemisphere CVA. He was seen by his general practitioner but not admitted to hospital. There was little physical impairment but FR did have some problems with his speech. His GP referred him for speech and language therapy and he was seen 3 months after the CVA.

FR had a mild to moderate impairment of spoken language. His speech was hesitant and he had difficulties expressing complex sequences of ideas. FR's wife commented that "he can't explain things to me". One effect of the aphasic difficulties was that FR relied on his wife to speak for him. She described taking more responsibility for him in activities that involved speaking with others, and reported that she now initiated most of the talk at home. FR reported a loss of confidence in his ability to communicate. He worried about meeting people in the street and would avoid situations where he needed to speak.

FR's word-finding skills were assessed using a test of spoken naming (PALPA 53, Spoken Naming; Kay, Lesser, & Coltheart, 1993). He named 32/40 items correctly, with a semantic error pattern. Reflecting caseload pressures, FR was not rated as a high priority for therapy when compared with clients with more severe aphasia. On the basis of the identified symptom of anomia, FR was given general word-finding tasks to carry out at home with his wife. These tasks were presented within the context of worksheets, and were explained and demonstrated by the therapist. A variety of semantic activities were assigned, including category naming tasks (e.g., *Name as many vegetables as you can*) and naming to definition (e.g., *Something which is worn on your wrist and is used to tell the time. What is it?*). All tasks focused on FR's ability to produce the spoken word; FR's wife would read out the questions and record his responses on the sheets.

FR's progress within therapy was reviewed monthly. This contact provided the therapist with additional opportunities to demonstrate tasks. Although no record was kept of the amount of time spent on therapy activities, FR and his wife reported undertaking short sessions three to four times a week, with each exercise being repeated several times over the month. Evidence of this was seen in the written record of FR's responses.

On reassessment after 6 months of this general therapy, FR's performance on the spoken version of PALPA 53 had not changed (31/40). More importantly, both FR and his wife reported no real change in his ability to communicate.

THEORETICALLY MOTIVATED ASSESSMENT

FR's lack of improvement following symptom-based therapy was thought to reflect the failure of therapy tasks to address the underlying cause of his expressive difficulties. It was felt that, with more targeted intervention, FR had the potential to make language gains, particularly given the level of commitment that he and his wife had demonstrated in completing exercises at home.

FR underwent a period of detailed theoretically motivated assessment, the aim of which was to identify the processing impairment underlying his expressive difficulties using a cognitive neuropsychological framework. A cross-modal model (see Lesser & Milroy, 1993, p. 57) was used as a framework to assess single word processing, whilst a model of sentence production (Bock, 1987) developed from Garrett's work (1980, 1984) was valuable when examining connected speech.

ASSESSMENT OF SINGLE WORD PROCESSING

A number of assessments were undertaken to investigate single word processing. A first step was to compare spoken and written naming in order to distinguish between a central semantic impairment (indicated by impaired performance in both modalities) and an impairment involving the phonological output lexicon (reflected in a modality-specific impairment). FR therefore completed the written version of PALPA 53, naming 34/40 items correctly and producing 6 semantic errors. His impaired performance in both spoken and written modalities, along with the semantic error pattern, suggested a central semantic impairment.

Further assessment of semantic abilities was carried out. Specifically, a written synonym judgement task (PALPA 50) was given in order to examine central processing of high and low imageability items. Whilst FR performed well on high imageability word pairs (28/30 correct), there were marked problems with low image-ability items (17/30).

Assessment of single word processing pointed to a central semantic impairment that particularly implicated low imageability items. However, FR's problems with spontaneous speech appeared out of proportion to his performance on assessments of single word processing. Assessment of sentence-level processing was undertaken to shed light on this discrepancy.

ASSESSMENT OF SENTENCE-LEVEL PROCESSING

An accessible introduction to the processes involved in sentence production, and potential levels of breakdown, is provided by Marshall, Black, and Byng (1999). Of particular relevance here is their account of verb semantics and the creation of sentence structure (pp. 5–6). In brief, a verb's semantic representation contains information about the number of entities involved in the specified activity. This is referred to as its argument structure. Verbs may assign one argument (e.g., *the baby is waving*), two arguments (e.g., *the cat is biting the chair*) or three arguments (e.g., *The girl is giving the book to the boy*). The verb's semantic representation also specifies the thematic role taken by each of these entities. For example, in the sentence "*the cat is biting the chair*", the cat has the thematic role of agent (the entity instigating the action) and the chair has the thematic role of patient (the entity affected by the event). Furthermore, verbs provide information that governs mapping between thematic role and grammatical relations. An example of such information is that in active sentences, agents occupy the subject position.

Whitworth (1996a) has proposed that a deficit in assigning thematic roles to lexical items in sentences can manifest itself as a word retrieval deficit characterised by omission of arguments in a sentence. If impaired processing of thematic roles does underlie a word retrieval deficit, production of words in sentences (requiring thematic role

assignment) should be poorer than single word naming (which only requires retrieval of one lexical item). The Thematic Roles in Production assessment (TRIP; Whitworth, 1996a) permits comparison of the retrieval of the same lexical items within both single word and sentence contexts using spoken picture naming and picture description. It includes 35 pictures of nouns as well as 85 pictures of events that represent a range of sentences with one-, two-, and three-argument structures. Picture description is modelled by the therapist for all items and the person with aphasia is then asked to describe the pictures. The TRIP is carried out over two sessions, in two matched halves.

In order to compare FR's lexical retrieval in sentences to that of single words, the TRIP was administered.[1] Table 8.1 summarises his performance.

TABLE 8.1

Summary of FR's scores on the TRIP assessment

Single word picture naming	Score
Target nouns produced	32/35 (91%)
Sentence production	Score
Target nouns produced for 1-argument structures	14/15 (93%)
Target nouns produced for 2-argument structures	26/38 (68%)
Target nouns produced for 3-argument structures	19/27 (70%)
Target verbs produced for 1-argument structures	14/15 (93%)
Target verbs produced for 2-argument structures	14/19 (74%)
Target verbs produced for 3-argument structures	3/9 (33%)
Thematic completeness of 1-argument structures	14/15 (93%)
Thematic completeness of 2-argument structures	10/19 (53%)
Thematic completeness of 3-argument structures	2/9 (22%)

As can be seen from the table, FR experienced difficulty with this assessment as stimuli became more complex. His ability to retrieve nouns declined with an increase in argument structure; the verb analysis also shows poorer retrieval of verbs that take a greater number of thematic roles. These two findings are reflected in the analysis of thematic completeness, which shows a pattern of decreasing completeness as the argument structure within test items increased. Table 8.2 provides examples of the types of error that FR produced.

FR's performance on the TRIP suggested impaired thematic role processing as a source of his expressive difficulties. Byng (1988) has proposed that impaired mapping of thematic roles will also manifest itself in comprehension. Assessment was therefore undertaken to examine FR's comprehension of thematic roles using PALPA 55 (Sentence–Picture Matching, auditory version), a test that permits comparison of reversible and non-reversible sentences and involves selection of one picture from a choice of three (target; reversal distractor; lexical distractor). In this test, selection of the target picture for non-reversible sentences (e.g., *the girl is washing the dog*) can be made on the basis of comprehension of the lexical items and real-world knowledge alone (i.e., that dogs do not wash girls). In contrast, in order to achieve a correct response for reversible sentences (e.g., *the horse is kicking the man*), an intact ability to map syntactic to semantic representation (i.e., to assign thematic roles) is required to discriminate between the target and the reversal distractor (*the man is kicking the horse*).

FR's performance highlighted a marked discrepancy between non-reversible sentences (15/16, 94%) and reversible sentences (9/20, 45%). All errors on the reversible sentences involved selection of the reversal distractor. Assuming that FR was able to eliminate the lexical distractor (which his error pattern for the reversible sentences and good performance on the non-reversible sentences suggested was likely), his selection was at chance level. His response to this assessment therefore supported the hypothesis that he had a central impairment of thematic role processing.

The final assessment of sentence processing was to examine FR's realisation of thematic roles in conversational speech by undertaking a sentence structure analysis. The purpose of this assessment was twofold. First, it permitted a check of whether the deficits manifest in structured assessment tasks did indeed reflect the difficulties experienced in everyday speech. Second, it provided a way of examining whether therapy based on these detailed assessments would result in meaningful improvement.

As noted earlier in this chapter, FR initiated very little speech and relied on his wife to do most

TABLE 8.2

Examples of FR's production on the TRIP assessment

Target sentence	*FR's production*	*Error type*
The baby is waving	the baby er boy is swimming is er-	Semantic error
The woman is showing the door to the dog	the boy is show er er watching the door showing the door	Omission of thematic role
The girl's giving the book to the boy	The boy's giving the book to the girl	Thematic role reversal
The cat is biting the chair	The chair is er scratching the chair	Repeated thematic role Semantic error
The children are giving the hat to the man	the man is holding the hat (4) to the little girl	Anomalous structure

of the talking. Collecting a sample of his conversational speech therefore proved difficult, and the couple failed to make a recording when left with a tape recorder at home. The sample was therefore obtained on one of the therapist's visits, with the therapist, FR, and his wife all contributing. An analysis of predicate-argument structure, based upon a simplified version of the analysis described by Byng and Black (1989), was undertaken on 70 consecutive phrases and clauses produced by FR. Repetitions of previous turns were not included in the analysis. Below is a sample from the conversation:

1   *Wife:*   Tell her what you are going to do for dinner.
2   *FR:*   I don't know really.
3   *Wife:*   Oh now!
4   *FR:*   She's got all the dinner ready. I mean put the (1) er (1) potatoes on the top (1) er gravy on er simple.
5   *Wife:*   How do you do the potatoes?
6   *FR:*   (1) er m- mashed pota- (2) er um what do they call then er um
7   *Wife:*   Instant potatoes.
8   *FR:*   Instant potatoes.
9   *Wife:*   Well how do you prepare them?
10   *FR:*   erm (2) milk and (1) water um er smash of butter (2) on the top.
11   *Wife:*   What do you do with the milk and water?
12   *FR:*   Milk and (2) w- um milk and water.
13   *Wife:*   What do you do with it?
14   *FR:*   I don't know.
15   *Wife:*   You boil it in a pan and then add the- (1)
16   *FR:*   Add the stock.
17   *Wife:*   Add the (1.0) add the potatoes.
18   *FR:*   Oh the potatoes yes aye.
19   *Th:*   So you're being left to your own devices for dinner?
20   *FR:*   For my dinner yes.
21   *Wife:*   He can make dinner just this pack is different.
22   *FR:*   I could make dinner. I generally cook my own (2) my own breakfast you know. Bacon and egg (2) and tomatoes (2) and sau- er sausage er cornflakes.

This sample shows how FR's wife used test questions to engage in conversation with FR (e.g., Turns 1, 5, and 9). Prior to the use of questions, FR had produced minimal responses to the therapist's questions about his recent activities. A number of patterns emerged within FR's talk that not only demonstrated means of contributing turns, but also illustrated the restricted nature of his output. He frequently repeated back words and structures produced by the previous speaker (e.g., T12, T20) and listed lexical items in order to take a turn (e.g., T22). Hesitations pervaded his contributions (e.g., T4, T10, T22). There was a limited range of verbs and a heavy reliance on the copula. Semantic errors, some of which were corrected and some of which were not, were also identifiable (e.g., T6 to T7).

Table 8.3 summarises the results of the structural analysis. Only 63% of the structures attempted were structurally complete with all arguments realised. Overall, FR relied upon phrases (41%) with very low clausal embedding (3%).

TABLE 8.3	
Summary of structural analysis undertaken on FR's spontaneous speech	
Structure	*Number produced as a percentage of all utterances*
Phrases	29 (41%)
1-argument clause—complete	1 (1%)
1-argument clause—incomplete	1 (1%)
2-argument clause—complete	22 (31%)
2-argument clause—incomplete	11 (16%)
3-argument clause—complete	1 (1%)
3-argument clause—incomplete	2 (3%)
Structures with embedded clauses	3 (4%)
Overall number of structurally complete clauses	24 (63%)

THEORETICALLY MOTIVATED, THEMATIC ROLE THERAPY

On the basis of this detailed assessment, thematic role therapy was carried out. It was predicted that this therapy would result in FR's improvement in sentence production and comprehension of reversible sentences, with no change in comprehension of low imageability words.

Whitworth's (1996b) therapy programme for remediation of anomia arising from impaired thematic role processing was used. The aim of this programme is to reactivate the ability to retrieve words in connected speech. The programme is input-oriented, with no spoken production being required. Instead, the client is asked to assign prepared labels to thematic roles within the written sentences provided. There are 13 graded stages. The client is required to achieve a minimum standard of performance at each stage before moving to the next. (For details, refer to Whitworth, 1996b.)

Each stage uses colour-coded cards to represent the verb and different thematic roles. At the start of the programme, the concept of verb is introduced in relation to *"what is happening?"* within a sentence. The programme then works through a range of one-, two-, and three-argument structures. Various thematic roles are introduced as they arise within the programme. Each thematic role has a "user-friendly" term, a sentence cue, and a question prompt. For example, the thematic role of agent is called *"actor"*, with the sentence cue of *"who is doing it?"* and the question prompt of *"who?"*. The thematic role is presented within the context of a sentence and the meaning of the role is discussed with respect to its relation to the verb. A demonstration sentence is given and the therapist places the colour-coded thematic role card under the relevant word in this sentence.

Ten practice sentences are then provided. The client is required to identify the verb, and place the corresponding colour-coded card under it, and then identify the thematic roles, again placing colour-coded cards in appropriate positions

beneath the sentence. Following identification of the targets, the therapist then asks questions that further discriminate these (e.g., *"who is doing it?"* for the agent). The therapist also discusses the obligatory nature of each role in the sentence, highlighting the incompleteness of the sentence should the role be omitted. When a mistake is made, the therapist identifies the locus of the error, and the sentence cues are used to assist the client in correction. Once the client is able to code 8 out of 10 sentences accurately, a second set of 10 practice sentences are worked through with the therapist providing feedback and support as necessary. When the same degree of accuracy is reached, the client is given a set of 10 evaluation sentences. If an 80% accuracy level is not achieved on these sentences, instruction using the two practice sets is repeated and the client reassessed with a second set of evaluation items. This cycle continues until the client reaches the 80% standard on evaluation sentences and moves on to the next level in the programme.

FR undertook this therapy programme within weekly, 1-hour therapy sessions in his own home. His wife observed all of these and used the therapist's model to work with FR between sessions. In each session, the therapist would introduce a stage within the programme and work with FR on the practice sets of sentences. The evaluation sets of sentences for that stage were given at the start of the next session; when FR passed the 80% criterion, the next stage was introduced. Except for stages 10, 13, and 14, no stage took more than 1 week to complete. During the programme there were two 1-week breaks for holidays and a month's break whilst FR went into hospital for a carotid endarterectomy. The programme was therefore completed over a 5-month period and included 16 hours of therapist-administered intervention.

Initially, FR was not keen on the therapy tasks and lacked confidence in his ability to undertake this type of work. He had left school at 14 and equated the therapy with school work, for which he felt he did not have an aptitude. He also questioned the input-oriented nature of the therapy, given that his major concern was to improve his speech. He did, however, persevere. As FR progressed within the programme, he gradually grew in confidence and reported a sense of achievement in working through the different levels.

REASSESSMENT

A number of the assessments undertaken before therapy were administered immediately after it, in order to evaluate the impact of intervention upon FR's performance. On the spoken version of PALPA 53 (Spoken Picture Naming) there was some slight improvement from 31/40 pre-therapy to 35/40 post-therapy. FR retained the semantic error pattern. There was no change in his performance on PALPA 50 (Written Synonym Judgement) and the previous pattern of more impaired processing of low imageability (19/30) than high imageability items (27/30) was still apparent. These latter results were in keeping with the pre-

dicted outcome of thematic role therapy; that is, that intervention focusing upon thematic roles would have no effect upon FR's comprehension of low imageability words.

In contrast, thematic role therapy had apparently achieved the desired effect of improving FR's word retrieval within connected speech. Figure 8.1 summarises changes in his retrieval of nouns as revealed by administration of the TRIP assessment immediately after completion of the therapy programme, and at 6 weeks post-therapy. FR demonstrated significantly improved noun retrieval in two-argument sentences after intervention (McNemar test, $p = .003$); a significant improvement within three element sentences was evident at six weeks (McNemar test, $p = .035$).

The post-therapy verb analysis also revealed improvements in FR's realisation of verbs taking two and three thematic roles. Again, these changes were still apparent at 6 weeks (see Figure 8.2).

Improvements in these two areas were reflected

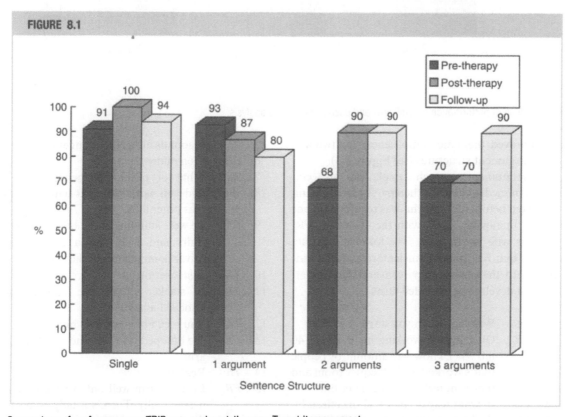

FIGURE 8.1

Comparison of performance on TRIP pre- and post-therapy: Target items correct.

FIGURE 8.2

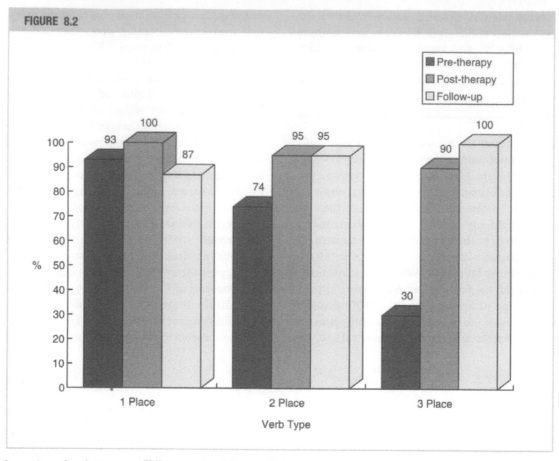

Comparison of performance on TRIP pre- and post-therapy: Verb analysis.

in improved thematic completeness for two-and three-argument structures (see Figure 8.3).

A spontaneous speech sample was also collected immediately after therapy. As for the sample taken before therapy, this was recorded on one of the therapist's visits with the therapist, FR, and his wife taking part. The following extract reveals that FR made a much more active contribution to the post-therapy conversation, initiating and developing extended turns.

1   *Th:*   Was that when you started work?
2   *FR:*   Oh I started working in 19 19 um 40 um 59. I know any amount of people that's worked in the lacquer room and they erm feel the effects later on.
3   *Th:*   In what way do they feel the effects?
4   *FR:*   Well erm breathing and that's it really.

5   *Th:*   It sounds altogether dangerous.
6   *FR:*   Seen many accidents.
7   *Th:*   What sort of thing happened?
8   *Wife:* Did you work out what happened to that other lad?
9   *FR:*   we were standing at the bottom of the stairs and there was a um stacker driver coming around the corner.
10 *Th:*   A stacker driver?
11 *FR:*   A stacker driver aye and er he knocked a lad down.
12 *Th:*   You mean bumped into him?
13 *FR:*   aye bumped into him and he's lost his arm
14 *Th:*   Really?
15 *FR:*   Lost his arm well only that far. Witnesses really. There's a lady come to the door for um-

FIGURE 8.3

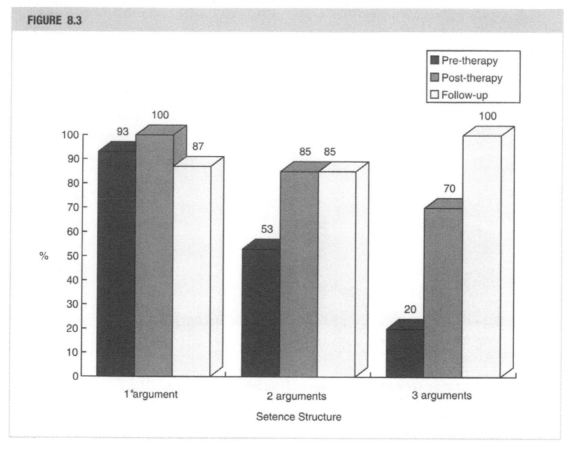

Comparison of performance on TRIP pre- and post-therapy: Thematic completeness analysis.

16 *Wife:* Was it the insurance company or commercial plastics? I don't know

17 *FR:* Well the lady came to ask what h-what really happened you know

18 *Th:* Right.

19 *FR:* Nothing happened really. Talked and talked and stacker driver came 'round the corner and bumped his arm. He's not lost arm but it's affected you know. He doesn't he can't use his arm.

Comparison of the pre- and post-therapy conversations also demonstrated a marked change in interactional patterns. In the first conversation, FR produced minimal answers to the therapist's questions; indeed, he barely initiated contributions other than to respond to direct questions from his wife. In contrast, in the post-therapy conversation, FR can be seen to initiate turns that develop the topic (e.g., T6, T13, and T19). A change in his wife's interactional style was also evident in the second conversation. The test questions previously employed to elicit FR's language were not apparent in this exchange; when she did ask FR questions, these appeared to be asking for novel information rather than that already known to her.

Figure 8.4 summarises the findings of the structural analysis of FR's conversation before and after therapy. The increased complexity of spoken output noted in other post-therapy assessments was mirrored here. For example, there was a reduction in the number of single phrases used conversationally, from 41% pre-therapy to 14% post-therapy; the number of

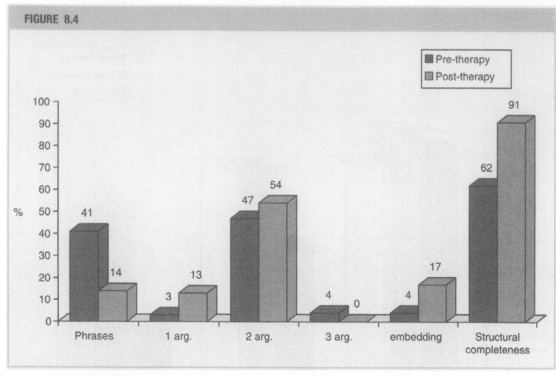

FIGURE 8.4

Spontaneous speech sample: Comparison of structures produced pre- and post-therapy.

embedded clauses increased from 4% to 17% over the same period. Therapy also seemed to have had an effect upon the adequacy of FR's contributions, with an increase in structural completeness from 62% to 91%.

Finally, FR was reassessed on PALPA 55 (Sentence–Picture Matching). Again, therapy had achieved a positive outcome, and this outcome was in line with that expected of thematic role therapy. Although reversal errors were still apparent at times, FR's comprehension of reversible sentences had improved from 9/20 (45%) to 15/20 (75%) in response to intervention.

In summary, reassessment identified improved word finding in connected speech on elicited assessment tasks (i.e., the TRIP) and in spontaneous speech. This suggested that this therapy programme, which focused on developing meta-linguistic knowledge of thematic roles, had reactivated FR's ability to retrieve words in sentences. As predicted, gains were also made in comprehension of reversible sentences, structures that require thematic role processing. In contrast

(and also as predicted), no change in semantic processing of low imageability items was found.

FR'S VIEWS OF THE EFFECT OF THERAPY

After completing the therapy programme, FR reported that his speech was more fluent and less hesitant. He felt better able to go beyond communicating basic messages to expressing more complex ideas. Whilst FR described increased confidence in communicating, he viewed this change as an improvement rather than an elimination of his aphasic difficulties.

DISCUSSION

The symptom-based therapy for anomia carried out with FR under normal caseload pressures involved 5 sessions of speech and language therapy: 1 session for assessment and 4 monthly reviews. This therapy was supported by twice-weekly home practice. Theoretically motivated therapy required more resources: 9 sessions of assessment and reassessment, 16 sessions for therapy and, again, regular work by FR and his wife.

The theoretically motivated therapy was more effective than the symptom-based therapy. FR showed specific improvement on the area targeted, and there was evidence from the spontaneous speech sample and FR's own report that therapy had had an impact on his everyday use of language. It could be argued that this improvement simply reflected the amount of therapeutic input provided and that an equivalent amount of symptom-based therapy would also have been effective. This possibility cannot be rejected: to do this it would have been necessary to have delivered the same number of hours to both therapy programmes. Our own view, however, is that the difference between these interventions does not reflect the quantity of therapy afforded but rather the degree to which the underlying impairment was targeted.

In a climate of limited resources, pressure is placed upon therapists to offer limited and potentially insufficient input to all. Correspondingly, there is a danger of merely focusing on surface symptoms with the risk of intervention being ineffective. This was the case for FR's initial period of therapy. In contrast, the results of the second phase of therapy demonstrated that, when theoretically motivated, aphasia therapy can be effective; this study highlights the need for the investment of resources in careful assessment and interpretation of assessment findings. Whilst we have focused on a cognitive neuropsychological approach to therapy here, the same principle is likely to apply to any framework of therapy. If therapy is going to be effective, it requires a sound base of assessment in order that a clear rationale for therapy be developed.

Having examined the question of whether to offer symptom-based or theoretically motivated therapy, we are left with the thorny issue of how we ration services or how we convince purchasers of the need for more resources for aphasia therapy. In relation to the latter issue, demonstration of the effectiveness of speech and language therapy for this client group is a vital first step. This project was a valuable exercise. It highlighted that, in aphasia therapy, short cuts may waste rather than save resources. Happily, it allowed us to persuade service managers to increase the clinical sessions available to aphasic clients.

NOTE

1 A pilot version of TRIP was used and, in its presentation to FR, five items were accidently omitted. Scores are presented as percentages in addition to the raw scores to facilitate comparison.

REFERENCES

Bock, K. (1987). Co-ordinating words and syntax in speech plans. In A.W. Ellis (Ed.), *Progress in the psychology of language 3*. London: Lawrence Erlbaum Associates Ltd.

Byng, S. (1988). Sentence processing deficits: Theory and therapy. *Cognitive Neuropsychology, 5*, 629–676.

Byng, S., & Black, M. (1989). Some aspects of sentence production in aphasia. *Aphasiology, 3*, 241–263.

Garrett, M.F. (1980). Levels of processing in sentence production. In B. Butterworth (Ed.), *Language production, Vol. 1*. London: Academic Press.

Garrett, F. (1984). The organisation of processing structure for language production: Applications to aphasic speech. In D. Caplan, A.R. Lecours, & A. Smith (Eds.), *Biological perspectives on language*. Cambridge, MA: MIT Press.

Kay, J., Lesser, R., & Coltheart, M. (1992). *Psycholinguistic assessment of language processing in aphasia*. London: Lawrence Erlbaum Associates Ltd.

Lesser, R., & Milroy, L. (1993). *Linguistics and aphasia:*

Psycholinguistic and pragmatic aspects of intervention. London: Longman.

Marshall, J., Black, M., & Byng, S. (1999). *Working with sentences: A handbook for therapists*. Bicester, UK: Winslow.

Whitworth, A. (1996a). *Thematic roles in production*. London: Whurr.

Whitworth, A. (1996b). *Mapping thematic roles onto syntactic frames*. Newcastle upon Tyne, UK: NUSE.

9

Therapy for life: Challenging the boundaries of aphasia therapy

Carole Pound

INTRODUCTION

This chapter documents the author's involvement with Tony, a young man with aphasia, over a 5-year period. I describe two key phases of therapy: the first, when Tony and I worked together in a neuro-rehabilitation centre, approximately 9 to 12 months after his stroke; the second, when I supervised Tony's therapy programme at a university-based aphasia centre between 3 and 5 years after his stroke. The chapter describes the therapeutic content and direction of these two periods of intervention and the changes and outcomes that ensued. These outcomes will be described from the perspective of the treating therapist (and student clinicians) and from the

viewpoint of Tony himself. Tony's reflections on therapy and change have been extracted from in-depth interviews conducted with him at 2½ and 5 years into his journey as a person living with aphasia. The reflections of a succession of student therapists are taken from their clinical notes.

My personal reflections grew from working with Tony in one-to-one sessions at the rehabilitation centre, and then within the group setting at the City Dysphasic Group. They are also the result of some uncomfortable listening to Tony's everyday experience of aphasia, ongoing observation of his interactions inside and outside the therapy groups, and a range of supervisory sessions with students that aimed to support and challenge them as they struggled to change Tony's language, confidence and lifestyle.

THE CONTEXT OF THERAPY

The two phases of therapy that I discuss here were carried out in different places. The first, individualised one-to-one therapy, was carried out at a neuro-rehabilitation unit when Tony was between 9 and 12 months post-stroke. He attended the centre 5 days a week as an out-patient. There he received an integrated package of physiotherapy, occupational therapy and an average of eight 40-minute sessions of speech and language therapy each week. The second therapy, taking place approximately 36 to 54 months after Tony's stroke, was received at the City Dysphasic Group (CDG). This centre, based at City University in London, specialised in intensive, long-term therapy and support for people living with aphasia. Clients typically attended the centre 2 days a week, for group therapy, supplemented by a weekly individual session. Therapy was predominantly carried out by student Speech and Language Therapists from City University, under the supervision of experienced aphasia therapists. The therapy was provided in termly blocks of approximately 10 weeks' duration; 1 year at CDG therefore represented approximately 32 weeks of intervention.

Tony began attending the CDG 18 months after his stroke. Prior to the second phase of therapy described in this chapter, Tony participated enthusiastically in a range of language- and communication-based activities with the group. These are not described in detail in this chapter but are identified as Phase 2a in the appendices.

Whilst the therapies described here take the form of neatly circumscribed tasks and activities in a clear(ish) and logical progression, inevitably this risks cleaning up the day-to-day mess of managing therapy and marrying it to people and lives. At the time of developing these therapies (the early 1990s), a guiding but to some extent confusing framework was the WHO classification of impairment, disability and handicap (now superceded by impairment, activities and participation).

Much of the therapy described in Phase 1—all of the language processing work and the exhortations to manage his impairment by developing better communication strategies—clearly focus on changing Tony's impairment. The confidence-based work in Phase 2 would appear to fit more neatly within participation-based goals. Frameworks, such as impairment and participation, are helpful in giving sense and order to clinicians struggling with unwieldy impairments and real lives. What these frameworks failed to sufficiently address for me was the interaction between Tony's feelings about his impairment, his reactions to a massively changed identity and his concerns about re-entering a disabling and disablist society. Another overarching framework that informed this therapy journey was the impairment/disability distinction from disability studies. By encouraging a more explicit focus on disabling barriers in the social environment and how to support people to construct a more robust disabled identity, this disability studies approach provided an appealing framework for acknowledging the importance of aphasia as impairment whilst foregrounding life rather than language.

TONY

Tony was a 38-year-old unemployed electrical engineer at the time of his stroke. Previously well, he suffered a left temporoparietal infarction that resulted in severe receptive and expressive aphasia and a right-sided weakness. Tony was single and living in a flat, which he part-owned. Due to management difficulties with the co-owner of the flat after his stroke, Tony moved in with his elderly mother, where he stayed throughout the 5 years covered here. Tony had two brothers, whom he saw rarely, and a sister living outside London. She was in regular contact and played a supportive role in helping Tony with correspondence and benefit issues. Whilst both Tony's mother and sister seemed very supportive, Tony always gave the impression that his rehabilitation was his business and he was not keen to involve them in therapy sessions or discussions.

Prior to his stroke, Tony had a wide circle of friends and enjoyed socialising with them at pubs and clubs. He was an avid sportsman, participating in football, boxing, tennis and watersports. Occupationally he had been involved in a range of engineering jobs, most recently as a jukebox engineer. His work had involved him working independently as well as managing others and, as he described it, being a bit of a jack-of-all-trades.

Relatives described Tony as a cheerful, sociable, sporty bloke who enjoyed a good laugh and also had a sensitive, reflective side to his personality. These characteristics were clearly evident on his initial presentation to the rehabilitation unit. Also in clear evidence was Tony's intense motivation to work on his aphasic impairments and a very high degree of anxiety, embarrassment and bewilderment about the extent and nature of his communication disability.

Initial impressions

Physically, Tony had made a good recovery and on admission to the rehabilitation centre he had only a very mild weakness of his right arm and some altered sensation in his right side. Both of these difficulties, however, continued to profoundly affect his ability to resume former sporting pursuits. Hearing and vision were unimpaired.

Cognitively, there were no obvious difficulties. Tony showed good non-verbal problem solving and reasoning. Orientation and memory for day-to-day events was good, although he could only recall two digits in an auditory digit span task. Tony showed good insight into the presence and impact of his language difficulties and a high level of motivation to work at and change his ability to use and understand words.

Socially, he was cheerful, friendly and apparently laid back in a blokish sort of way! He made full use of his social speech and non-verbal skills and used a number of effective strategies to conceal the severity of his difficulties with receptive and expressive language.

Language and communication

Tony was able to follow simple, everyday conversation in context, though he required frequent repetitions and clarifications for any conversation that lacked context or some form of visual support. His comprehension difficulties multiplied with increased speed of presentation and any level of background noise. Cognitive/emotional interference such as fatigue or anxiety also affected his understanding significantly. His ability to follow written information was impaired but markedly superior to his auditory skills.

Expressively Tony had bursts of fluent, socially appropriate words and phrases. However he had severe word-finding difficulties when he tried to produce any more specific language. Conversation beyond social exchanges tended to be empty and lacking in content, on the rare occasion that Tony attempted it. Whilst there was some evidence that Tony had partial access to phonological knowledge of target words, his attempts at spoken output tended to be few and far between, constrained or aborted by repeated sub-vocal rehearsals, self-inhibitions and acute embarrassment at errors. Tony was hyper-aware of errors in output but unable to self-correct at a segmental level.

ASSESSMENT RESULTS

Results of language assessments on Tony's admission to the rehabilitation unit are presented in Tables 9.1 and 9.2. Examples of errors in output at this time appear in Figure 9.1.

In summary, test results and observations of everyday language performance showed that Tony had relatively well-preserved semantics, although some difficulties accessing semantic knowledge via the auditory channel were evident. There appeared to be some residual difficulties in early acoustic analysis of words and sounds, confirmed by the marked impact of interference, speed, accent and stimulus length upon ability. Comprehension was facilitated by repetition, reduced speed of presentation, lip-reading and the provision of context.

Tony performed much better on tasks requiring written as opposed to spoken output. Errors were qualitatively similar across all forms of output. A pattern of hesitation and considerable sub-vocal

TABLE 9.1

Results of assessments of language processing: Input

Type of input	Spoken	Written
Minimal pairs (real words)[a]	49/50	
Lexical decision	91%	
Kay's word to picture match (unpublished)	36/40	38/40
Synonym judgement		
High imageability	30/38	35/38
Low imageability	20/38	34/38
Test for Reception of Grammar[b] (Bishop, 1983)	57/80	

[a] Hesitant responses, needing repetition of stimuli, lip-reading.
[b] Reading comprehension better, but affected by increased grammatical complexity at the sentence level.

TABLE 9.2

Results of assessments of language processing: Output

PALPA 53 (Kay, Lesser, & Coltheart, 1992)	
Spoken naming	12/40
Written naming	36/40
Oral reading	11/40
Repetition	26/40
Tests of internal phonology	
Rhyming pictures (match to 1/4)	17/20
Written homophone judgement[a]	32/40
Pseudohomophone detection	25/30

[a] Influence of orthographic similarity.

FIGURE 9.1

i) Simplification
Cluster reduction: screw – /sku/; mountain – /mautin/
Assimilation: glove – /blub/

ii) Complication
cathedral – / skae .../ ; vegetable – / ref tival/
tobacco – / taeg baek /

iii) Other phonologically related
telephone – / feliw n/ ; belt – / bilt /

iv) Lexical/semantic
lemon – orange ; dog – cat
swing – circle ; bread – belt

v) perseveration

Errors produced in output tasks: Qualitatively similar across different tests of spoken output.

knowledge. There was some evidence that more reliably available orthographic knowledge influenced spoken output (e.g., scissors—/skizez/) and, in reading aloud, there were examples of over-regularisation indicating at least some ability to convert graphemes to phonemes.

Tony's ability to self-monitor spoken output was relatively good at a gross word level but more limited at a sound level. Whilst he was able to recognise that he was making errors in production, he had difficulty locating these sounds and segments within words. Attempts at self-correction were therefore rather random. At a sound level, monitoring of word-initial consonants was superior to that of word-final phonemes, which in turn were more reliably monitored than vowels or second consonants in clusters.

PHASE 1 THERAPY

Phase 1 therapy plan
A therapy plan was designed, based on the assessment results. It had the following aims.

1. To develop a self-cuing strategy to facilitate spoken word production of content words, by capitalising on Tony's relatively

rehearsal was apparent prior to any voiced attempt at production. Repeated attempts at a target tended to slowly approximate and ultimately facilitate output. Difficulties with speech became more obvious with increased word length and phonological complexity, but error patterns suggested rather good access to phonological preserved orthographic knowledge and his partial ability to convert graphemes to phonemes. This strand of therapy also aimed to heighten Tony's awareness of phonological segmentation as a prerequisite for self-monitoring therapy and activities.

2. To improve self-monitoring of phonological errors as a precursor to therapy addressing self-correction. Self-monitoring therapy would emphasise: listening and acoustic analysis activities in both tasks and conversation; encouraging production vs. over-inhibition of output; developing listening (and feedback) strategies.

3. To encourage selective listening in sentence-length material to improve comprehension in everyday conversation. This strand of therapy emphasised using contextual information, concentrating on key words and gist (in contrast to Tony's focus on too much detail and upon understanding every word) and use of listening strategies.

4. To improve Tony's general levels of comfort and confidence in attempting spoken output and giving reliable feedback to speakers about his true level of understanding and communicative needs.

Phase 1 therapy activities

Keyword strategy to facilitate content words in output

The prime aim of this therapy was to enable Tony to develop a self-cuing strategy to facilitate spoken production of content words. Components of the therapy programmme were based on the grapheme-to-phoneme conversion work of De Partz (1986) and the extension of this work to the production of self-generated phonemic cues (Nickels, 1992, 1995). The use of written words and graphemes not only built on Tony's strengths with orthographic material but also helped provide him with a stable, visual peg to aid spoken output.

Tasks that underpinned this programme of therapy included:

- preliminary listening tasks to raise phonological awareness

- selecting first phoneme (from an array of 5 and then 10 graphemes) given a spoken word: s g th d sh —"shoe"; "goal"; "soup"

- generating a list of keywords that corresponded to phonemes (short, concrete, high frequency, regularly spelt nouns, which Tony could write and pronounce with ease)

- memorising keywords and replacing any that were inconsistently remembered or produced (e.g., with a shorter, more familiar or higher frequency item)

- repeating the keyword three times, then isolating and producing the initial sound, then saying the keyword once more

- following the previous repetition and initial phoneme segmentation task, generating one to three different words beginning with the same initial phoneme (semantic and/or written word cues provided by therapist as required)

- picture naming via the following sequence:
  - producing the target word in its written form
  - saying the keyword beginning with the same initial phoneme
  - segmenting and producing the initial phoneme from the keyword
  - attempting the new target word by self-cuing with this initial phoneme

- producing minimal sets using rapidly swapped scrabble tiles + the keyword chart backup
  - ban   can   ran   Dan   fan
  - swim   skim   slim

- Tony was also encouraged to practise grapheme-to-phoneme conversion, segmentation and blending skills in a range of home assignments (set at different points within the programme), which included:
  - word generation to a given phoneme (e.g., three words beginning with /d/, /s/, etc.)
  - generate three words that rhyme (e.g. cat → bat, —, —)
  - segmentation of a written word into its component number of phonemes, and then attempt production (e.g. c/augh/t/ = 3, r/u/bb/i/sh = 5)

— segmentation of sounds within written/pictured word, then attempt blending of sounds to produce word.

The following hierarchies of difficulty were considered within all tasks: short to long words; regular to exception words; high to low frequency words.

A small-scale, controlled study of Tony's response to this therapy revealed changes in his ability to name pictures (see Table 9.3).

Single content word production in connected speech

Certain tasks were then assigned to encourage the carryover of content word production into connected and spontaneous speech. These included:

- content word count: for example, Tony was asked to tell me about his weekend; his response was recorded and the number of content words counted
- composite picture description
- story recall from a picture sequence or video clip (e.g., Mr Bean, Laurel and Hardy).

These tasks served as an additional opportunity to remind Tony of more practical uses of the keyword strategy and to raise his awareness of improvement, with word counts acting as objective measurements of success and change. On some occasions, priming of target vocabulary (in the form of category-based verbal fluency exercises—e.g., name 10 football teams; station names; racecourses) was carried out.

TABLE 9.3		
Pictures named correctly before and after "keyword" therapy (n = 30)		
	Pre-therapy	*Post-therapy*
Target words	11	29
Control words	12	17

Listening, input and monitoring tasks

Listening and phoneme monitoring/segmentation tasks followed those described by Jones (1989) and Harding and Pound (2000).

- Scrabble tiles—spot the change:
  CVC HAT: "cat"; "rat"; "chat"; "hat"
  "ham"; "hag"; "hash"; "hat"
  "heart"; "hurt"; "hot"; "hat"

In this task, a CVC word was presented to Tony using Scrabble tiles. He was asked to listen to the therapist producing a CVC word, which was either the target or a minimally similar CVC word (see line 1, above). He was then asked to indicate whether the therapist's word matched the Scrabble tiles or not. Initially Tony would be alerted to whether change might occur in word initial, word final or vowel position. Subsequently the position of change became more random. The task then progressed to incorporate the following:

- spot the change *and* correct from multiple-choice tiles
- as above *and* offer spoken attempt after correction, using keyword strategy to prompt output where necessary
- spot the deliberate paraphasic error, given a picture of an object (e.g.
  Therapist: "is it a . . . hat . . . cat . . . back . . . boat ?"
  Tony: "No it's a . . .")

As before, hierarchies of difficulty were incorporated within these tasks: from word initial to word final to vowel change and from single to bi- to polysyllabic words.

Sentence comprehension and word monitoring in sentence contexts

In order to provide Tony with practice in monitoring and comprehending single words in context, tasks were constructed in which he was asked to listen for a given word in a sentence spoken by the therapist, and then to indicate whether the spoken sentence matched simultaneously presented written material. The written material, and the demands of this task, were systematically varied:

- therapist provides written sentence with position of potential change marked (e.g., the train arriving at Platform 1 is a *Wimbledon* train, the winner of the 2.30 race at *Chepstow* is Jack the Lad)
- therapist provides written sentence but no indication of location of change
- using close semantic/phonological distractors for items changed
- Tony then asked to select correct item from multiple-choice written array.

Confidence in spoken output and feedback on levels of comprehension

After initial discussion, these themes were not addressed in isolation but threaded through the various language tasks described above. For example, in tasks emphasising listening and sound or word analysis Tony was encouraged to ask if he required repetition or to explicitly state that he hadn't "heard" or understood. In tasks requiring spoken output the emphasis was on thinking about it and then "having a go". This was in marked contrast to his usual behaviour of rehearsing subvocally multiple times, but sometimes avoiding saying anything, in the "keep mistakes to a minimum" strategy. Therapist feedback within these tasks served primarily to affirm the closeness of his attempts to the target form. Writing and Scrabble tiles were used to rapidly flag up errors.

PHASE 1 THERAPY OUTCOMES

Changes in output

Reassessment at the end of this 3-month block of therapy revealed a number of changes in output at the single word level. These changes are summarised in Table 9.4.

Aside from these quantitative differences, Tony was able to use the keyword strategy to cue spoken output in conversations within therapy sessions, in other communications around the centre and, to a lesser degree, outside the rehabilitation unit. Tony and his therapists, friends and

TABLE 9.4

Outcomes of Phase 1 therapy: Output

PALPA 53	Pre-therapy	Post-therapy
Spoken naming	12/40	36/40
Written naming	36/40	39/40
Oral reading	11/40	39/40
Repetition	26/40	38/40

FIGURE 9.2

Mr Bean—Royal Film Performance

It was about the ...queen or something like that...I don't know why he's doing it...and there's...guests... He had his...shoes em...he got ...what is it ...ss..spit on his...clean or something...He got...what's it called ...he was going like this (mimes testing breath) ...his breath...He got a ...thimble (thread)...the...must be a...handkerchief...he didn't have one that's why ...he got em...card...the em... fold...for his nails...thimble no.../zim...zim / ..zip ...He em..butted that queen or whatever it is.　　　(7 minutes)

Narrative description after Phase 1 therapy.

family all reported an increase in the fluency and content of his conversation; a story narrative recorded at this time (Figure 9.2) adds weight to these reports. Another marker of change was that, at the beginning of therapy, Tony did not attempt any picture description, whereas at the end he did so readily.

Changes in input

Changes in Tony's receptive abilities were marked by his increased awareness and understanding of his auditory comprehension impairment. With this improved insight came an almost visible increase in panic and low confidence. Tony's improved performance within tasks requiring listening and phonological segmentation of words, together with an improved ability to repeat, did suggest some small changes in comprehension. Within the structured and prompted sessions, there was also evidence of some increase in his use of listening strategies. Endless "therapist nagging" had led to Tony asking more frequently for repetitions and clarification. These requests, however, were almost entirely limited to therapy tasks rather than more natural conversation, where Tony clearly remained profoundly reluctant to signal any failure to understand speech.

Reflections on change

The therapist's view
As Tony's therapist I was encouraged by the positive impact of specific, theoretically motivated therapy programmes on his language impairments, particularly those affecting spoken output. Moreover, I had clear proof of the effectiveness of my therapy in the form of:

- changes on assessment scores
- growing generalisation of the keyword strategy to the production of untreated words
- reported generalisation of strategy use beyond the clinical setting
- related improvements in self-monitoring and self-correction.

These positives helped to alleviate some of my disappointment and frustration at Tony's continuing over-inhibition of output, apparently associated with a fear of producing "mistakes".

In relation to Tony's comprehension difficulties, I had the impression of some subtle changes in his ability to perceive and monitor individual sounds. I also had a clear sense of his future and potential to use certain strategies to minimise the communication disability associated with impaired auditory skills.

Without doubt the issue that concerned me most was the inability of any of these therapies to impact upon Tony's profound loss of confidence and level of distress. I sensed that beneath the cheerful, sociable, joking exterior there was a well of anxiety, embarrassment and low self-esteem. I felt I had followed Tony's lead in focusing on language rather than emotions but I was aware that I had not begun to access Tony's thoughts and feelings about himself and his life. He showed no signs of opening up this type of discussion with me or with other therapists, or with trained counsellors.

Tony was still only 1 year into his life with aphasia. Although there was little local therapy on offer when he left the rehabilitation centre I was relieved that Tony would be accessing further, hopefully long-term therapy, at the City Dysphasic Group. Tony had enthusiastically agreed to be referred to CDG and my hope was that over time these confidence issues could be addressed as the focus rather than the periphery of therapy.

The excerpts below are from interviews with Tony. They provide his own retrospective accounts of this first phase of therapy and afford an interesting contrast to the view from my side of the therapy table.

Tony's reflections on language therapy
When we were doing that sort of like word things ... yeah word ... keywords like ... like that's to me I thought Oh God this is stupid you know ... it's sort of ... but I have to you know ... all the time.

it was um ... I could say cat and dog and pub and things like that ... it was um ... it wasn't what I wanted to say ... you know what I mean ... it's um when I starting to sort of panicking ... I suppose its um Oh Christ um ... I can't ... I'll never never gonna be normal sort of thing. . .

Tony's reflections on contact with others with strokes and disabilities
When questioned about how other patients at the rehabilitation centre had affected him during this period, Tony reflected on his feelings of panic that the others were all "better" than him. Paradoxically, Tony did not identify himself with being "handicapped", reserving this term for his descriptions of fellow "inmates".

Tony's reflections on confidence and identity
By the time Tony was coming to the rehabilitation centre he was reporting a loss of contact with former friends and a growing sense of isolation.

I was like in my own shell sort of thing.

I'm just sort of like a boring man sort of thing, you know, like I'd come down here, I said "oh yes" I said "pub" sort of thing, I said a word . . . know what I mean . . . like to me oh that's alright but um actually I was so uptight.

This change in identity was compounded by a loss of interests and work prospects.

Nothing at all outdoors I couldn't . . ., I'd look at the television but I couldn't hear that . . . I'd probably walk down the p . . . er pub but er you know I . . . no-one sort of they wouldn't talk to me there.

Thoughts on leaving rehabilitation, future prospects

Despite what felt like a sensitively handled preparation for discharge with follow-up appointments to address potential work assessments, and reassurances from the therapy team regarding future improvements, Tony's reflections on that time show the depth of his anxiety and foreboding:

. . . when it stopped it sort of like went oh my God you know . . . its um . . . I didn't know what was going on you know . . . its like I said it was er . . . I was sc . .sc. . after that er slow with learning . . . cos for me I could ss . . . I could know that I could do some more . . . I thought oh my God does that mean it's gonna be the same? Am I gonna get better or better or better or stopped? And that's sort of like I think the worst that you never know.

PHASE 2 THERAPY

Tony joined the City Dysphasia Group 18 months after his stroke. The phase of therapy described in this section occurred when I took up a new job working at CDG and resumed therapeutic contact with him. Tony was now 3 years post-stroke. His life outside CDG had taken an upturn in the

amount of time he now spent on the golf course and doing gardening jobs for friends. But his reflections on who he was remained dominated by phrases such as the following:

I'm just like a loser . . . a yes man . . . cos I don't know what's sort of like going on so I just put a yes and hope its right . . . its like a boring man sort of thing.

I used to have pride . . . that's to me like jobs and things but it's it's a bit gone now.

I noticed considerable improvements in his spoken and written output from our earlier time together. He was still troubled by significant auditory comprehension difficulties, though as before, he rarely signalled these to others.

Reflections from Tony on the intervening time frame suggest that his earlier time at CDG was dominated by anxieties about "being the worst", and ongoing feelings that "I've got some kind of disease". However, over time, and thanks no doubt to his engaging, shy, but sociable manner, he settled in as a reliable and committed attender, well liked by staff, students and clients at the group.

Comments and reflections from student therapists during Tony's first 18 months at the group (Phase 2a) highlighted Tony's ongoing commitment to language therapy coupled with the student therapists' feelings of frustration that the therapy wasn't quite hitting the mark:

Tony is obviously not well adjusted to his communication problems and other difficult circumstances. He needs to learn to face his problems before he is able to benefit from more therapy. It may be beneficial to have some counselling . . . but this is not really possible, therefore it may be more beneficial to do more structured therapy.

It was clear that Tony had established himself as a popular and helpful member of the CDG community. It was also clear that his confidence remained barely changed. He was still committed to working hard on his language.

Tony: Um . . . er . . . actually to me I think it was er my verbs . . . in the group they took verbs all the time.

C.P.: Did that seem important to be working on them ?

Tony: Oh it really . . . it 'cos I didn't know what . . . like from school I didn't know what a verb was . . . but I do now . . . it was sort of like drummed in me brain.

C.P.: How did you feel about doing all these drills?

Tony: Brilliant . . . its like I was actually I was doing something now.

Another attempt to encourage him to see the resident stroke counsellor at the beginning of this period met with failure, with Tony expressing the view that what he needed were friends to talk to and be with rather than an occasional hour with a counsellor. His comments to students at around this time suggested he might, however, be ready for a change in the emphasis and direction of therapy : "I think to begin with its all confidence which is my problem"; "the therapy . . . its . . . its something missing".

Phase 2 therapy plan

Notes from a first period of therapy at City Dysphasic Group (not described here), when Tony was between 18 months and 3 years post-stroke, suggest that therapeutic input initially concentrated on and to some extent fed Tony's constant requests for activities addressing his language impairments. In contrast, the phase of therapy described here might be more appropriately entitled "Learning to live with aphasia". Whilst real-life issues and facing the future with aphasia had often been touched on in the past, particularly in group work, they had perhaps not been afforded the structure, status nor the time allocation of other language and communication work. Perhaps the fragmented and diluted way in which therapy had addressed these issues in the groups, the lack of a clear framework or evidence base in our work with long-term aphasia, and the understandable preference for student clinicians to work on "safe" language issues rather than

unwieldy psychosocial issues, underpinned my feeling (and Tony's) that we had somehow not hit the mark.

Tony's low confidence but determined focus on language was almost a perfect match for our own low confidence in really helping his life. We were both lured to more work on verbs and prepositions. This was crystallised for me when, in a goal-setting session, I asked Tony what he would really like to work towards in the next phase of therapy, and he said: "*Well really verbs and conjunctions and prepositions*". Goal setting was focused and explicit, involving discussions of what further language work could and could not achieve in the context of Tonys life goals—getting a job, being one of the lads again.

The overarching aims of this phase of therapy then had a much more direct focus on:

1. Developing Tony's confidence in living with and accommodating his aphasia.
2. Identifying and affirming life and work skills and exploring options for return to work.
3. Exploring, developing and using strategies, gadgets, and gizmos that might help Tony acknowledge and circumvent some of his auditory comprehension difficulties.

Phase 2: The context of therapy

Therapy again took the form of predominantly group sessions (three 90-minute sessions per week in a group with six to eight members) with once-weekly individual sessions. Group sessions would tend to be themed in line with group decisions about priorities for the group, e.g., assertiveness and aphasia; developing a video; access to work and education; understanding aphasia.

These themes were also supported in a range of ways outside the formal therapy sessions. For example, Tony was encouraged to take a more active "helping" role within CDG. To some extent this was through working with therapy staff and students to help set up rooms and video equipment. It also took the form of supporting new group members to travel to CDG, if they lived near Tony, and in playing a teaching role with students and visitors.

An overview of the themes covered in individual and group sessions during this period is given below.

Individual sessions

- Ongoing discussion of Tony's short- and longer-term hopes and aspirations and the barriers and facilitators to achieving these
- identification and review of confidence and self-identity in given contexts (e.g., an interview with the Disability Employment Advisor)
- identification of strengths, skills and needs and how to present these to relevant others (e.g., developing a CV, rehearsing interviews).

Group sessions

- Aphasia and disability—addressing the meaning, consequences and challenges of living with aphasia; discussion and project work highlighting individual needs, coping strategies and coping styles
- communication and life skills—developing skills and strategies in assertiveness, goal setting, telephone use
- roles within a group—raising awareness of individuals' roles and contributions to group interactions through observation and feedback
- awareness raising—directed at self, group and others; educating others about individuals' communication needs in order to promote accessible and enabling environments.

Phase 2 therapy activities

Unlike the first phase of therapy, aims and activities had a less clear one-to-one relationship. Themes of confidence, identity and internal/external barriers to participation wove in and out of group and individual sessions and also through changing relationships with different group members and student clinicians. These changes were not always easy to track. The groupings of therapy activities described below is a retrospective clarification of some key strands of therapy.

Self-perception

In order to challenge the negative self-image of Tony and other group members, group and individual work was undertaken addressing questions such as "who am I?" and "how do I come across to others?". Within group sessions this work involved comparing members' perceptions of themselves to that of others. Specific tasks included:

- identifying qualities and characteristics in other people (e.g., celebrities, most admired people) to generate a vocabulary for styles and attributes
- identifying admired and salient qualities in group members at a personal and communicative level
- completing self- and peer-ratings on given and group-generated personality traits, communication skills, etc.
- recording one's own personal list of qualities and reflecting as a group on any areas of mismatch.

The discussions and peer feedback generated by these activities were an important component of Tony's therapy. Other members' identification of Tony as a skilled listener, facilitator and negotiator both enhanced his level of confidence and helped to challenge some of his perceptions of his own communication. These observations and discussions fed individual work around developing a CV and using this to support confident self-presentation in interview practice (see below).

Confidence building and developing a robust self-image

Compiling a curriculum vitae and developing interview skills

This activity served a number of purposes, including Tony's preparation for work. The creation of the CV included:

- highlighting and elaborating Tony's overt work strengths and skills
- reviewing and stating implicit, less obvious personal and interpersonal skills

- linking, rather than separating, past and present abilities (e.g., former work skills, current contributions within group)
- highlighting new skills and experiences, the positive contributions of stroke and change
- reviewing Tony's life history, enabling reflections on losses, gains, change and the emergence of an identity that incorporates the experience of disability
- documenting all of these strengths and skills in a written, recorded form as the basis for both affirmation and negotiation.

Work on developing a CV formed the basis of preparing for an interview with the Disability Employment Advisor. However, a number of confidence-building opportunities arose:

- preparing and articulating strengths, skills and needs
- elaborating and supporting statements about personal strengths
- self-affirmations—statements and role play, being careful to monitor and discuss emotional response and provide concrete justification and example
- self-evaluation of video—rating performance in mock interview on given scales (e.g., general content, self-presentation, clarity in expressing needs, assertiveness in asking for clarifications, etc.).

Confidence hierarchies

Establishing Tony and other group members' personal comfort and discomfort zones in communication situations proved a useful activity to revisit at the beginning of each therapy term. This naturally fed other goal-setting activities and the content and evolution of particular groups, e.g., the assertiveness and aphasia group. A key issue in therapy was balancing sufficient time for reflection on attitudes (own and others'), telling and hearing personal stories of identity and identifying both internal and external barriers to feeling and participating more confidently. The following framework of activities supported this work:

- group brainstorms to identify communicatively easy or difficult situations and people

- rating situations and/or people on a 1–5 visual analogue scale (i.e., 1 = *very easy*, 5 = *extremely difficult/communication not attempted*)
- using specific examples from these hierarchies to tell a story, taking care to paint the whole picture (e.g., a detailed description of the situation, the person, Tony's personal feelings, reactions and behaviours in this context)
- eliciting and recording concrete reasons why a situation or person is easy/difficult communicatively (i.e., beginning to locate the source of the problem outside Tony)
- brainstorming strategies for dealing with the situation/person, and identifying a manageable first step
- role playing a given situation, using prepared script/cue cards to avoid excessive communication demands
- feedback on what happened in the role play and any feelings that arose in the role play
- problem solving as a group communication and emotional/stress management strategies that have arisen
- further role play, experimenting with different responses from the communication partner
- assignments and goal setting for encounters beyond the therapy room
- monitoring of goals and further problem solving of any difficulties.

Questionnaires and their completion provided another means of trying to separate out different strands of confidence, and perform ongoing reality checks of pre- and post-stroke responses and tendencies. Examples of suitable questionnaires can be found in Thelander, Hoen, and Worsley (1994; e.g., Ryff's "How I feel about myself" scale) or can be more personalised.

Another important confidence-builder for Tony was discussion and review of interim reports and goal plans. Formal review of written and explicit confidence goals for the term supported the stepwise addressing of what had until now proved a massive but ill-defined enemy. Changes were identified and next steps articulated. But unlike before and after numerical scores, subtle, qualitative or environmentally dependent factors reinforced the concept of therapy as a journey rather than as something more discrete, where success is determined by both the skills of the therapist and the commitment of the patient. These types of evaluative discussions seemed to reinforce a sense of partnership in tackling difficult problems together.

Assertiveness skills

Another, complementary strand of Tony's therapy addressed the development of assertiveness skills. This group-based course ran over two 6-week blocks and addressed a range of skills and issues: definitions and awareness; aphasia and assertiveness; personal styles; and "learning the tools". Methods predominantly comprised group discussion, practice and role play, and observation and feedback. Tony, along with other group members and students, was given the opportunity to experiment with new styles, for example talking about himself in a "boastful" style, which was quite at odds with his exceptionally modest usual style of presentation. Group members provided one another feedback. They identified and role-played relevant situations for them. Many of the baseline activities were taken from Holland and Ward (1990). (See also Pound, Parr, Lindsay, & Woolf, 2000.)

During this time Tony also participated in a range of group and centre activities that reinforced some of the more structured work outlined above. Activities addressed themes of understanding aphasia without continuously apologising for it, thinking about barriers imposed by the ignorance of others rather than the shortcomings of one's own language. Some specific examples were:

- developing a group video about living and coping with aphasia—identifying personal and social barriers to feeling okay about yourself and participating on equal terms; scripting who you are and how aphasia is (and isn't) a key part of your life
- preparation for a visit by a British Telecom disability products salesperson—identifying the shortcomings of commercially available

items for people who are deaf or visually impaired; the terror of automated telephone answering systems
- a variety of "teaching" and "hear it from the expert" type activities—training volunteers and students to be better conversation partners drawing on the work of Kagan and Gailey (1993) and Lyon et al. (1997), talking to centre visitors about the nature of stroke and aphasia and the need for long-term therapy and support, supporting the development of publicity and information materials.

Avoiding work on impairments

Although some group sessions had a more obvious focus on discussing language impairment and communication strategies, it seemed important with Tony to try, as far as possible, to avoid explicit impairment-level therapy. This was *not* because I had the feeling that Tony could no longer make specific gains with language remediation programmes. It was because, in my opinion, impairment-focused work seemed to bring the huge risk of undermining the fragile but steady gains in confidence made through disability-level therapies.

This therapy "tactic" of avoiding work on impairments was perhaps most obviously addressed in the regular goal-setting sessions. These were not easy and I quickly learned that they were not always safe in the hands of inexperienced student clinicians, desperate to help and desperate to find something nice and tangible to work on and to track improvements. Over time they became easier as Tony saw the impact of improved confidence on conversation. Hope for the future gradually became dissociated from the number of prepositions he could write accurately or verbs he could produce. Negotiating therapy goals involved careful listening and questioning and assertive bargaining. My attempts to value Tony's insider experience and expertise in aphasia and to use my experience and expertise in a supportive but not overtly controlling way was difficult and variable in its execution.

In sum, Tony's individual goal plan during this time more explicitly reflected "living with" as opposed to "fixing" his disability. Inevitably this moved away from traditional roles involving the language therapist as sole expert and the traditional assumptions that a "response" was right or wrong. Although Tony was naturally happier looking to the therapist for answers, the aim of the therapetic partnerships Tony engaged in at this time was to promote therapeutic collaborations based on shared thinking, problem solving and mutual growth.

Phase 2—reflections on change

Therapists' reflections

Increased confidence in communication skills
Review of the clinical notes, discussions with student clinicians and my own personal reflections at last concur on a qualitative change in Tony's confidence and sense of self-worth. Tony appeared less anxious about his interactions. He showed evidence that he could select and use strategies to facilitate his communication. For example, he used a text pager to make golfing appointments without the fear of getting dates and times wrong. There was also a noticeable increase in Tony's contribution to groupwork, particularly (and most surprisingly) within discussions of the emotional impact of stroke and aphasia. His increased confidence and assertiveness in expressing his strengths and needs was also well documented.

Role and identity
Within group sessions, informal interactions at CDG and in lunchtime pub outings, Tony showed a new-found ease and social confidence. He seemed to enjoy helping others both at CDG and beyond, and placed a particular value on the new friendships he had developed, in contrast to feeling the need to disassociate himself from other "handicapped" people. Leisure activities were playing a much bigger role in his life and he had new hopes and aspirations relating to these, for example improving his golf swing and developing his computing skills. Finally, there was, in my opinion, an important shift to identifying aphasia as a disability, not a "stigma". Tony seemed more

able to acknowledge his difference and that much of his struggle to live with aphasia came from an ignorant and non-enabling society rather than from personal weakness.

Exploring options for living with aphasia
A further measure of Tony's resourcefulness, and his acceptance of strategies as enabling rather than "cheating", are the range of aids he had begun to use or to research. These included:

- an electronic thesaurus
- a fax machine to convey more complex or numerical information
- a British Telecom text pager
- a person to help with form-filling and advocacy.

His priorities in therapy now had a disability-based rather than impairment-based focus and the comments of student therapists confirmed the changes in progress and direction.

> Tony has progressed very well—he can now state his employment needs and also his personal strengths and skills ... the project work has been particularly beneficial for Tony as he has had the opportunity to confront disability issues in parallel with working as a valued member of a team, offering ideas and opinions, which has enabled him to develop more confidence.

> Tony is beginning to discuss and perhaps "accept" his feelings regarding his dysphasia and to realise that there is a partnership between the other clients and the student and that he has an important role within that.

Tony's perspective on change

Identity and relationships
The following discussion with Tony reflects his perceived changes in his identity and relationships.

Tony: I'm diff- ... I'm in a way I'm ... better really ... I'm sort of um I'm a bit of ...

bit of a noisy person (laughs) . . . I can talk to other people more . . . let's say a new friends came down there and before I wouldn't talk to him but now I say "oh hello there" and I'll . . . I'll actually talk to their name.

C.P.: So its changed the way you are with other people. You perhaps spend more time with new people?

Tony: Oh yeah. I re- . . . I wish I did have my friends again but er . . . it's like you got that sort of . . . stigma with that stroke . . . d'you know what I mean? They know me from my stroke . . . um that's gone see he knows I've had a stroke and that's his problem?

C.P.: It's like sort of a new identity almost?

Tony: Yeah

C.P.: It sounds like you quite like it as well in some ways?

Tony: No I have to really (laughs) . . . it's nice . . . probably better

The notion of moving from an observer of life and social outsider to a more confident and active participant is summarised in Tony's reflection, "Before I was a trainspotter . . . now I'm like a traindriver".

Feelings

The slow emergence of, and reflection on feelings is another recurring theme, as is the possibility that this type of introspection was only feasible after a certain amount of language-based therapy. Tony's comments appear to have implications for the timing of intervention and the issue of discharge:

Tony: I think like I'm very slow . . . I need practice for other feelings . . . it's weird like er . . . my brain won't um . . . my feelings sort of thing it's gone . . . now I'm sort of . . . I got more feelings now . . .

C.P.: So your feelings were sort of shut off just like your speech got cut off?

Tony: Yes before it was like just a boring person, now it's I'm sort of got more feelings now, yeah. . . .

C.P.: So you think there's a link between the brain and these feelings?

Tony: um . . . it's like . . . from when I had the stroke it's been to me . . . it's like there's no petrol from it, it's gone . . . like I need some more petrol for me brain to keep it going, you know what I mean, it's going up.

Role of therapy

Tony's thoughts on the importance of long-term therapy are very clear: "Wow it's priceless really innit?" "I've still got more but um . . . the last bit there it makes me even better . . . I can do more things now, know what I mean?"

As are his thoughts on short-term contracts: "Cor blimey it'd be really hard . . . I don't think it would work".

In contrast to his comments of the past, there is a clear acknowledgement of the role of his aphasic peers in contributing to the process of therapy: "It's good with other people who've had er strokes . . . They help us to talk mmm".

Language changes

Whilst Tony had minimal work on his language impairments in this final phase, he has no doubt that this period brought about improvements in *"hearing what's going on and talking"*. This emerged both in the interview and in the visual analogue scale identifying perceived change in language (Appendix 9.3).

General reflections on how to capture change

There is widespread agreement amongst clinicians that our tools for measuring change in the areas discussed are both underdeveloped and unsophisticated (see, for example, Pound et al., 2000; Thelander et al., 1994). The evaluations specified below may appear somewhat insufficient in their attempt to capture the complexity of human experience and psychological change. They are inevitably largely subjective and possibly of dubious influence in the cut and thrust of evidence-based medicine. However, they are a first attempt at trying to capture something meaningful within an eclectic framework (Van der Gaag, 1993) and may give clinicians ideas for developing a portfolio of tools and scales suited to their own and their clients' needs.

Means of evaluating change

- Confidence ratings—the use of repeated scaling on personally relevant areas of communicative confidence (see Appendix 9.1).
- Individual group evaluations—probing pre- and post-course understanding of (for example) the meaning of assertiveness and clients' ability to identify specific assertiveness techniques.
- Goal planning and monitoring of achievement—timely goal setting and monitoring of the achievement of individual goals.
- The "tree of life" diagram—a concrete and visual tool for identifying and discussing changes in emotional state, as well as the factors and feelings underpinning these changes. In the given example (see Appendix 9.2), Tony selected figures 1 as indicative of his state at the end of Phase 1, and the two figures marked 2a, "*at the bottom and looking to other people for help, what's going on?*", as indicative of his anxieties and expectations after his first 18 months at CDG. When asked which characters best represented his position after the confidence- and identity-building therapies of Phase 2, he replied after a long pause "*Well I'm all of them now*", singling out particularly those marked (2).
- Visual analogue scales—the use of timelines to identify and quantify changes in an individual's perception of both communicative and psychological/emotional status (see Appendix 9.3).
- In-depth interviews—the measures which have given perhaps the most telling insights of change are the *in-depth qualitative interviews* used to support the views presented in this case study. Whilst these are time-consuming in terms of the interview itself, and subsequent transcription and analysis, the value of in-depth interviewing in presenting the "insider" rather than the therapist perspective cannot be underestimated. Tapping the potential of this technique to inform more flexible and sophisticated evaluations, and in measuring change, presents an exciting challenge.

QUESTIONS AND CHALLENGES

In conclusion, my journey through therapy with Tony has raised a number of questions. These are by no means unique to Tony and me. They are ones that challenge many therapists grappling with issues related to aphasia and long-term disability.

1. Should we expect the roles and skills of the Speech and Language Therapist to cover issues involved in living with a disability? Issues surrounding language and life may seem inextricably linked, but how many of us feel equipped to respond to life issues in the way that we respond to requests to work on language processing and communication skills? Should we leave life and social goals to other colleagues within the rehabilitation team or should we listen harder to the links that clients make and develop our skills accordingly?

2. How can we effectively offer and integrate impairment and disability work within a package of therapy? For example, how can we spell out the benefits of group therapy addressing identity and confidence with the same clarity as one-to-one therapy that focuses, for example, upon speech and writing? What does it mean, within client-led therapy, to refuse to continue work on language when there is still room for change but no hope for the yearned-for restoration to a pre-aphasic self? Is our concept of therapy, its benefits and limitations, sufficiently developed to allow us to articulate this clearly when setting out the "menu" of therapy options (Elman, 1998)?

3. Should we assume that disability-level work has its most appropriate timing after impairment-based therapy? In Tony's case, disability-level work took on a prominent role in his last phase of therapy, after

impairment-based therapy had brought about change and some acknowledgement that it could not provide the solution to aphasia. His post-therapy interview suggested that he had wanted and needed to feel more in control of his language before considering work on his life. But to what degree does a traditional approach to therapy prime expectations and values that suggest that therapy for a language impairment is somehow preferable early on, whilst disability-level therapy is merely a consideration prior to discharge?

4. How, within a programme of long-term therapy such as Tony's, can therapist and client avoid falling into the dependency trap? Whilst many therapists working within resource-starved services may view this as a luxury that short-term contracts do not allow them to experience, responsive, long-term therapy will always raise issues of blurred boundaries and difficult endings. Are there more tangible ways in which the therapeutic process can move towards the moment of leaving therapy, a time when the limitations of intervention and the challenge of facing the future with imperfection will be inescapable?

5. If group-based disability therapies facilitate the process of living more comfortably with aphasia, how can we track the changes they promote in an authentic, meaningful way? The ways of measuring change in response to some of the group programmes described are clearly open to criticism. Undeniably, they lack the focus of routinely used impairment-based measures. Whilst we need to research and develop valid, reliable tools to measure confidence, identity and well-being, should the current unavailability of such tools prevent us from doing disability-level therapies? Perhaps asking and listening to clients in an in-depth and ongoing way offers a starting point for documenting the aphasic person's experience of change.

6. How can we combat the advent of short-term contracts and the dysphagia-induced squeeze on adult services that prevent clinicians from providing longer-term treatment?

ACKNOWLEDGMENTS

With special thanks to Tony for teaching me many challenging, stimulating lessons about the complexities of life, aphasia and therapy. Thanks also to all of the group members, students and clinicians at the City Dysphasic Group whose ideas, discussions and clinical notes have formed the basis of this paper, and to Susie Parr, Chris Ireland and Sally Byng for their helpful comments and insights during the preparation of this paper.

POSTSCRIPT

Shortly after the final phase of therapy, Tony left the group to start part-time work. This evolved into a full-time job with the same employer, where Tony worked for a number of years until his death in 2002.

REFERENCES

Bishop, D. (1983) *Test for reception of grammar*. London, UK: Psychological Corporation.

De Partz, M.-P. (1986). Re-education of a deep dyslexic patient: Rationale of the method and results. *Cognitive Neuropsychology*, *3*, 149–177.

Elman, R.J. (1998). Diversity in aphasiology: Let us embrace it. *Aphasiology*, *12*, 456–457.

Finkelstein, V., & French, S. (1993) Towards a psychology of disability. In J. Swain, V. Finkelstein, S. French, & M. Oliver (Eds.), *Disabling barriers—enabling environments*. London: Sage.

Harding, D., & Pound, C. (2000). Needs, function, and measurement: Juggling with multiple language impairment. In S. Byng, K. Swinburn, & C. Pound (Eds.), *The aphasia therapy file*. Hove, UK: Psychology Press.

Holland, S. & Ward, C. (1990). *Assertiveness: A practical approach.* Oxford, UK: Winslow Press.

Jones, E. (1989). A year in the life of EVJ and PC. In *Proceedings of the British Aphasiology Therapy Symposium,* Madingley, Cambridge.

Kagan, A., & Gailey, G. (1993). Functional is not enough: Training conversation partners for aphasic adults. In A. Holland & M. Forbes (Eds.), *Aphasia treatment: World perspectives.* San Diego, CA: Singular Press.

Kay, J., Lesser, R., & Coltheart, M. (1992). *Psycholinguistic assessment of language processing in aphasia.* London: Lawrence Erlbaum Associates Ltd.

Lyon, J.G., Cariski, D., Keisler, L., Rosenbek, J., Levine, R., Kumpula, J., Ryff, C., Coyne, S., & Levine, J. (1997). Communication partners: Enhancing participation in life and communication for adults with aphasia in natural settings. *Aphasiology, 11,* 693–708.

Nickels, L. (1992). The autocue? Self-generated phonemic cues in the treatment of a disorder of reading and naming. *Cognitive Neuropsychology, 9,* 155–182.

Nickels, L. (1995). Reading too little into reading? Strategies in the rehabilitation of acquired dyslexia. *European Journal of Disorders of Communication, 30,* 37–50.

Pound, C., Parr, S., Lindsay, J., & Woolf, C. (2000). *Beyond aphasia—therapies for living with communication disability.* Bicester, UK: Speechmark.

Ryff, C.D. (1995). Psychological well-being in adult life. *Current Directions in Psychological Science, 4,* 99–104.

Thelander, M.J., Hoen, B., & Worsley, J. (1994). *York–Durham Aphasia Center: Report on the evaluation of effectiveness of a community program for adults.* Toronto, Canada: York–Durham Aphasia Center.

Van der Gaag, A. (1993). *Audit: A manual for speech and language therapists.* London: Royal College of Speech and Language Therapists.

APPENDICES

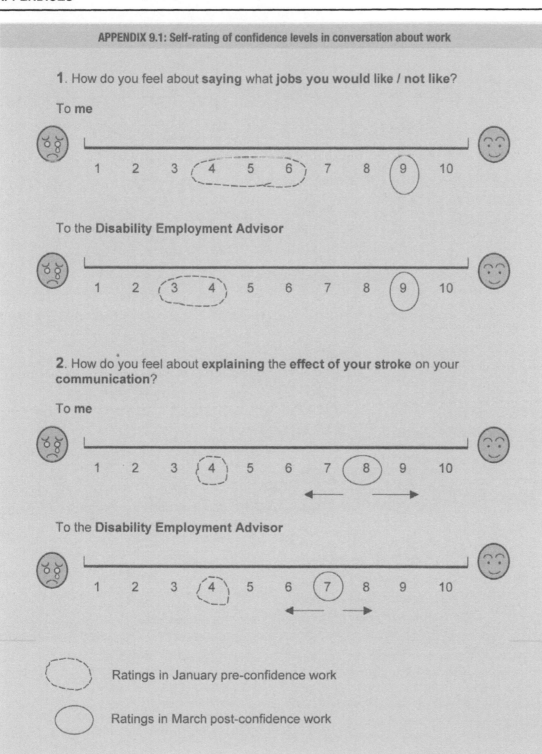

APPENDIX 9.1: Self-rating of confidence levels in conversation about work

1. How do you feel about **saying** what **jobs you would like / not like**?

To **me**

1   2   3   4   5   6   7   8   9   10

To the **Disability Employment Advisor**

1   2   3   4   5   6   7   8   9   10

2. How do you feel about **explaining** the **effect of your stroke** on your **communication**?

To **me**

1   2   3   4   5   6   7   8   9   10

To the **Disability Employment Advisor**

1   2   3   4   5   6   7   8   9   10

Ratings in January pre-confidence work

Ratings in March post-confidence work

APPENDIX 9.2: Changes in Tony's perception of self over time

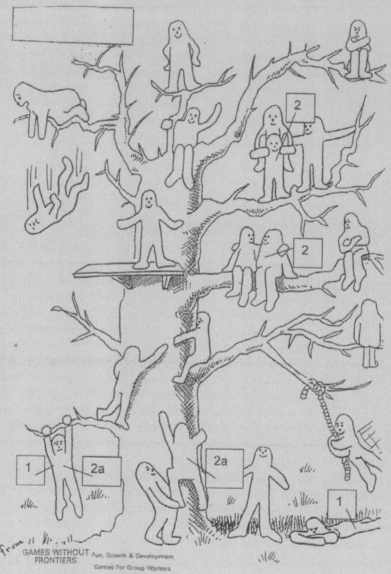

GAMES WITHOUT FRONTIERS Fun, Growth & Development
Games For Group Workers

1 – at end of Phase 1 of therapy

2a – at end of Phase 2a of therapy

2 – at end of Phase 2 of therapy . . . "Well . . . I'm all of them now"

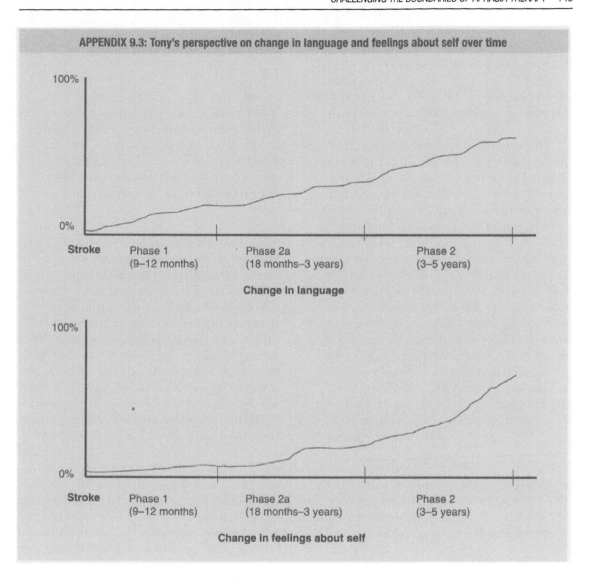

APPENDIX 9.3: Tony's perspective on change in language and feelings about self over time

Change in language

Change in feelings about self

10

Replicating therapy—more than just more of the same?

Jo Robson and Simon Horton

INTRODUCTION

What do we mean by "replicating therapy"? What do we expect to have to do to be able to replicate therapy, and what issues emerge from attempts to do so? Replicating "successful" therapy is seen as vital in two major respects—both as a means of establishing that the therapy is a genuinely effective form of treatment for a particular disorder, and to give the opportunity to address theoretical issues and areas of uncertainty arising from the original study (Nickels, Byng, & Black, 1989). Replication may take the form of trying the therapy with a different client or clients (in the case of single case studies), or trying the therapy with a group of clients.

Single case methodology—where a particular clinician poses detailed questions about the use of a particular therapy with a particular client—has been advocated as a useful means of exploring the effects of aphasia therapy (Howard, 1986; Pring, 1986). However, it does pose the practising clinician a number of problems. His or her interest in the study is often primarily motivated by the practical question: "Will this help my client too?" rather than interest in the exploration of theoretical issues, fascinating though they may be. As such, clinicians want to know whether the study informs the choice of therapy offered to a wider population.

Single case studies have a number of difficulties in addressing this issue.

- Clinicians may want to identify suitable candidates for therapies described in case studies relatively easily, using quick and readily available assessment tools. This is difficult when authors provide a detailed description of the idiosyncrasies using extensive (and often novel) language testing procedures.

- Given the diversity present in the population of people with aphasia it is unlikely that the clinician will be in contact with a client who matches exactly the profile of the original speaker. Yet single case studies rarely suggest which features of a client's presentation were critical for the therapy to be appropriate.
- Single case studies rarely identify the key skills or combinations of skills that enable the client to respond to the treatment offered. While it may be clear which deficit was targeted by the treatment, the nature of the skills exploited in therapy (and therefore fundamental to its success) are often less carefully specified.
- The description of the therapy may be restricted to an outline of the tasks undertaken, possibly extending to some description of the cues and feedback offered, failing to offer detail of how the tasks were carried out.

It has been suggested that the process of doing therapy may need to be more precisely specified (Horton & Byng, 2000a). For example, single case studies may need to describe more carefully how therapy tasks exploited residual skills, the precise processing mechanisms by which the language deficit was targeted, and the way in which this was reflected in the interaction between therapist and client.

What sort of details are needed for clinicians to be able to apply therapy approaches that have been developed in single case studies to the wider population of people with aphasia? What issues are important for discussion and what vocabulary is needed to describe them?

In this chapter we will explore some of the issues surrounding the replication of therapy in relation to a particular therapy programme—writing therapy. We will first discuss a single case study using writing therapy with a person with jargon aphasia (Part one). Then we talk about replicating a single case study across a small group of clients (Part two), and how a comparison between the work done by the two authors with the same client can shed light on the nature of therapy treatment and its application in practice (Part three). These three sections will be used to illustrate issues entailed in "doing therapy", and how the enactment of therapy may be described and analysed in terms of its various constituents for purposes of cross-clinician and cross-client replication.

PART ONE: A SINGLE CASE STUDY OF WRITING THERAPY

A programme of writing therapy was carried out with RMM (Robson, Pring, Marshall, Morrison, & Chiat, 1998), a speaker of undifferentiated jargon. Her speech was almost entirely lacking in recognisable words and, at the outset of therapy, meaningful writing was not attainable. Investigation of RMM's writing skills across a number of tasks demonstrated that, while unable to produce meaningful output spontaneously, she did retain some residual knowledge of the orthographic forms she was attempting to access. A period of picture naming therapy was successful in establishing a small vocabulary of single written words. Despite these having been selected for their functional relevance, RMM failed to make use of them in communicative settings. We undertook a further period of specific therapy, termed "message therapy". Message therapy aimed to show RMM how her new-found writing abilities could be used to convey a range of communicative messages. Following therapy RMM showed significant gains on a message assessment and also demonstrated functional use of her writing in everyday situations.

The single case study undertaken with RMM was interesting for a number of reasons. It demonstrated that relatively subtle language skills at the outset of therapy were a positive indicator for treatment. The study explored issues concerning the transfer of communicative skills to functional use and argued that this process may need to be facilitated by specifically designed therapy. Finally, the study reported the successful outcome of therapy with a client with severe jargon aphasia, a population often thought to be poor candidates for impairment-based therapy.

PART TWO: A GROUP STUDY USING RESIDUAL ORTHOGRAPHIC SKILLS IN A GROUP OF JARGON SPEAKERS

Although encouraging, the study represented a successful outcome with only a single client. The question of whether the efficacy of this therapy with this particular client could be shown to be effective in more general terms was then addressed in a group study (Robson, Marshall, Chiat, & Pring, 2001). This second study had three aims:

- to investigate whether residual orthographic skills were present in a group of jargon speakers
- to investigate whether these skills could be successfully exploited in written naming therapy
- to explore how skills acquired in therapy were used communicatively and whether message therapy could successfully facilitate the transfer of skills for functional use.

Ten subjects with jargon aphasia were recruited to the project. Selection criteria stated that clients should present with a minimum 6-month history of jargon aphasia and be medically stable at the time of referral. Clients should present with speech that was made unintelligible by the presence of non-words. Comprehension skills should be sufficient for the client to participate in formal assessment and therapy.

In the initial phase of the study, clients completed three assessments designed to investigate their written language skills. To facilitate comparison across conditions, the three tasks used the same vocabulary of 32 picturable nouns.

- Written picture naming assessment: Clients were presented with a line drawing and asked to write the correct name for the picture.
- Anagram sorting: Clients were given a picture stimulus together with the relevant letter tiles for the target word. Clients were asked to sort the letters into the correct order.
- Delayed copying: Clients were presented with a written stimulus. Stimuli comprised

either a real word or a non-word, created by rearranging the letters of the real word. Clients were shown the target and allowed to look at it until they indicated they were ready to start. The stimulus was then removed and clients were asked to write the word (or non-word) from memory.

The rationale behind the use of the three tasks was as follows. Written picture naming should give an indication of the clients' ability to retrieve and produce written word forms. Anagram sorting investigates the presence of covert skills. This task requires access to stored orthographic representations without written production. A pattern of poor picture naming with superior anagram sorting skills indicates that the client can access orthographic information despite being unable to support written naming. The delayed copying task also provides an opportunity to explore covert word knowledge. Presumably the task can be completed relying solely on visual memory skills. This predicts an equal pattern of performance across word and non-word stimuli. Clients who are additionally able to access orthographic information when completing the task should show an advantage for real word copying.

The findings from the background assessments are given in Table 10.1. All ten clients had impaired writing skills. No client obtained even a 50% success rate on the written naming task. The group's poor performance with written picture naming supports the suggestion that preserved written skills in jargon aphasia may be relatively subtle. Encouragingly, both the anagram and delayed copying assessments suggest that covert word knowledge is nonetheless present. Superior performance in these conditions indicated that clients were able to exploit residual orthographic knowledge when completing the tasks.

The results of the assessments show that the original single case study finding of residual writing skills in jargon aphasia has been replicated in a larger number of speakers. For this population of aphasic people, often thought to be poor candidates for impairment-based therapy, there is a suggestion that despite severely disrupted written output, covert orthographic knowledge that has

TABLE 10.1

Percentage success in each of three 34-item therapy tasks for each of 10 participants

	Written naming	Anagram sorting	Delayed copying for real words	Delayed copying for non-words
JH	4	19	30	18
GR	8	10	24	14
AK	0	11	2	1
BB	0	17	5	2
CM	0	13	0	0
SW	3	14	9	0
AM	14	30	31	23
DH	8	17	17	1
LT	0	8	10	5
DY	0	9	0	1

potential to be exploited in therapy may be present.

The criteria for recruitment to the study produced a group of jargon speakers who were far from homogeneous. For example, clients completed the spoken word-to-picture matching task from the Psycholinguistic Assessment of Language Processing in Aphasia (PALPA; Kay, Lesser, & Coltheart, 1992), and across the group performance ranged from 13/40 to 36/40. Similarly, the nature of the clients' spoken jargon showed considerable diversity.

The clients therefore showed considerable variability in their surface presentations. Despite this, covert writing skills were evident across the group. The replication of this original finding therefore appeared not to depend on specifying exactly the clients' surface symptoms (essentially their disabilities), but rather on looking for the right underlying abilities.

Six clients—all presenting with severely restricted spoken language—were selected based on an optimistic prognosis for writing therapy. Despite relatively poor written naming, all had showed some ability to access covert word knowledge during the background assessments. In view of their severely restricted spoken language, it

was thought that the acquisition of a small written vocabulary would potentially facilitate everyday communication.

The clients who were offered picture naming therapy showed evidence of covert writing skills on at least one of the background assessments. They also needed to be able to benefit from the acquisition of functional writing skills.

The suitability of clients to participate in this period of therapy was thus determined by the pattern of skills with which they presented and by their potential to benefit from the anticipated outcome of therapy. This contrasts with the more typical approach of selecting clients on the basis of their impairments and deficits. The criteria used in this study were perhaps more positive, focusing on baseline skills and the potential to benefit from therapy.

Three of the six clients were offered a subsequent period of message therapy. Clients were offered message therapy if they had maintained the significant gains made during the original period of therapy but failed to show communicative use of writing. Clients were also required to have a carer who was available to support therapy, and with whom writing might be used communicatively.

The nature of therapy: Therapy stimuli

Each client selected a personal vocabulary of 40 items. These were chosen in collaboration with the client's main communication partner. Words were selected for their potential value in daily conversation and were chosen from topics that frequently gave rise to communication breakdown. Twenty words were to be practised in therapy; the remaining items acted as controls.

The criteria stated that selected items should be of personal interest to the client and should reflect their communicative needs. Criteria imposed by the project were simply that words should be nouns (either proper or common nouns) that could be targeted by a picture stimulus. This resulted in the development of diverse vocabularies for the six clients participating in therapy. Vocabulary topics included family members and friends, towns, shops, places commonly visited, garden plants, food, drink and words associated with favourite hobbies. Stimuli included line drawings, photographs and maps.

The variability in the therapy stimuli was made possible by the use of criteria that defined the vocabulary largely in functional terms. This allowed the development of highly personalised materials despite the context of a group study, and may well have contributed to the enthusiasm demonstrated by the clients during therapy.

The range of stimuli used in the message assessment also reflected the diversity of the therapy vocabularies. Messages ranged from: "We are going to spend a day in the capital", to: "Our best player has a knee injury". Therapy items from the earlier (picture naming) therapy were once again practised during message therapy. Control items continued to be unpractised.

Two writing assessments were carried out to ascertain a baseline of performance for picture naming and sensitivity to using written words for conveying messages. In the first assessment the participants were asked to write the name of pictures. In the second assessment they were shown a written message targeting one item from their particular therapy vocabulary. Messages were devised to represent the sort of messages the clients themselves might wish to communicate. For instance, one of the items in DY's vocabulary was "Norwich". The message targeting this item was: "I want to go into the city". The client was shown the written message and this was also read aloud. The client was then asked to write one word that could help convey this message to a listener.

Following the initial assessment, the six clients received 12 sessions of picture naming therapy. Three of the six clients then received six additional sessions of message therapy. Where possible, communicative partners were encouraged to be actively involved in the message therapy.

In contrast to many studies of aphasia therapy treatment, the therapy here was defined in terms of "processing goals"—in other words, in terms of the nature of the processing that we hoped to promote in the client's language system. The two processing goals were:

- to enable the client to access stored (and possibly latent) semantic and orthographic information about the target item, and therefore reinforce representation of target related information
- to prime or support the production of the lexical form.

These processing goals led to a basic "decide and produce" format for therapy tasks whereby a decision was followed by production of the target form.

Having devised therapy tasks in terms of their potential to realise these processing goals, it became possible to use a range of different tasks, rather than attempting to reproduce exactly the same tasks across the group of participants. Tasks were tailored to the particular needs and abilities of individual clients and applied flexibly within sessions, while at the same time maintaining the same processing goals.

The "decide and produce" format supported a wide range of surface activities in the picture naming therapy. For instance, decisions might be based on either the semantic or orthographic properties of the target pictures. Semantic decisions included written word-to-picture matching (with semantic distracters), associated word-to-picture matching (again with semantic distracters), categorisation judgements, odd-one-out judgements and generating semantic information about the target. In contrast, orthographic decisions concerned the properties of the written word form. Here tasks could involve matching pictures to their first letters, identifying initial letters from an alphabet chart and categorising words according to their length.

Production tasks were similarly varied. These required that the client should produce part, or all, of the target word form. Tasks therefore included writing the first letter of the word, inserting missing letters into the target word form, completing anagrams, delayed copying, cued written naming and uncued written picture naming.

The message therapy also had a "decide and produce" format. In the "decide" component, clients were asked to match one of the treated words to a stimulus word, phrase or message. Stimuli were either presented singly or with more than one stimulus for each treated word. Single word stimuli included synonyms and associated words. Phrases and messages were limited to short sentences. Thus stimuli for the therapy item "Norwich" might include: "Norfolk" (word level), "city centre" (phrase level) and "I went into the city at the weekend" (message level). Clients identified the correct word for a message by selecting it from a choice of written words, by selecting a picture or by writing the target word from memory. On all occasions where a choice was offered, the distracters comprised semantically related items from the pool of therapy words.

The second component of each activity required written production of the target word. This could involve delayed copying, written picture naming and writing the word from memory.

The message therapy tasks had two purposes. First, they aimed to make explicit the ways in which a single word can be used to convey a range of messages. Second, the repeated practice of the therapy words served to facilitate their written production.

Results of the group study

Both the written naming and message assessments were repeated immediately after picture naming therapy and at follow-up 1 month later. At the end of the message therapy the picture naming and message assessments were also repeated.

Progress was measured in two ways: first, in terms of the number of completely correct responses, and second, in terms of the number of target letters correctly produced by the client. This additional measure was adopted to reflect the large number of partially correct responses produced in the post-therapy and follow-up assessments. Although technically incorrect, these responses were often sufficiently accurate to identify the intended target. Written approximations were therefore analysed for the number of letters from the target word realised in the response. No credit was given for additional occurrences of a letter where this was not required by the target word. Letter position information was ignored.

Counting partially correct responses offered a more sensitive measure of the very real gains

made in therapy. The ability to produce even partial information about a target word is a genuinely useful communication skill. Partial responses that successfully identify the writer's intended target are as communicatively valuable as responses that are completely correct. Therefore the use of such responses to measure progress reflected the intention to explore the communicative use of writing in jargon aphasia.

Picture naming outcomes

All six clients showed significant gains on this assessment immediately after picture naming therapy. These gains were maintained 1 month later for four of the six clients. No client showed evidence of generalisation to items not treated in therapy. For the three clients who were given message therapy, two of the three clients continued to make improvements in their recall of written picture names. For both of these clients the gains were evident in the number of therapy items written completely correctly. A third client continued to make progress in the accuracy of her partially correct responses, although this increase failed to reach significance. As before, no client showed evidence of generalisation to the control items.

Message assessment

Only one client showed an improved ability to complete the message assessment (after picture naming therapy), and these gains were maintained at follow-up. Unfortunately, this was not matched by evidence of communicative writing outside assessment tasks. One other client who failed to show progress on the message assessment did, nevertheless, show communicative use of writing in functional settings.

After message therapy all three clients showed significantly improved performance on the message assessment. For one client this was evident in terms of the number of correct responses. For the remaining two clients the gains were seen in the accuracy of their partial attempts at the target words. The change was highly significant for each client and confirmed the observation that these responses were most useful for the communicative partner.

Despite the severely restricted writing skills

exhibited at baseline, all clients made significant progress during therapy. These abilities were maintained at follow-up for most clients. All clients found the message assessment harder to complete and significant gains were present for only one client. Despite the progress seen during picture naming therapy, only one client was observed to make communicative use of their writing during conversation.

The group thus largely replicated the outcome seen in the single case study. Like RMM, most of the group clients made significant gains in written naming, but were unable to complete the message assessment and showed no functional use of writing.

The outcome of the message therapy replicated the results obtained in the initial single case study. In other words, message therapy resulted in improved performance on the message assessment. In the original study, the gains seen at the end of message therapy were accompanied by the emergence of communicative writing in functional contexts. Was this result also replicated in the group?

At the end of message therapy, sessions were adapted to include time for general conversation between therapist and client. This offered the three clients the opportunity to make use of their writing in a communicative context. Conversations were not contrived to target the practised vocabulary, and covered topics such as activities undertaken during the week, contemporary sporting competitions, holidays and the family.

All three clients demonstrated the ability to make spontaneous use of their writing during these conversations. On some occasions this involved the production of treated words—for example, one wrote a friend's name to indicate that this person was particularly easy to communicate with. On other occasions clients attempted to write words that had not been practised in therapy. For example, one wrote "SUN" when discussing newspapers. These examples suggest that clients are now able to attempt written words that have not been targeted in treatment. Other examples suggested that clients were now using their writing in ways that were more creative than had been practised during message

therapy. On some occasions this involved combining single words into more connected output. For example, one wrote fragments of the days of the week and then used these to indicate when she had carried out a particular activity. On another occasion she wrote "EVA" (a practised word) together with "AUS" (August, unpractised) to communicate that she was going to visit this person in August. Other examples indicated that clients could produce creative combinations of writing and drawing. For example, one drew a picture of a box and wrote "K" to indicate what her husband liked to eat for breakfast.

These examples of communicative writing occurred during therapy sessions. Reports from carers indicated that clients were also employing their writing with other conversational partners. Encouragingly, a comment made by one client's husband more than 3 months after the completion of the therapy programme indicated that these skills were well maintained: "She writes things down to help out understanding, it could be parts of words".

Observations from the therapists and comments from the communication partners therefore indicate that clients are now making spontaneous and functional use of their writing. Indeed, the resourcefulness of clients in using their writing creatively often exceeded the expectations of the therapists. The finding replicates the outcome of the original study, which found that communicative writing was associated with the successful completion of a period of message therapy.

PART THREE: TWO THERAPISTS WITH THE SAME CLIENT—IS IT THE SAME THERAPY?

As described above, replication of therapy treatment from the single case to the group study, and across the different clients within the group study, was seen in terms of processing goals, thus allowing flexibility in the application of tasks.

A third perspective on replication can be seen for one participant in the group study, DY, whose therapy was shared by the two authors. This gives a contrasting perspective to the concept of replication, in that with DY, both authors were attempting to enact therapy in exactly the same way. This raises interesting questions about whether this is actually possible, and about how to isolate, describe and analyse the relevant constituents of therapy.

Horton and Byng (2000b) developed a framework for structuring therapy data in terms of the discourse, rather than in terms of tasks and materials. This structure was developed in order to allow comparable events to be isolated within and between therapy sessions. This structure focuses on the "technical" aspects of doing therapy and is not concerned with the affective relationship between therapist and client. Technical therefore means those features of the therapist–client relationship that specifically address the language work together. This discourse framework is not dissimilar to ones developed by other investigators looking at child language and other related therapies (e.g., Panagos, 1996).

The structures in the data—called "enactment processes"—are defined as sets of interactions that can be isolated in terms of their: (a) topical uniformity, (b) interactional structure, (c) use of particular vocabulary and materials, and (d) that may be identified by their sequential position in the interaction.

An analysis of the therapy interactions between each of the authors (SH and JR) and DY, their client, suggests that the main difference between them involved the following three enactment processes:

- *elicitation*, which is to do with setting the task in motion, the configuration of materials and the language and cognitive processing demanded of the client
- *response management*, which is to do with therapist and client actions contingent on the client's response
- *summary*, which is to do with how therapist and/or client summarise both the client's "performance" and the purpose of the therapy.

By detailing a number of "factors" within each enactment process, it becomes clear that the two

therapists who were ostensibly carrying out the same tasks with the same client showed considerable variability in the way in which they implemented therapy activities. For example, comparing the two elicitation enactment processes below, in transcriptions 1 and 2 (where SH and JR are both "doing the same task"):[1]

Transcript 1: Session 1, between SH and DY

SH: mhm ((writes choice of words underneath picture)) I'm doing you three to choose from now

DY: right

SH: ((shows picture with choice of three words beneath))

Transcript 2: Session 2, between JR and DY

JR: okay I'm going to give you a choice of words to read. One will be right and one will be wrong see if you can spit spot which one's right okay so this one and ((writes words)) okay which one of those two is right for that one

Elicitations clearly differ considerably between the two therapists. This could be attributed to "therapeutic style" in these instances, but the use of different numbers of distracters (three by SH and two by JR) suggest that the two therapies are actually making different cognitive and language processing demands of the client.

Similarly, comparison between *response management* in transcripts 3 and 4 suggests that the client may be bringing different things to, and taking different things from, the two sessions:[2]

Transcript 3: Session 1, between SH and DY

DY: ((writes first letter))

SH: mhm

DY: ((crosses out anagram letter))

SH: spot on

DY: ((writes second letter and crosses out anagram letter))

SH: mhm no prizes for the last letter

DY: ((writes third letter and crosses out anagram letter))

Transcript 4: Session 2, between JR and DY

DY: ((writes letters in frame))
JR: are you happy
DY: yeah I think so
JR: yeah I think that looks right let's have a look ((uncovers target))
DY: ((looks at target)) yeah
JR: brilliant

SH evaluated each letter of DY's contribution, whereas JR not only waited until DY had finished writing the word ("bus") but also offered a self-evaluation route, which allowed additional language and cognitive processing opportunities. It is again clear that the task as implemented by SH places different demands on DY from that implemented by JR.

Finally, comparisons between *summary* in transcripts 5 and 6 below tend to highlight differences in the personal style of the therapists:[3]

Transcript 5: Session 1, between SH and DY

DY: bus the <u>bus</u>
SH: yeah (.) catch the bus
DY: the bus (.) yes
SH: there's probably buses going up and down here right now
DY: the bus ((laughs))

Transcript 6: Session 2, between JR and DY

DY: bus bus
JR: well done yeah bus good good so you managed to copy it when everything or to write it when everything was covered that's excellent well done (.) it is easier when they're shorter isn't it
DY: yes it is yeah
JR: yeah yeah

SH tried to contextualise the item both linguistically (e.g., "catch the bus") and by referring to the real world outside the therapy room ("there's probably buses going up and down here right now"), while JR alluded to the therapy itself ("you managed to copy it") and invited DY to share in the summary ("it is easier when they're shorter isn't it").

One would have to analyse many instances of summary enactment processes to be able to comment on whether overall "stylistic" tendencies affect the outcomes.

The illustrations above highlight how difficult it is to genuinely replicate the complex processes involved in language therapy. It also suggests that these features of therapy may need to be more carefully described by future therapy studies, and certainly borne in mind by therapists in their enactment of therapy treatments.

CONCLUSIONS

A variety of issues around the notion of replication have been addressed in reporting this study as a whole, and in detailing the work of the authors with one of the participants, DY. These have been issues to do with the following.

1. *The type of client who may benefit from a particular therapy, and how this may be established.* Here clients were chosen for the study not in terms of their deficit-related symptoms, but in relation to their underlying residual abilities. Of course the abilities investigated were closely related to the processing that was to be targeted in therapy.

2. *Which items to target in the therapy.* Here stimuli were targeted in terms of their potential value to the client, rather than in terms of, for example, frequency or word length. One might conjecture that targeting such items might cause difficulties setting up some of the therapy tasks—for example, where the client has to choose between semantically related items. In practice, however, items tended to fall into categories, and manipulating items in a variety of ways in order to provide material for therapy tasks proved relatively simple.

3. *Defining what was done in therapy.* Therapy activities were defined in terms of the language processing they were intended to promote. Therapy tasks were devised in order to put the processing goals into operation. Thus a range of therapy tasks was used

within the two periods of therapy. Different tasks were used with different clients, while the processing goals of the activities remained the same. This illustrates how defining tasks in terms of processing goals makes it possible to exploit a much wider range of activities than when tasks are described at a more mechanical level, for instance in terms of what the client has to do with the materials. Defining therapy in this way not only provides a welcome level of diversity for both the client and the clinician; it also makes it possible to tailor therapy to the particular needs of individual clients while still investigating whether the positive outcome of a particular therapy approach can be replicated across different clients.

4. *Defining how therapy was actually carried out*. The purpose of describing therapy features such as *elicitation, response management* and *summary* (as well as sub-factors entailed within these processes) may be more subtle than simply to ensure that different therapists do exactly the same thing. Rather, it should be possible to ensure that the inevitable variability across therapists does not contradict the underlying processing goals of the therapy. In other words, by defining elicitation techniques it should be possible to ensure that the task really does promote the language processing originally intended, be this access to the lexicon, semantic processing or whatever. Similarly, response management techniques should be devised to ensure that the client again engages in the language processing intended by the therapy. Thus the techniques used to elicit and manage responses and the summaries provided to the client should be consistent with the underlying goal of therapy and should contribute to its achievement.

In summary, the terms used by the project to define clients, therapy stimuli and treatment intervention adopted a slightly different focus from those usually employed by single case studies. Clients were selected on their ability to benefit from therapy, stimuli by their potential value to the client, and therapy activities by the language processing they were intended to promote. These criteria attempt to approach the key issues involved in replicating therapy from a new angle. It is suggested that using such definitions will make it easier for therapists to answer their original question: "Will this help my client too?"

ACKNOWLEDGMENTS

The group study was carried out with the support of grant 17/97 from the Stroke Association.

Work on enactment processes was carried out with support of grant 18/98 from the Stroke Association.

NOTES

1 The "task" was a written word-to-picture [bus] match with distracter words. Here the transcriber's description is in double brackets thus ((writes words)).
2 Here DY is required to write the name of a picture [bus] into a "word frame", using an anagram cue.
3 Both extracts come at the very end of work on this particular item ("bus"). Underlining indicates emphatic stress; (.) indicates a micropause.

REFERENCES

Horton, S., & Byng, S. (2000a). Examining interaction in language therapy. *International Journal of Language and Communication Disorders, 35,* 355–375.

Horton, S., & Byng, S. (2000b). *Defining a therapy intervention for language impairments: Working towards effective learning outcomes.* Paper presented at the 9th International Aphasia Rehabilitation Conference, Rotterdam, August 2000.

Howard, D. (1986). Beyond randomised controlled trials: The case for effective case studies of the effects of treatment in aphasia. *British Journal of Disorders of Communication, 21*, 89–102.

Kay, J., Lesser, R., & Coltheart, M. (1992). *Psycholinguistic assessment of language processing in aphasia*. Hove, UK: Lawrence Erlbaum Associates Ltd.

Nickels, L., Byng, S., & Black, M. (1989). *Replicating treatment for a sentence processing deficit: A comparison of two patients*. Paper presented at the British Aphasiology Society Biennial Conference, Reading, UK.

Panagos, J.M. (1996). Speech therapy discourse, the input to learning. In M.D. Smith & J.D. Damico (Eds.), *Childhood language disorders*. New York: Thieme Medical Publishers.

Pring, T. (1986). Evaluating the effects of speech therapy for aphasics and volunteers: Developing the single case methodology. *British Journal of Disorders of Communication, 21*, 103–115.

Robson, J., Marshall, J., Chiat, S., & Pring, T. (2001). Enhancing communication in jargon aphasia: A small group study of writing therapy. *International Journal of Language and Communication Disorders, 36*, 471–488.

Robson, J., Pring, T., Marshall, J., Morrison, S., & Chiat, S. (1998). Written communication in undifferentiated jargon aphasia: A therapy study. *International Journal of Language and Communication Disorders, 33*, 305–328.

Revealing competence and rethinking identity in severe aphasia using drawing and a communication book

Carol Sacchett and Jayne Lindsay

INTRODUCTION

People with severe aphasia respond poorly to impairment-based therapy designed to improve language function (Marshall, Tompkins, & Phillips, 1982; Sarno, Silverman, & Sands, 1970). Instead, therapies with this group have promoted the use of alternative communication modalities such as gesture (McIntosh & Dakin, 1989), pantomime (Rao, 1986) or a visual symbol system (Funnell & Allport, 1989). In this vein, inter-est has grown in using drawing as an alternative or augmentative communication tool, with some success being reported. Improvements have been documented in both drawing skill (Kearns & Yoder, 1992; Morgan & Helm-Estabrooks, 1987) and communicative drawing (Lyon & Sims, 1989; Trupe, 1986).

Drawing Together is a research project that has investigated the development of communicative drawing in a group of seven people with severe, long-term aphasia (Sacchett, Byng, Marshall, & Pound, 1999). The overall results of the project were very encouraging. In the group as a whole, significant improvements were documented in subjects' ability to draw "generatively" (i.e. from memory), which is one of the prerequisites of communicative drawing.

These results must be viewed with caution. First, it is well-known that group results can be misleading. Second, statistically significant improvements do not necessarily imply a clinically significant change. Doing better on a test, even a so-called "functional" assessment, is no measure of a person's real-life performance.

To counter both of these charges, one individual, FM, has been selected from amongst the project participants for more in-depth study. The main focus of this chapter will be on how using drawing to communicate impacted on his life. Specific therapy techniques will be described that developed and refined FM's new skills and assisted in the transfer of these skills into real-life conversational settings.

A particular focus will be on the development of a communication book, through which FM was enabled to regain an element of control over his life and reassert his identity. Accounts of the use of communication books in the literature typically discuss only the communicative benefits they confer, despite recommendations that they should include information of personal relevance to the users (Fox & Fried-Oken, 1996; Hux, Beukelman, & Garrett, 1994). Our chapter therefore goes beyond this traditional view to encompass consideration of identity or "self" and the potential of therapy to "reveal the competence" of people with aphasia (Kagan & Gailey, 1993).

DRAWING TOGETHER THERAPY PROJECT

This was a 1-year therapy study, funded by The Stroke Association, which had the following aims:

- to develop and evaluate therapy to promote communicative drawing in people with severe chronic aphasia
- to examine generalisation to functional use

of communicative drawing in real-life settings and generalisation to other modalities.

Why drawing?

Drawing has two main advantages over other non-verbal channels of communication. First, it is a visual channel in which information is represented iconically. Therefore it does not require any ability to process symbols, a skill that is often compromised in severe aphasia. Second, drawing provides a fixed, permanent record of an exchange, which can be modified by both parties. Therefore it does not make demands on short-term memory or sequential ability, unlike, say, gesture, which is both transitory and sequential (Lyon, 1995). However, drawing should not be viewed as an isolated skill. On the contrary, the most successful therapy studies referred to earlier have incorporated drawing within the framework of a Total Communication approach (Lyon & Sims, 1989; Trupe, 1986). Drawing is not, therefore, a substitute for language or other forms of communication. Rather, it can be regarded as a useful augmentative tool to assist in the communicative process.

What is communicative drawing?

Communicative drawing refers to the use of drawing to exchange information and ideas. The success of communicative drawing depends on a number of factors. It depends to some extent on the accuracy or quality of the representation but, contrary to popular belief, this is one of the least important factors. In certain circumstances, too much emphasis on accuracy can actually interfere with the communication process (Bauer & Kaiser, 1995). The time taken to produce a "perfect" drawing, which often will include details that are not communicatively relevant, far outweighs the efficiency of the communication attempt. Communicative drawing therefore does depend on the ability to draw "economically", i.e. to include enough detail, *and only enough*, to get the message across. It also depends on the ability to produce drawings from memory, i.e. to generate an idea, call up a visual representation for that idea and translate this into a drawing (Van Sommers, 1989). In this chapter, this skill is referred to as "generative drawing".

Finally, and perhaps most importantly, communicative drawing depends on the ability of communication partners to derive meaning from the produced drawings even if these are not immediately recognisable. This is a skill that needs to be developed, and therapy for communicative drawing will only be successful if the interpretation skills of key interactants are also targeted (Lyon, 1995) and if attempts at interpretation meet with useful and appropriate responses.

A fundamental aspect of communicative drawing therapy, therefore, is the need for the therapist to use drawing him- or herself, both in conveying and interpreting messages. Only by using drawing oneself can one persuade others of its communicative value. It "levels the playing field" and provides an excellent opportunity to model strategies for clarification and interpretation.

Participants in the *Drawing Together* project were selected on the basis of a short screening assessment and an interview with the prospective participant and his/her main carer. Selection criteria are detailed in Appendix 11.1. A number of qualitative and quantitative evaluation measures were then carried out with selected participants prior to the start of therapy. Below is a description of FM and a presentation of his performance on the evaluation measures.

FM's BACKGROUND

Medical details

At the time of his referral to the *Drawing Together* project, FM was 47 years old. He had had a left-hemisphere sub-arachnoid haemorrhage 2 years previously whilst in the USA (September 1994). Investigations revealed two cerebral aneurysms, one on the left carotid artery and the other on the posterior cerebral artery. He underwent craniotomy with successful clipping of the posterior communicating artery aneurysm, but intra-operative bleeding prevented clipping of the second aneurysm. He had a "stormy post-operative passage", requiring ventilation and tracheostomy, and also developed hydrocephalus, requiring a ventricular peritoneal shunt.

FM has a right hemiplegia and reduced sensation on the right side. He is able to transfer independently and can walk with a stick for short distances. At home he spends most of the time in an electric wheelchair, which he uses independently. His right arm remains non-functional and there is some apraxia in the left arm. He was previously right-handed.

Personal and social history

Prior to his stroke, FM had been a well-known musician, both as a performer and songwriter. He has his own recording and mixing studio in his flat in London. His wife reports that "his whole life revolved around music". Social contacts were all people in the music industry, and he had few other interests. He had travelled widely with his music and had many contacts throughout the world. Although he spent much of his time alone writing music, his wife describes him as an "extremely articulate" person before the stroke. He was also described as "fiercely Glaswegian", a supporter of Celtic football club.

Previous speech language therapy

FM received some rehabilitation in a London hospital between July and August 1995, and had been provided with an ORAC communication aid programmed to say 16 common object names. However, he made no attempt to use it in everyday life. This was followed by a period of intensive in-patient rehabilitation at a Regional Rehabilitation Unit. Speech and Language Therapy during this period included work aimed at improving communication through establishing a clear "no" response and the use of gesture and drawing to augment speech. Some progress was reported and it was felt that augmentative communication channels could be developed. To this end he was referred to the *Drawing Together* therapy project. He was also referred to his local community therapist for ongoing therapy and support.

FM: INITIAL ASSESSMENT RESULTS

Language function

The results of these standardised assessments are presented in Table 11.1. They provide a snapshot of FM's abilities at the single word level.

These results suggest that FM's semantics were minimally impaired at the single word level for high imageability items. Spoken and written naming abilities were severely restricted. In conversation at that time, spoken output was limited to "Aye", certain expletives and occasional poorly intelligible single words. Mainly he produced a string of unintelligible phonemes /dedededede/. He was able to call his wife's name reliably. Written output was limited to some numbers and occasional first letters of words. Comprehension of more complex material was not assessed, but observations suggested that FM was able to follow simple conversation well.

Non-verbal communication

Various measures were used to assess FM's non-verbal communication abilities. His ability to understand picture semantics was assessed on the Pyramids & Palm Trees test. His score of 47/52 represents a performance just below normal. His gesture production was assessed in response to a number of black-and-white line drawings of

TABLE 11.1

Results of pre-therapy assessments of single word language processing

Test	Score
PALPA Spoken word to picture match	39/40
PALPA Written word to picture match	38/40
PALPA Auditory synonym judgement	20/30 LI
PALPA Spoken picture naming	0/40
PALPA Written picture naming	0/40

common items. FM was asked to "Show me what you do with it" or "Show me what it does". This assessment was carried out twice before the start of therapy. On the first occasion FM scored 3/35 and on the second he scored 2/10. His poor performance was attributed in part to his manual apraxia. FM was therefore unable to use gestures communicatively, although in conversation he had developed one or two idiosyncratic gestures, such as punching the air with his fist. FM's use of facial expressions, although not formally assessed, was observed to be appropriate.

FM's drawing abilities were also assessed. He was able to copy simple drawings well. He could draw common objects to command but recognisability was sometimes compromised. Generative drawing was assessed on a test specifically designed for the project, which assesses subjects' ability to generate and draw absent items (Sacchett et al., 1999). The results of this assessment indicated that the majority of FM's drawings were not recognisable out of context (only 18/120 were of his drawings were recognisable). Recognisability improved dramatically when interpreters knew the context in which the drawing was produced (score 86/120), but nevertheless remained low.

FM's difficulty in making recognisable drawings was mainly due to two aspects of his drawing production. First, at an executive level, his manual dyspraxia made drawing certain shapes difficult. He tended to draw curves rather than straight lines. This gave his drawings a very idiosyncratic character. Second, he tended to include many unnecessary details that detracted from the communicative value of the drawing.

Communicative use

To establish the range and type of communication skills and strategies used by FM in his daily life, a qualitative measure, the Pragmatics Profile (Dewart & Summers, 1996), was selected. This involved a structured interview with FM's wife in which actual communicative behaviour in different situations is probed. This assessment does not yield "results" as such, but will be of interest when we examine transfer of skills and effects of therapy on FM's life.

THERAPY PROGRAMME

During the 12-week therapy period, FM received one individual session of about 1 hour's duration at his home, and one 2-hour group session, per week. His wife always participated in the individual session and was able to observe the group session on a video link-up. The following description of therapy will be focus on FM's individual therapy. Group therapy aims mirrored those of individual therapy, with the additional aim of providing a supportive environment in which to practise and develop emergent skills.

Therapy aims
Therapy was focused on overcoming barriers to successful communication. The main "barriers" to FM's successful communicative drawing were identified on the basis of pre-therapy evaluations, observation and discussion with FM and his wife. These are detailed below:

- poor recognisability of drawings, due to idiosyncratic style
- "uneconomic" drawing: tendency to add unnecessary detail; difficulty focusing on important aspects of message
- poor awareness of needs of communication partner: failure to attend to /respond to questions; inconsistent Yes/No response
- limited ability to use clarification strategies such as gesture, identification of important parts of the drawing
- limited use of interpretation strategies by wife: tendency to try to guess FM's drawing, rather than requesting clarification; reluctance to use drawing herself.

There were also a number of positive factors that would influence the success of therapy. First, both FM and his wife were highly motivated to participate in the project. The active participation of his wife, in particular, would be crucial to the transfer of skills into everyday life. Second, FM had already been exposed to the concept of non-verbal communication and had shown some willingness to use drawing to communicate. Third,

FM's auditory comprehension was relatively good, which enabled him to understand therapy tasks and rationales and allowed for a higher level of message-giving.

Therapy tasks were chosen that aimed to reduce or eliminate the above barriers, whilst capitalising on the positive factors, and the following outcome goals were set for FM:

- FM will use drawing alongside other communication modalities to convey novel information in real-life conversational situations
- FM will include only communicatively important details in his drawings: distinguishing visual features, relevant verb arguments etc. (economic drawing)
- FM will demonstrate improved awareness of his communication partner (AM), by responding consistently to attempts at interpretation and by using appropriate clarification strategies
- AM will practise relevant and effective interpretation strategies.

Therapy strategies
Throughout the therapy programme, equal emphasis was given to modelling and feedback of useful strategies to aid in interpretation of messages. It was important that FM and his wife themselves identified which strategies they would find useful and would be willing/able to use. An observation checklist was provided for AM (Appendix 11.2) and a number of specific interpretation strategies were selected for her to practise (Appendix 11.3).

FM's awareness of other people's interpretation attempts also needed targeting. He tended to get so carried away by his drawing that he failed to attend to questions and failed to check that the interpreter was following the conversation. Specifically he had to:

- listen to all questions
- answer all questions with a definite YES or NO
- allow the "listener" time to interpret each element of a message
- use clarification strategies such as gesture, pointing out the important bits, enlargement.

Therapy tasks

Task selection was responsive rather than pre-scriptive. In other words it did not follow a rigid, hierarchical programme, but remained flexible and dependent on FM's week-by-week perform-ance. Structured tasks were used only to demon-strate and practise useful strategies which could then be employed in conversations, and were always used in conjunction with less formal "conversations".

Therapy schedule

Economic drawing

The focus of therapy in the first 2 weeks of ther-apy was on improving awareness of the need to include *useful* distinctive features of items in drawings. The absence of distinctive features is a common characteristic of drawings produced by people with aphasia (Gainotti & Tiacci, 1970; Swindell, Holland, Fromm, & Greenhouse, 1988; Warrington, James, & Kinsbourne, 1966). How-ever in FM's case, it was not the *absence* of detail, but rather the inclusion of unnecessary details, which interfered with the effectiveness of his drawings. The reason for this is unclear. Absence of detail has been attributed to a deficit in con-ceptual or semantic processing (Gainotti, Silveri, Villa, & Caltagirone, 1983; Kirk & Kertesz, 1989). As we have seen, FM's semantics, at least at the single word level, were intact. However, the semantic assessments undertaken did not require FM to generate a visual image of items, as these were already supplied in the tests. The cognitive processes required to draw items from memory have been described in detail by Van Sommers (1989). They include access to visual representa-tions, i.e., stored knowledge about what objects look like, followed by a number of output pro-cesses. Exactly what "knowledge" is stored in the visual representation system is not specified. However, it seems likely that it would include details about the physical structure of objects, specifically those physical features that are neces-sary to distinguish a particular object from other similar exemplars. It was hypothesised that FM was unable to determine which were the *distinct-ive* features of an object as opposed to incidental features about its appearance. Therapy tasks therefore focused on distinguishing between and drawing items with shared visual features, for example base shape. At this stage the tasks selected did not necessarily require generative drawing. Drawings were mainly produced to command or in response to a picture stimulus. However, the tasks selected did involve turn-taking and conveying novel information, which mirrors natural conversation to some extent. Examples of tasks used in weeks 1 and 2 of ther-apy included the following:

- *Adding details to base shape*: FM was given a geometric shape, in this case a circle, and asked to add details to turn it into different objects, e.g., a ring, a coin and a plate.
- *PACE task, visually similar objects*: FM had to convey unknown items by drawing, pay-ing particular attention to distinguishing visual features. FM's drawing of an orange below shows that he now includes some dis-tinguishing features in his drawings, and is beginning also to use other clarification strategies, such as gesture and writing.

When asked to draw an orange, FM's drawing is shown in Figure 11.1. The talk accompanying the picture FM drew went as follows:

CS guesses "apple". FM gestures "eat".
FM writes ORA. CS guesses "orange". F says "Aye"!

Transfer to real-life conversation

The focus of therapy in the third to seventh weeks of the programme was to bring drawing into a conversational setting. Since we do not generally converse about single items, it seemed necessary at this stage to develop FM's ability to convey more complex messages. Single-item drawing tasks were therefore replaced by tasks requiring FM to con-vey actions, events or states. Although a number of drawing therapy studies have reported improvements in the ability of aphasic people to draw complex concepts (Lyon & Sims, 1989; Trupe, 1986), there has been little attempt to clarify the processes required to achieve this skill.

FM's drawings of events were similar in style to

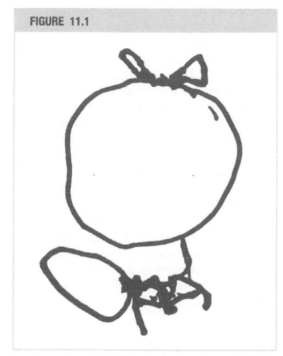

FIGURE 11.1

Drawing produced in PACE task, stimulus picture: ORANGE.

essary information to convey a complex message, by means of developing a strategy of separating the message into key communicatively significant elements (WHO—WHAT—WHERE). The task went as follows:

> This was a PACE-type task. The picture stimuli depicted simple actions, then later actions involving movement and direction were used. FM was required to think about the communicatively significant elements of the event and was trained to draw these elements separately, rather than simultaneously as portrayed in the stimulus picture. This strategy is demonstrated in the figure below (Figure 11.2), which FM produced in response to a stimulus picture showing a woman giving a boy some tablets. The most important aspect of this event, in FM's opinion, is the tablets, and these have been enlarged to show their significance. FM has also successfully depicted the sender/receiver roles by drawing an arrow.

Figure 11.3 details a conversation between FM and the therapist about his weekend activities. FM's initial drawing portrays the whole event simultaneously, but he is subsequently able to select the most important aspects of the event and convey these clearly. Many of the strategies used in interactive drawing as described by Lyon (1995) are demonstrated in this exchange, such as enlargement (Drawing 2), adding details (Drawings 3a and 3b), and use of drawing by the therapist herself.

those of Mr X, a globally aphasic man described by Bauer and Kaiser (1995). Like Mr X, FM tried to represent the whole event in one complex simultaneous drawing. It was unclear which elements of the drawing contained information relevant to the communication of the event. Also, the boundaries of different referents in the event were not defined. For example, in a drawing of man holding a cat, it was impossible to differentiate the cat from the man's hand, which covered it.

Bauer and Kaiser attribute Mr X's difficulties in drawing complex situations to an inability to draw in a "*listener-oriented*" way. In other words, he was unable to determine which aspects of a message were crucial to its being understood by an interactant and to focus on those aspects in his drawings. They recommend that a goal of therapy should be "conventionalising means of representation and techniques of communication".

Some structured therapy tasks were therefore developed with the aims of: (a) developing a "convention" for depicting action and movement and (b) improving FM's ability to sort out the nec-

Development of complexity of messages

The focus of therapy between weeks 7 to 12 was to develop FM's ability to give complex messages and hold complex conversations. He had successfully grasped the strategy of separating key elements of the message when using a picture stimulus of a single event.

To achieve generative, and therefore truly communicative, drawing, it was important to reduce reliance on a picture stimulus. Tasks were therefore introduced that required FM to convey a verbally presented problem or situation to his wife. It was also necessary at this stage to extend the use of the hitherto successful strategy of separating a message into key elements to convey messages involving more than one activity/event or describing a sequence of events over time.

Initially FM had great difficulty separating messages into key elements. As was the case earlier in his therapy, he tended to try to convey the whole message simultaneously in a single drawing, rather than separating it into communicatively relevant elements. Attempts at interpretation were met with slavish repetition of the original drawing, going over and over the same details, regardless of whether he was being understood.

FM's difficulty in selecting the important information from a longer, more complex message may have been due in part to the increased demands on his auditory comprehension and auditory memory. It seemed that FM had an additional difficulty in analysing and organising

the sequential aspect of longer messages, or in separating the whole situation or problem into a number of clearly definable events.

It was therefore decided to reduce the demands of the tasks by only giving him one piece of information at a time to convey, and by instructing him to make sure AM had successfully understood it before giving the next piece. To promote this a cartoon-strip format was introduced, in which each piece of information is drawn in a separate box. This technique has been successfully used in previous therapy programmes. Most notably, Morgan and Helm-Estabrooks' (1987) programme, *Back to the Drawing Board*, trained two adults with severe aphasia to draw one-, two- and three-panelled cartoons from memory. They report improvements in the ability of these two people to depict sequential events and details critical to those events.

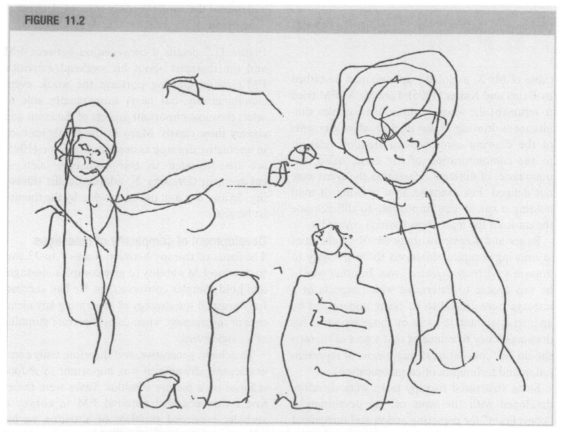

FIGURE 11.2

Drawing produced in PACE task, stimulus picture: A woman giving a boy some tablets.

FIGURE 11.3

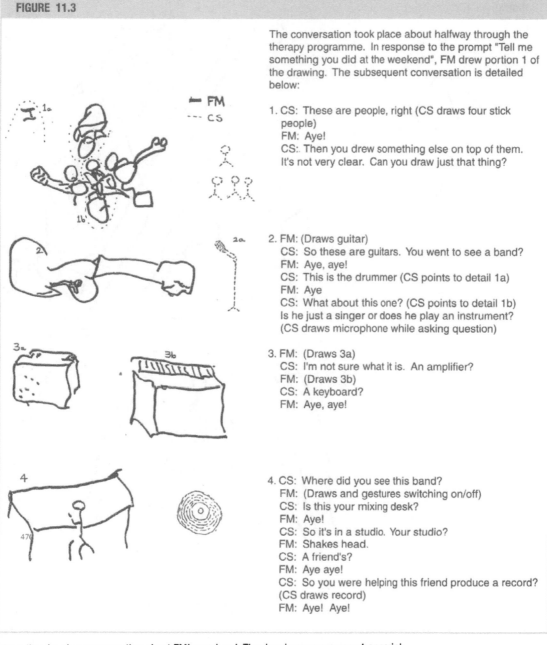

The conversation took place about halfway through the therapy programme. In response to the prompt "Tell me something you did at the weekend", FM drew portion 1 of the drawing. The subsequent conversation is detailed below:

1. CS: These are people, right (CS draws four stick people)
   FM: Aye!
   CS: Then you drew something else on top of them. It's not very clear. Can you draw just that thing?

2. FM: (Draws guitar)
   CS: So these are guitars. You went to see a band?
   FM: Aye, aye!
   CS: This is the drummer (CS points to detail 1a)
   FM: Aye
   CS: What about this one? (CS points to detail 1b) Is he just a singer or does he play an instrument? (CS draws microphone while asking question)

3. FM: (Draws 3a)
   CS: I'm not sure what it is. An amplifier?
   FM: (Draws 3b)
   CS: A keyboard?
   FM: Aye, aye!

4. CS: Where did you see this band?
   FM: (Draws and gestures switching on/off)
   CS: Is this your mixing desk?
   FM: Aye!
   CS: So it's in a studio. Your studio?
   FM: Shakes head.
   CS: A friend's?
   FM: Aye aye!
   CS: So you were helping this friend produce a record? (CS draws record)
   FM: Aye! Aye!

Interactive drawing: conversation about FM's weekend. The drawings accompany transcript.

Figure 11.4 contains examples of tasks used to aid FM in working with complex information. The examples in the figure are of tasks designed to convey complex situations. FM was presented with a complex problem or situation auditorily. The therapist then helped FM to work through the situation, determining the sequence of events and deciding what elements were significant in each event. FM then had to convey the problem to AM via drawing, within a total communication

FIGURE 11.4

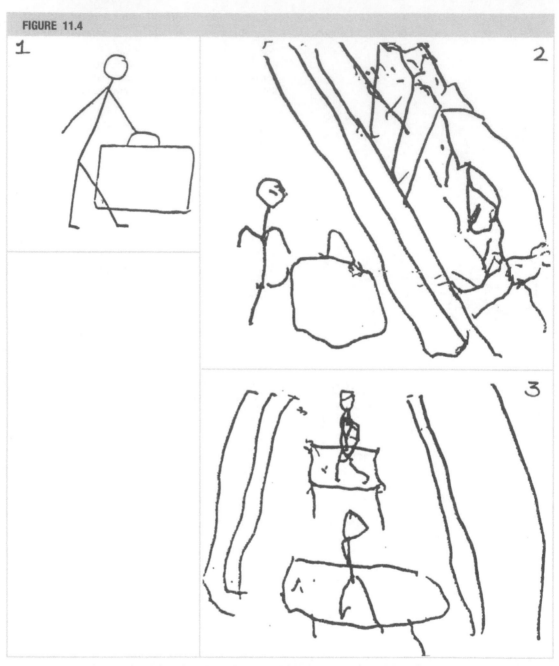

Story completion demonstrating cartoon strip format: Panel 1, therapist's drawing; Panel 2, FM's drawing of a man waiting on a platform and a train; Panel 3, FM's drawing of a man sitting inside the train carriage. (Note the change in orientation to a birds'-eye view inside the carriage.)

framework. The individual events making up the whole situation/problem were presented sequentially in separate boxes. The strip cartoon format was used to develop FM's ability to generate his own ideas and depict them in drawings. FM was required to complete a "story" started by the therapist's drawing.

Figure 11.4 illustrates the result of the process activity. Panel 1 is the therapist's drawing. Panels 2 and 3 are FM's completion of the story. Panel 2 shows the man waiting on a platform and a train. Panel 3 shows the man sitting inside the train carriage. Note the change in orientation to a bird's-eye view inside the carriage.

OUTCOMES

Outcomes will be described in terms of the four outcome goals set for FM.

FM will use drawing alongside other communication modalities to convey novel information in real-life conversational situations

As can be seen from the examples used in describing the therapy, by the end of 12 weeks of therapy FM was able to convey complex information in conversations. Transfer of this skill into real-life situations and for a variety of purposes was reported by his wife in the repeated Pragmatics Profile. He uses drawing to convey problems, ask questions, make his needs and feelings known and make requests, as shown by the following excerpts:

Q: How would F let you know if he wanted something? Supposing it was something that he couldn't actually point to . . . does he do anything else?

A: Yeah draw me a picture.

Q: Can you think of an example?

A: Oh yes, yes. He wanted these six tapes posted so he drew me a picture . . . of six tapes. Cassette tapes. And a stamp on the corner so that I knew that he wanted them sent off.

Q: Can you think of an example where you've got the wrong end of the stick and then F has drawn you something which has put you in the picture?

A: . . . Oh about his pills. They've changed the packaging on his pills and he kept saying to me they were the wrong ones and I said they're not 'cos they're exactly the same. And then he drew the old type and the new type 'cos I didn't know what he was talking about.

Q: Right, right. And then you got what it was?

A: And then I had to explain they are still the same, it's just a different box.

Q: And was he happy with that?

A: Yes.

FM will include only communicatively important details in his drawings

A look at FM's drawings over the therapy period will show that in terms of quality, they have not changed much. Out of context, FM's drawings would still be difficult to recognise. Indeed, this is borne out by his results on the *generative drawing* assessment referred to earlier (Table 11.1). Comparison of FM's pre- and post-therapy recognisability scores shows that there has been little change when the context is unknown to the rater. However, when the context is known, the recognisability rating post therapy is higher, but not significantly so (see Table 11.2).

So, if FM's drawings were no more recognisable at the end of the therapy period, how was this outcome achieved? Two points must be borne in mind. First, the generative drawing assessment only looked at FM's drawings of single objects.

TABLE 11.2

Pre- and post-therapy scores on the recognisability of FM drawings

Rating condition	*Pre-therapy score*	*Post-therapy score*
Context unknown	18/120	17/120
Context known	86/120	97/120

The therapy, on the other hand, focused on developing FM's ability to convey complex messages, which is more useful conversationally. As discussed, this depends to a large extent on the ability to select appropriate important elements of a message and convey these in a way that facilitates interpretation. Towards the end of therapy, FM was indeed able to do this.

Second, this result underlines the fact that ease of interpretation of messages conveyed by drawing relies on more than the quality of the drawings produced and their ease of recognition. Certainly the examples cited above from FM's wife suggest that he has little difficulty in getting his messages across, despite the fact that his drawing *ability* itself has not changed. The reasons for this may become clear when we consider the next two outcomes, which will be discussed together.

FM will demonstrate improved awareness of his communication partner by responding consistently to attempts at interpretation and by using appropriate clarification strategies, and AM will practise relevant and effective interpretation strategies

The examples given in the therapy section provide clear examples of both FM's improved clarification skills and AM's improved interpretation skills. FM was successfully using strategies such as allowing the interpreter time, listening and responding to questions and providing additional information using gesture or enlargement of important parts of the drawing.

For her part, AM's interpretation skills had improved considerably over the therapy period, as indicated by therapy notes written at that time:

A is very aware of F's intentions . . . and also of his Y/N response, which is not always clear to me. She uses strategies of asking F to point out important bits and enlarge them, checks F's Y/N response.

AM was observed to be asking more "homing in" questions rather than just guessing randomly. She was also more willing to ask FM for clarification. She remained reluctant to use drawing herself, or to write key words down, feeling that these did not add to the communicative value of interactions with FM.

DISCUSSION

To summarise, there was a marked improvement in FM's ability to use drawing communicatively and in AM's ability to interpret his messages during the course of the *Drawing Together* project. This improvement was not limited to the clinical setting, as FM used drawing spontaneously and successfully for a variety of purposes in real-life conversations both with his wife and with friends. This result now begs the question: Can this improvement be attributed to the therapy he received?

A comparison of FM's pre- and post-therapy performance provides clear evidence that no spontaneous recovery was taking place (Table 11.2). There was no significant change in any of the language measures. However, a significant improvement in gesture production did occur. This can be attributed to the fact that, in therapy, one of the clarification strategies that FM was encouraged to use was "Show me what you do with it?" It could therefore be argued that, through exposure to this therapy, FM's attitude to using alternative communication methods was changed. He could now see the value of non-verbal communication and recognised its potential to "reveal his competence" as a creative communicator.

Additionally, therapy tasks had targeted the development of specific strategies required to achieve successful communicative drawing of complex events. Whilst there is no before and after measure of FM's ability to make use of these strategies, there is ample evidence from his performance that an improvement in these skills has taken place. Specifically, FM had been trained to separate a single event into its key elements and to draw these from a "listener-oriented" perspective. In other words, he is aware of the communicative significance of various elements of the event, and is able to "work towards the interactant's understanding" (Bauer & Kaiser, 1995). He had also been trained to use the strategy of separating a complex situation into a number of single events, and to convey these using a cartoon-strip format. Bauer and Kaiser suggest that, because cartoon strips are sequential and propositionally organised, their production makes higher demands on verbal skills such as verbal mediation and/or encourages increased connections between graphic and verbal skills. As FM's semantic ability and auditory comprehension were both good, it is possible that he was able, with assistance, to harness these abilities to aid his processing and depiction of events.

In retrospect, assessment of his event processing and sentence comprehension abilities both pre- and post-therapy would have yielded some useful information in this respect. However, at the start of the therapy programme there was no indication that FM's drawing skills would improve to such an extent. FM had had some exposure to drawing as a communicative medium prior to the start of this therapy programme and no such gains were reported. It does not therefore seem unreasonable to claim that the improvements in FM's communicative drawing abilities can be attributed to the therapy he received during the *Drawing Together* therapy project. There was no doubt in FM's wife's mind that this change was a direct result of the therapy programme. In the Pragmatics Profile interview, she said:

Q: You've said you know he would draw something. Is that something that's changed or is that something that he would always have done?

A: No. Something that's changed dramatically.

Q: Right, right. At about what stage during the project did he start to do that?

A: About the third or fourth week.

Q: And is it something that's happened because you've suggested that he might draw or does he do that spontaneously?

A: No, he'll do it spontaneously ... He's into drawing, F is, ... really into drawing.

The remainder of the chapter will describe FM's continuing therapy; in particular, how he was

enabled to refine his non-verbal skills and build on them to achieve life-enhancing goals. In particular, we will describe the work to develop a communication book with FM.

DEVELOPING THE COMMUNICATION BOOK

A second strand of therapy has been the development of a personalised communication book. Whilst it will become apparent that the book has conferred benefits beyond "getting the message across", it was primarily introduced to supplement existing communication skills. A communication book was seen to have the advantage of providing a readily interpretable vocabulary, even to naïve communication partners; through inclusion of information such as the names of friends and commonly visited places, the book could also be used to communicate about items and events that were difficult to draw.

FM appeared to possess a number of key visual, motoric and linguistic abilities that would allow him to make good use of a communication book (Hux et al., 1994; Kraat, 1990; Pyatak Fletcher, 1997). He clearly understood pictured information, could point to pictured items upon request and to demonstrate preferences and could select from a semantically grouped array. Indeed, he was already using maps and pictographic information (including symbols from other people's communication books) in group therapy sessions. FM was keen to interact with those around him, and was understandably frustrated when they could not understand his drawings or attempts to gesture. His ability to read some single words for meaning meant that symbols or pictures in any communication book could be supplemented by simple written information, further enhancing its intelligibility to new or unskilled communication partners.

FM expressed great interest in developing his own communication book. FM's wife, however, was sceptical about the usefulness of this, noting that FM had been similarly keen to try the ORAC communication aid (Mardis Limited) but now did not use it. Despite the considerable effort that went into programming the ORAC, FM used it on very few occasions. When asked about the ORAC, FM gestured that he found the aid too heavy to transport. He also indicated that several of the vocabulary items were not useful.

Negotiating the therapeutic relationship

Work started on the communication book in May 1997. Initial sessions were devoted to developing a rapport with FM and his wife. As the student Speech Language Therapist was keen for FM to assert his needs in therapy, and to establish a collaborative model of working, the following goal guided her early interventions: FM will set his own goals for therapy, in partnership with AM and his keyworking student.

This client-centred approach was seen not only to be useful in selecting relevant goals, but also in maintaining FM's interest in therapy. This approach was also felt to reinforce a shared responsibility for change; AM's support and involvement was deemed key to any generalisation of skill from the clinic to the home.

As part of the goal-setting procedure, FM was provided with pictographs representing the different forms of therapy that the centre where he was receiving therapy could reasonably provide: FM was encouraged to refer to these pictographs, and produce his own drawings, in three-way discussions of potential therapies. The student's notes at this stage reveal her frequent use of Total Communication to facilitate FM's comprehension; she also produced drawings and wrote single words "on-line" to illustrate her understanding of FM's communication, and to summarise decisions reached. The following goals were subsequently agreed upon:

Long-term goal:
- FM will use Total Communication in natural conversations with a variety of communication partners.

Short-term goals:
- FM will use Total Communication in his interactions with current communication partners
- FM will develop a Communication Book

that meets his needs, in collaboration with his wife and his keyworker.

After this period of introductions and goal setting, several therapy sessions were spent discussing relevant sections and vocabulary for the communication book. These discussions included consideration of FM's weekly timetable, current interests, usual topics of conversation and conversation partners. Initially, after FM indicated that he wanted to include all of the items from another group member's book within his own, a discussion of the relevance of this information, and the benefits of personalised communication, took place.

Sections on the following topics were agreed upon: *food*, *drink* and *everyday objects* (e.g., sweets; Walkman). It was also decided that, in order to facilitate both FM and others' access to the book, each vocabulary item would be represented by a drawing and a word. FM insisted that he would prepare all of the drawings.

While FM continued to express his interest in developing the communication book, he failed to bring any of his drawings to the session. Liaison with AM revealed that FM did not think that his drawings were "good enough" to appear in the book. Therapy took a new slant after she found some computer clipart and loosely arranged it in FM's communication book over the course of a weekend. This clipart included some symbols that FM had wanted to include in his book (e.g., favourite foods and drinks), and others that FM subsequently identified as less useful.

Refining and personalising communication

Whilst AM's actions helped to overcome a short-term problem (i.e., FM's difficulty in preparing items for the book), they were somewhat contrary to the student SLT's desire for FM to assume responsibility for his therapy and, ultimately, for the development of his communication book. Rather than reject AM's contribution, the student SLT renegotiated the immediate focus of her therapy with FM: that is, FM would indicate which of the symbols should stay in the book, indicate how these symbols would be categorised and advise on the overall layout. The student's notes reveal a rekindling of FM's interest in therapy after this renegotiation.

The ensuing period of therapy not only helped to refine and personalise FM's communication book, but also enhanced its potential as a means of interacting with, and influencing, others. As highlighted by Hux et al. (1994) (and elaborated elsewhere by Kagan & Gailey, 1993, and Simmons-Mackie & Damico, 1995), interpersonal communication transcends the mere transmission of information to encompass social affiliation and the making and maintenance of friendships. Correspondingly, Hux et al. stress the need for communication books to move beyond the more traditional lists of personal possessions to include vocabulary that *shares information* (e.g., names of family members, friends, pastimes and favourite places) and *fosters social closeness* (e.g., biographical information and personal photographs). Changes to the communication book during this period included:

- specification of previously generic information (e.g. the inclusion of the label of FM's favourite tipple, in addition to more "neutral" symbols for *drink*)
- addition of information under the categories: sport; events; transport; weather/seasons; days/months; therapy
- addition of maps of the world, and of the USA
- photographs of friends, family and favourite places (e.g., his holiday villa in Spain)
- photographs and symbols pertaining to Celtic Football Club.

An important stage in the development and use of the book was the inclusion of information relevant to FM's musical affairs, particularly his back catalogue; as noted previously, AM was facing increasing demands to distribute these songs. AM was aware that FM held strong views about which songs should be released but, in the absence of a quick and reliable means of discussion, felt some pressure to make decisions on her own. Small photocopies of FM's album covers were therefore included in the book to allow them to discuss his published work. His catalogue of

(approximately) 500 unpublished songs proved harder to accommodate; however, categorisation of these songs according to type (e.g., love song, country song, etc.) and the inclusion of suitable symbols has facilitated communication.

Other, related information that now appears in the book includes:

- names and photographs of fellow musicians
- names and photographs of lyricists
- symbols depicting certain recording labels/publishing companies
- symbols pertaining to studio equipment
- pictures of musical instruments.

The following examples, cited by AM, show how the book has transformed FM's ability to control aspects of his work.

- FM wants to tell his wife which of his musical tracks he wants to forward to an agent. Previously FM would gesture "vaguely" and AM would make a series of (often unsuccessful) guesses. FM would find the track by listening, one by one, to his library of audiotapes. Now, for published work, FM points to one of the album covers in his communication book, and/or a publishers' symbol and the photograph of someone he wrote it with. For unpublished work, FM can point to the song type and/or the photograph of a collaborator.
- FM wants to tell his wife to phone JM (a singer-songwriter in California). Previously, he would gesture "phone" and point to a map of the USA. AM would then name all of the contacts they have in the USA until she reached JM. Now FM gestures "phone", and then points to JM's photograph in the book. Before JM's photograph was included in the book, FM used the symbols "*man*", "*singer*", "*writer*", as well as a map, to communicate about him.

FM continued to express great interest in refining his book, and more recently worked with a new therapist to do so. Again, the focus was upon increasing its personal relevance and interactive potential; developments include information about growing up in Glasgow (e.g., maps of the city and photographs) and about previously unmentioned family members (e.g., a grandfather who played for Rangers). FM and the student negotiated that he would work with his Music Therapist to include more information about recording equipment. FM also expressed a desire to devise some pages that could function as "stories" in their own right (i.e., that go beyond the bounds of categorised information); these include childhood memories and tales from early days in the music industry.

OUTCOMES OF THERAPY, AND CONCLUSION

Whilst FM's progress through therapy has not been accompanied by significant changes in language function, or upon formal testing of drawing ability, it is clear that he has made gains communicatively. AM, his most frequent communication partner, has noted differences in the quality of his drawn output: he now produces pictures "that you can actually understand". She reports that he is beginning to communicate with people who could not comprehend him previously, and she is now confident enough in his skills to leave him alone with others. AM has noted that FM can now convey complex messages, often using a combination of strategies (e.g., the communication book to specify the person he is talking about, and then drawing to "fill in the story"); indeed, the presence and use of the communication book is an outcome in its own right.

Changes in FM's communication are also beginning to result in changes in his everyday life: for example, the inclusion of album covers in his communication book has allowed him to convey decisions about the distribution of his music. He can use photographs in his book to specify which lyricists he would like to work with and, indeed, has started to collaborate musically once more.

It is in his communication about musical matters that one can see another benefit of therapy emerge: that of regained identity. FM's communication book contains many clues to his status and profession: backstage passes, pictures of fellow musicians and famous friends, album covers. He often uses these parts of his book when introducing himself. FM's reference to himself as a Celtic supporter and Glaswegian further assists in asserting his identity. AM sees the success of the communication book over the ORAC in these terms: the book is "about FM as a person" (although she also admits that the book is appealing because it holds more information). Her occasional comment that the communication book is becoming "FM, This Is Your Life" may well be close to the mark.

Ultimately, changes in FM's communication have assisted in revealing his competence. His severe aphasia has, for some time, served to conceal the "active mind". As FM has become more able to communicate, he has revealed his ability to make decisions in keeping with his premorbid abilities: for example, he remains acutely aware of which singers suit his songs, and distributes his work accordingly.

AM has recently disclosed that FM is about to agree a contract regarding the re-release of his albums. As part of this process, he needs to decide which publishing company will take charge of his music and whether he should undertake a 3- or 5-year agreement. AM expects that FM will use his drawing and/or communication book to assist in this process. In her estimation, he is "back in control of his songs". The therapies detailed in this chapter, in their layering of interactive tasks, and their provision of means of communication that transcend the transmission of basic needs, have been important in regaining this control.

REFERENCES

Bauer, A., & Kaiser, G. (1995). Drawing on drawings. *Aphasiology, 9*, 68–78.

Beukelman, D., & Mirenda, P. (1992). *Augmentative and alternative communication: Management of severe communication disorders in children and adults.* Baltimore, MD: Paul H. Brookes.

Dewart, H., & Summers, S. (1996). *Pragmatics profile*

of everyday communication skills in adults. London: NFER Nelson.

Fox, L.E., & Fried-Oken, M. (1996). AAC aphasiology: Partnership for future research. *Augmentative and Alternative Communication, 12,* 257–271.

Funnell, E., & Allport, A. (1989). Symbolically speaking: Communicating with Blissymbols in aphasia. *Aphasiology, 3,* 279–300.

Gainotti, G., Silveri, M.C., Villa, G., & Caltagirone, C. (1983). Drawing objects from memory in aphasia. *Brain, 106,* 613–622.

Gainotti, G., & Tiacci, C. (1970). Patterns of drawing disability in right and left hemispheric patients. *Neuropsychologia 8,* 379–384.

Hux, K., Beukelman, D., & Garrett, K. (1994). Augmentative and alternative communication for persons with aphasia. In R. Chapey (Ed.), *Language intervention strategies in adult aphasia* (4th ed.). Baltimore, MD: Williams & Wilkins.

Kagan, A., & Gailey, G.F. (1993). Functional is not enough: Training conversation partners for aphasic adults. In A. Holland & M. Forbes (Eds.), *Aphasia treatment: World perspectives.* London: Chapman & Hall.

Kearns, K., & Yoder, K. (1992). *Artistic activation therapy.* Paper presented at Clinical Aphasiology Conference, Durango, CO.

Kirk, K., & Kertesz, A. (1989). Hemispheric contributions to drawing. *Neuropsychologia, 27,* 881–886.

Kraat, A.W. (1990). Augmentative and alternative communication: Does it have a future in aphasia rehabilitation? *Aphasiology, 4,* 321–338.

Lawson, R., & Fawcus, M. (1999). Increasing effective communication using a total communication approach. In S. Byng, K. Swinburn, & C. Pound (Eds.), *The aphasia therapy file.* Hove, UK: Psychology Press.

Lyon, J.G. (1995). Drawing: Its value as a communication aid for adults with aphasia. *Aphasiology, 9,* 33–50 & 84–94.

Lyon, J.G., & Sims, E. (1989). Drawing: Its use as a communication aid with aphasic and normal adults. In T. Prescott (Ed.), *Clinical aphasiology proceedings, Vol 18.* San Diego, CA: College Hill Press.

Marshall, R.C., Tompkins, C.A., & Phillips, D.S. (1982). Improvement in treated aphasia: Examination of selected prognostic factors. *Folia Phoniatrica, 34,* 305–315.

McIntosh, J., & Dakin, G. (1989). The restoration of communication through Amer-Ind. In E.V. Jones (Ed.), *Advances in aphasia therapy in the clinical setting.* Cambridge: Proceedings of the British Aphasiology Society Therapy Symposium.

Morgan, A., & Helm-Estabrooks, N. (1987). Back to the drawing board: A treatment program for nonverbal aphasic adults. In R. Brookshire (Ed.), *Clinical aphasiology proceedings.* Minneapolis, MN: BBK Publishers.

Pound, C., Parr, S., Lindsay, J., & Woolf, C. (2000). *Beyond aphasia: Therapies for living with communication disability.* Bicester, UK: Winslow Press.

Pyatak Fletcher, P. (1997). AAC and adults with acquired disabilities. In S.L. Glennen & D.C. De Coste (Eds.), *The handbook of augmentative and alternative communication.* San Diego, CA: Singular Publishing Group.

Rao, P.R. (1986). The use of Amer-Ind code with aphasic adults. In R. Chapey (Ed.), *Language intervention strategies in adult aphasia* (2nd ed.). Baltimore, MD: Williams & Wilkins.

Sacchett, C., Byng, S., Marshall, J.F., & Pound, C. (1999). Drawing together: Evaluation of a therapy programme for severe aphasia. *International Journal of Language and Communication Disorders, 34,* 265–290.

Sarno, M.T., Silverman, M., & Sands, E. (1970). Speech therapy and language recovery in severe aphasia. *Aphasiology, 9,* 59–63.

Simmons-Mackie, N., & Damico, J. (1995). Communicative competence and aphasia: Evidence from compensatory strategies. In M. Lemme (Ed.), *Clinical aphasiology, Vol. 23.* Austin, TX: Pro-Ed.

Swindell, C.S., Holland, A.L., Fromm, D., & Greenhouse, J.B. (1988). Characteristics of recovery of drawing disability in left and right brain-damaged patients. *Brain and Cognition, 7,* 16–30.

Trupe, E.H. (1986). *Training severely aphasic patients to communicate by drawing.* Paper presented at the American Speech-Language-Hearing Association Convention, Detroit, MI.

Van Sommers, P. (1989). A system for drawing and drawing-related neuropsychology. *Cognitive Neuropsychology, 6,* 117–164.

Warrington, E.K., James, M., & Kinsbourne, M. (1966). Drawing disability in relation to laterality of cerebral lesion. *Brain, 89,* 53–82.

APPENDICES

APPENDIX 11.1: Selection criteria for *Drawing Together* therapy project

Minimum, 1 year post-onset
No clinical or neuro-radiographic evidence of bilateral or diffuse brain damage
No evidence of dementia or other degenerative condition
Little or no spoken or written output
An ability to recognise objects and pictures
An ability to copy simple line drawings
An ability to draw objects on command or gesture
An inability to draw generatively (i.e. from memory) or communicatively
Availability of carer willing and able to participate in the research

APPENDIX 11.2: Observation checklist for identification of useful interpretation strategies for FM

Observe the conversation between FM and CS closely. Note down things they do or say and try to decide whether those things were helpful or not and why. Using the handout "What to do if the drawing is not clear" try to decide what strategies CS used to help her to work out FM's message. To help you do this, there is a list of possible strategies.

1. Letting FM finish before starting to interpret.
2. Stating the general theme of the drawing.
3. Asking questions about the drawing before trying to guess.
4. Asking FM to point out the most important parts of the drawing.
5. Asking FM for clues such as gestures.
6. Asking FM to draw parts of the drawing bigger.
7. Asking FM to add details to his drawings.
8. Adding details herself to FM's drawings.
9. Asking yes/no questions or forced-choice questions about parts of the drawing.
10. Making sure FM answers questions.
11. Checking FM's answers by writing key words.
12. Drawing her "best guess" and getting FM to fix it.
13. Repeating every few minutes what she knows about the drawing and checking she is on the right track.

APPENDIX 11.3: Specific interpretation strategies for AM to practise

1. Ask "homing in" questions (yes/no) about the drawing before trying to guess what it. Make sure he gives you an answer!
2. Ask FM to show you the important bits. If you don't recognise them, ask him to draw just those bits again, bigger.
3. Ask FM for other clues, e.g., "Show me what you do with it." "Show me how big it is."
4. Add or change FM's drawing by drawing something yourself—your "best guess".
5. Write down key words about the drawing as you find things out. This helps you to remember questions you have already asked and helps to trace a breakdown in communication

12

Respecting the rights of a person with aphasia to their own life choices: A longitudinal case study

Sam Simpson

INTRODUCTION

In recent years I have become increasingly interested in the process of identity reconstruction following acquired communication disability. I have come to realise that people with aphasia cope differently. In particular, I have been repeatedly intrigued by the way in which a small number of people embrace the new circumstances they find themselves in post-injury, adapting to find a way to live with their communication dis-

ability and to incorporate it into who they now are as people. This is in stark contrast with others who appear to find this transition more difficult.

Having shared this clinical observation with a number of my peers, I was surprised to discover similar observations in support of my own. This commonality of experience led me to the literature, only to find that this somewhat elusive area had been little studied to date. This discovery spurred me on to undertake some research into the area myself. I thus set out to examine how the experience of aphasia impacts upon people's sense of self, and to identify and describe the factors that people with aphasia report which inhibit and facilitate the construction of a strong aphasic, personal identity (Simpson, unpublished data, 2000).

This research introduced me to the concept of narrative, which is gaining increasing importance in the field of sociology as a means for understanding people's attempts to deal with chronic illness and the changes in identity that this brings about in the context of personal biography (Nettleton, 1995). Thus, the term "narrative" refers to the "stories we live by", that is, stories that enable us to discern meaning from a particular experience by integrating it with others (Somers, 1994). People are conceptualised as story weavers (Stainton Rogers, 1991), navigating their journey of identity reconstruction through the knitting together of the past, present and future. More recently, "narrative medicine", pioneered by Kleinman (1988) and Frank (1995), has attracted the attention of mainstream medical practitioners, including general practitioners (Greenhalgh & Hurwitz, 1998) as a means of listening more attentively to clients and approaching their problems holistically in order to identify needs and prioritise goals more comprehensively. Increasingly, speech and language therapists have also become interested in the narrative concept (Barrow, 2000; Pound, 1999; Pound, Parr, Lindsay, & Woolf, 2000). Indeed, my research upheld the use of the narrative concept as the most comprehensive and overarching framework for illustrating the process of identity reconstruction in the context of aphasia at present.

In his book *The Wounded Story teller*, Frank (1995) proposed three "types of narrative", that is, three general story lines that can be recognised underlying the plots of stories following an illness disruption. These are the "restitution narrative", "chaos narrative" and "quest narrative". Frank suggested that whilst people tell their own unique stories, they in fact compose their stories by adapting and combining the three narrative types. His rationale for proposing these general types of narrative was to encourage closer attention to the stories that people tell and to provide a means of sifting the different narrative threads employed.

According to Frank, no actual story conforms exclusively to any of the three narratives, but will combine all three alternatively and repeatedly. Any given experience, however, can be described by the narrative type that predominates at that moment. The following is a brief summary of the three types of narrative proposed by Frank (1995).

- *Restitution*: The plot of this narrative has the basic story line "yesterday I was healthy, today I'm sick and tomorrow I'll be healthy again". Thus, illness is viewed as transitory with a focus on cure.
- *Chaos*: This is the opposite of restitution in that the plot imagines life never getting better. Thus illness is overwhelming and a person's life map is lost.
- *Quest*: In quest stories, the teller meets suffering head on in that they accept the illness and seek to use it. Illness is viewed as a "journey that becomes a quest"—that is, a search for alternative ways of being ill in the belief that there is something to be gained from the experience.

This model is attractive in its simplicity; however, it is important to remember that people require many diverse accounts in order to navigate the journey of identity reconstruction. The three narrative types proposed by Frank (1995) provide a useful set of guidelines for listening to and interpreting these accounts, however it is not the only set. Furthermore, each individual's cocktail of stories is both subjective and selective, as they are told and perceived differently depending on the listener, the context and the circumstances at the time of telling. Narratives thus emerge gradually and are co-constructed over time. Both what is said and how it is told are significant.

The value of narratives is not just restricted to clients and their families. Narratives also provide a tool with which we can listen to ourselves. Elwyn and Gwyn (1998) and Simmons-Mackie and Damico (2001) have drawn attention to our need to be aware of our preferred narratives and our patterns of response to the narratives we favour less. It is with this in mind that the author is consciously using the personal pronoun in this chapter. Any therapy relationship involves at least two people—the client and the therapist, both of whom bring their own life experiences and narratives with them (Clarkson, 1995). Consequently, this chapter intends to make my narrative as therapist explicit in order to demonstrate how it, too, has played an important part in the therapy process with Carlos, a 22-year-old man with mild to moderate aphasia.

This chapter will take a narrative-based approach for its framework. Specific attention will be paid to the key plots and themes in Carlos's lifestory and how these have changed over the past 2 years (Frank, 1995). This will be achieved by means of analysis of in-depth interviews carried out separately with Carlos and his parents. The majority of the quotations used in this chapter are taken directly from these interviews. A retrospective view is taken to explore the influence Carlos and his parents' narratives have had on the therapy approach and how they in turn have been influenced by it. In addition, attention will be given to the key factors that have influenced the decision-making process during both blocks of therapy.

This case study represents a typical case in a busy, clinical setting. The therapies took place at the the Wolfson Neurorehabilitation Centre (WNRC) a specialist, tertiary centre for people with a range of acquired neurological disorders. It offers intensive, interdisciplinary rehabilitation on both an in-patient and an out-patient basis and increasingly offers flexible packages of care over a longer timeframe. The following report is not cast in tight research terms. Rather, it is presented in terms of the issues it raises relating to working with younger people with aphasia, the identity and lifestyle issues that pertain to this age group, the practical application of a life participation model of aphasia therapy within a rehabilitation centre, the importance of access to interdisciplinary team working, the use of outcome measures as both evaluation and process tools and finally the provision of speech and language therapy in the longer term and the interfacing of community-based services, rehabilitation centres and aphasia centres.

CARLOS'S STORY

Carlos was born in South America and came to the UK for political reasons at the age of 10 years with his parents and younger sister. They left behind many friends and family members and on arrival in the UK were faced with the task of reconstructing a new lifestyle over here. This is of significance as it has given Carlos a strong sense of family. Since their arrival his parents have studied and worked to build up a successful and prosperous family business in London. This has resulted in a strong family culture of anything being possible provided you put in the effort.

Carlos received all of his secondary education in the UK and, following successful completion of his A-levels, started a business course at university. His reasons for this were as follows:

Int: Why had you chosen business?
Carlos: 'Cos my dad does . . . my dad was always doing business . . . and basically the only thing I was thinking is . . . money comes from business . . . if you do business you earn more . . . and the most thing I wanted was money, so . . . do business, even though it's boring, that's what you're going to earn . . . and that's basically the only reason . . .
Int: Why was money important for you, do you think?
Carlos: Because I think money is the most important thing . . . people say that money doesn't buy . . . things . . . doesn't buy everything . . . I think it does. I think you need money to be happy.

Carlos was in the second year of his degree course and was not finding the course as interesting as he had hoped. Similarly, he reported he was not a willing student, doing minimal independent study and all written assignments at the last minute. Academically, however, this was sufficient for him to get by.

Carlos was still living at home with his parents

and younger sister as he had decided it was more financially viable than living out and he was loath to give up all of his home comforts. He had a girlfriend and a large network of friends with whom he had an active social life (e.g. visiting people in halls, going to bars and clubs, the cinema and out for meals). He was passionate about football. He was an avid fan of a London football club and played regularly with his friends. He also enjoyed playing golf with his father.

Carlos prided himself on being bilingual. Spanish was the language that he used at home with his parents, whilst he spoke English with his sister and friends. He considered speaking Spanish an important expression of his South American roots.

Carlos described himself as being "a good friend", "kind", "laid back" and "confident" at this time. His parents described him as being "a normal 20-year-old", "ambitious", "very independent" and his "own person" (he adored his car and the freedom this gave him, for example, and did not drink or smoke in spite of peer pressure) in addition to being "very sporty".

Carlos described his future aspirations prior to his stroke as follows:

> I was gonna finish university, start working . . . I don't . . . wasn't sure where . . . somewhere earning loads of money, having a Porsche and owning a flat . . . buying a flat in London . . . and then get married when I was like 28, then have a couple of boys . . . and I'd be happy . . . that was it.

THERAPIST'S REFLECTIONS

I would like to share a number of thoughts that struck me when I first met Carlos and subsequently witnessed his pre-aphasia life story. The first relates to how image conscious he was and is. He affords much status to his appearance, hair and clothes as well as to his belongings. On admission he was extremely proud of his car, for example, and the latest multi-system music centre and wheel hubs he had had put in. He was also extremely conscious of his surgical scar and always wore a baseball cap to conceal it. I was struck by his relatively sheltered life history, especially in later years, and limited life experiences (e.g., lack of independent living skills). I was also conscious of the strong family culture of "effort always brings success" and the absolute importance of "positive thinking", which I sensed Carlos had inherited from his father in particular, yet had not actually had to validate for himself. It was clear that his father was an extremely influential figure in his life. Finally, Carlos's parents, sister and girlfriend were essentially his key sources of support for, although he had a large network of friends, it was apparent that these people came to him for support and advice, rather than the other way round.

Why did the above observations of Carlos come to my attention? I have learnt that I often do not attend to that which is similar to me, but will comment on contrast. So, whilst the above is not intended as a value judgement in any way, many of the points raised contrast with my sense of who I am as a person and my life story.

CARLOS'S INJURY

The medical account

In April 1998 Carlos was out playing golf with his father when he experienced a headache and sudden onset of confusion and aphasia. He was taken a local hospital, where a CT scan showed a large left temporo-parietal haemorrhage. Following transfer to his local neurosurgical hospital he underwent an emergency craniotomy for evacuation of the haematoma. A subsequent angiogram showed an arterio-venus malformation, which was removed surgically. He was discharged home after a few weeks with community speech and language therapy.

Carlos's account

Below are Carlos's (C's) descriptions of the time immediately after his injury:

C: Well, I wasn't . . . I wasn't really sure what had just happened . . . I don't know I was . . . I was . . . I was noticing that I couldn't talk properly . . . and I was . . . I was noticing that I couldn't walk . . . I couldn't walk properly, so I wasn't really sure what had just happened . . . and I was hoping that everything was gonna be alright . . .

Int: How did you notice that you couldn't talk properly?

C: Well, because people were . . . like my parents . . . were all . . . all they were doing was asking me the names and I was saying "Arsenal" and I thought "there's something wrong with that" . . . then . . . and when my girlfriend was asking me things like "How are you?" and inside I knew what to say, but I didn't know how to . . . actually say it . . .

Int: How . . . how did that make you feel?

C: Well, really, really, really, really bad because there wasn't any . . . I couldn't understand what had happened, why it happened to me . . . what have I done? . . . And could it get better? Maybe it was up to me, maybe it was up to someone else if . . . ?

Int: Up to you or up to someone else?

C: Oh, I don't know . . . whatever I had wrong with me . . . if someone knew how to teach me then would it . . . make me . . . OK . . . ? Make me go to a 100% right or . . .? If there's some . . . is it up to me to learn things to . . . to go back to how I was before or could people make me go back to how I was before or is there things that they can't do, it's just up to me or is . . . or is up to my own . . . brain . . . ?

When he returned home Carlos reports having been relieved to be back in his familiar surroundings and to have his family and girlfriend around him. The "World Cup", community speech and language therapy at home two to three times a week and "homework and stuff" featured highly in the subsequent weeks prior to his admission to the WNRC in July 1998.

FIRST ADMISSION TO THE WNRC

Carlos was admitted to the WNRC for the first time in July 1998 and attended as an out-patient on a daily basis for an initial 6-week block. During this time he received daily speech and language therapy (approximately 2 hours), daily physio-therapy, regular occupational therapy (i.e. three times a week) and screening by a trainee clinical neuropsychologist. The remainder of his admission was graded. Thus, from September to December 1998 he attended twice-weekly on an outpatient basis and from January 1999 through to the end of February on a once-fortnightly basis. Whilst he initially received input from a number of different disciplines, this diminished over time. He eventually was receiving primarily speech and language therapy with periodic monitoring of his physical exercise routine from his physiotherapist.

My philosophy and preferred model of therapy

As a speech and language therapist I work very much within a life participation model of therapy. Consequently, I have welcomed the integrated framework for therapy recently devised by Byng, Pound, and Parr (2000). This framework depicts the multidimensional nature of aphasia and the different levels and types of therapeutic input that can comprise aphasia therapy. The framework proposed by Byng et al. (see Figure 12.1), aims to meet the overarching goal of promoting healthy living with aphasia together with choice and autonomy. Within this, however, six main inter-connected subgoals of therapeutic intervention in aphasia are described. These subgoals are derived from a number of sources, including therapeutic tradition, the principles of the social model of disability and current developments in healthcare policy. The six specific goals of intervention include enhancing communication, identifying and dismantling barriers to social participation, adaptation of identity, promoting a healthy psy-chological state, health promotion/illness preven-tion and self-actualisation.

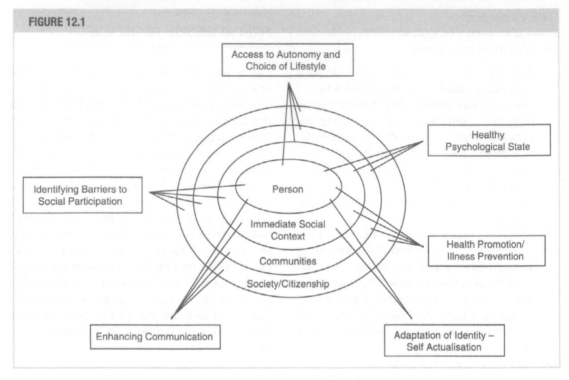

FIGURE 12.1

Living with aphasia: Goals of intervention (Byng et al., 2000).

The interconnectedness of the model is of significance as different goals may be addressed at the different levels of social functioning depicted. Thus, the goal of enhancing communication may be tackled directly with the individual, with their immediate communication partners, with the different communities and institutions the individual belongs to and at a broader societal level through advocacy and education. The interconnectedness of the goals, however, results in one major goal providing a means of addressing another. So, it follows that enhancing communication, for example, may in itself be the major goal of intervention, or may be a means of addressing the breaking down of barriers to social participation or adaptation of identity, etc. This framework will be used to organise assessment findings, intervention, and outcome of Carlos's first block of therapy at the WNRC.

ASSESSMENT FINDINGS ON INITIAL ADMISSION

Communication

When Carlos came to the WNRC his communication skills were his primary concern. His description of these included "not being able to understand all of it, but most of it", "not being able to speak properly", "taking ages to read one page" and "difficulty with some spellings". Formal and informal language assessment revealed moderate receptive aphasia and moderate expressive aphasia characterised by marked word-finding difficulties and agrammatism, moderate dyslexia and dysgraphia.

Social participation

On admission to the WNRC Carlos reported preferring his own company. He had narrowed his social circle down to his family, girlfriend and a couple of close friends and reported even avoiding conversations with them because of "not being able to say everything" he wanted to. He rarely left his house and then only when accompanied, spending much of his time trying to watch television, listening to music and weight lifting in the garage. His university course was being held open for the following year. Carlos had tried to play one game of golf with his father, but had been severely disappointed by the impact that his visual perceptual difficulties had had on his game. He was also unable to drive, which was another major concern for him.

The Becker's Assessment Scales of Handicap Relative's Questionnaire (now the Brain Injury Community Rehabilitation Outcome Scales—BICRO) completed by his parents on admission showed a pre-injury score of 77 as compared to a post-injury score of 126. Changes for the worse were noted in all areas (i.e. independence, activities, relationships and emotional behaviour).

Adaptation of identity
Analysis of Carlos's in-depth interview carried out in May 2000 revealed that immediately after his injury Carlos was primarily concerned by his physical disabilities, which conflicted directly with his view of himself as a sportsman:

C: I saw ... I saw myself ... sitting in a wheelchair and I thought "what is this? I'm not supposed to be in a wheelchair ... 'cos I'm supposed to be the guy who walks and plays football, so why am I in a wheelchair?"

His good physical recovery brought about new dilemmas as Carlos struggled to make sense of the hidden nature of his communication disability, however:

C: I haven't got my legs back how it used to be, but at least I can walk and I look ... if people look at me they think that it's ... that I look normal, so it's just my speech is not 100% still ... from ...

Int: Looking normal ... how important is that for you?
C: I don't know ... before I used to think it's ... it's good because then people just don't ... don't kn ... know that there's something wrong with you, but at the same time it's not good when ... when people look at me they think that I'm normal and then if I start talking and not talking properly then people ... the first thing people think is "what's wrong with him? What ... ?" They just ... they just say "weirdo". You know what I mean, it's like, you can't ... it's just ... "is he stupid or something?" So ... it's like, when I see people that ... who can't talk properly, but they ... they can't even like walk properly, then people really realise because they can't ... walk properly, then they can't talk, then it's the same thing, there's something wrong must have happened to them, but if they see me walking properly, running properly and then I can't talk and they probably think "what's wrong with him?"

This dilemma resulted in high avoidance of speaking situations and masking of his communication difficulties.

Of further concern to Carlos was the impact that his aphasia had on his ability to speak Spanish. Whilst both English and Spanish had initially been similarly affected, Carlos reported his English to be progressing at a rate that was significantly faster than his Spanish. Carlos would often refer to feeling increasingly frustrated with his sister's lack of interest in speaking Spanish at home with his parents. He compared this directly to his wanting to, but no longer being able to do so.

Psychological state
Whilst superficially Carlos generally tried to put up a good front and always presented with a big smile, it is apparent that internally he was struggling with many strong emotions:

Int: How did that make you feel inside?
C: Really, really bad 'cos ... it just get ... I just get really, really ... it's just not the same way

as I . . . as I used to be before . . . why is that? Why is it not like that? So, I kept remembering what's . . . was before . . . and now . . . before and now and which one is better? I would say before and why is it not like that and what have I done? And hoping that it would be like it was before . . . I used to get really angry . . .

Int: How would that show itself?

C: 'Cos I . . . I used to . . . argue with my parents a lot and sometimes just . . . just get angry . . . and just cry or something . . . a lot of crying (laughs)

Int: You're laughing . . . ?

C: 'Cos I'm so embarrassed . . . so much crying that I never used to do . . . you know, I'm like a girl now (laughs)

His parents also described Carlos as "unhappy" at this time, which they attributed primarily to his not being able to drive. They also made reference to his frustration and loss of faith due to his slow rate of progress in relation to his communication as compared to his physical recovery.

Autonomy and choice of lifestyle

Not being able to drive and the prospect of having to rely on his family, girlfriend and friends for lifts symbolised to Carlos his change in social status and lack of independence. He was also preoccupied with the fact that were he to return to university in September 1999 as he planned, he would be a year behind his friends. He frequently referred to "life being on hold" and "being left behind".

INTERVENTION

Interdisciplinary

I was Carlos's allocated chairperson during this first admission, which gave me two roles; overall co-ordinator of his rehabilitation process and his primary speech and language therapist. A summary of Carlos's goals during his first admission is given below.

Initial goals

- Carlos will have an established plan to structure his year off from September 1998 to July 1999 (including a combination of study, exercise, leisure and social activities) in preparation for his return to university in September 1999
- Carlos will have a 45-minute conversation with a familiar person, taking equal responsibility for keeping the conversation going (i.e., 50:50) as demonstrated by self/other report
- Carlos will have identified ways of explaining his communication difficulties to both familiar and unfamiliar people and dealing with their different reactions
- Carlos will have an established a healthy eating and sleeping routine.

Midway admission goals

- Carlos will give a 10-minute presentation on a topic of his choice to members of staff
- Carlos will read the sports section and at least two main articles in a newspaper once a week
- Carlos will self-correct 50% of his errors when writing and be using external aids and support to correct the rest.

Speech and language therapy

Carlos received speech and language therapy on both an individual and a group basis as well as in conjunction with other members of the team (e.g., OT, physio), his family (e.g., parents and sister) and friends. Sessions took place either in the Centre or in local community settings (e.g., Pizza Express, pubs, a local bowling alley). In addition, self-directed work was carried out on a regular basis (e.g., worksheets, reading and writing assignments, supported and unsupported community visits).

Carlos had clearly found his early impairment work beneficial in terms of raising his awareness of the extent of his aphasia:

Int: How helpful was speech therapy at home during that time?

C: I found it really helpful because all the little things that I didn't know that I didn't know . . . it was bad when I found out "Oh, my god, I can't even . . . I can't even say what a cat means . . ." It was bad, but at least I knew that I need help for even . . . at little things like that . . . do you know what I mean?

However, it is also apparent that for Carlos such work was reminiscent of school and highlighted to him the fact that his language levels were now similar to that of a younger child:

Yeah, it was like . . . it was like after hospital I have to go back to "homework" . . . I don't know, it was like . . . I had to . . . had to learn stuff like this and I had to do it, so . . . didn't like it obviously, but I had to do it and I didn't . . . the reason why I didn't like some of it as well is because it looked so easy, but it wasn't easy, you see what I mean? Just little words like cat and dogs and stuff . . . to me just looking at myself doing homework to do with cats and dogs and that's like . . . that's a joke and the thing is I'm thinking why am I . . . why do I have to do this now? I'm like 20, so why am I doing this stuff? And reading all those books . . . the fact that I couldn't read like when I was like what . . . ? One. Oh, man . . . it's just stupid things like that . . .

An overview of the therapy is detailed in Table 12.1 below, using the framework for living with aphasia therapy interventions proposed by Byng et al. (2000).

Avoidance reduction therapy

In addition to my work at the WNRC I also work part-time at the City Lit, an adult education institute that houses a national centre for adult stammering therapy. The majority of the work takes place in groups and the courses offered are based on Van Riper's Block Modification therapy (Van Riper, 1973) and Sheehan's Avoidance Reduction approach (Sheehan, 1970, 1975). Simply stated, the introductory courses enable clients to gain a greater understanding of the overt and covert aspects of their stammering, to work

towards becoming more desensitised and more open about stammering (requiring a reduction of avoidance strategies) in order to reveal their core stammering pattern and, thus, learn how to modify it and "stammer more fluently". Sheehan (1970, 1975) put forward a model of avoidance that was designed to increase people's understanding of the different forms avoidance can take. Practically speaking, this model also provides a useful framework for structuring work on avoidance reduction.

Avoidance reduction therapy in relation to Carlos

There seemed to be a striking mismatch between Carlos's abilities on admission and potential competence in comparison with his level of functioning and actual performance. The cumulative effect of avoidance and the negative consequences of the cycle of avoidance and fear are also well documented (Sheehan, 1970, 1975), so it was anticipated that unless Carlos's avoidance behaviours were tackled directly, they would continue to increase. This was also of primary concern to Carlos's parents, who were well aware of his risk of social isolation and depression. Furthermore, in terms of Carlos's potential for change and capacity to engage in the therapy process, it was going to be necessary for him to be able to take some risks and become more desensitised to his aphasia.

In my early sessions with Carlos I was struck by how often he reminded me of someone with an *interiorised stammering* pattern. This term refers to an individual who is highly sensitive to hearing themselves stammer and, thus, strives to conceal or "interiorise" it. Sheehan's model of avoidance represents an attempt to illustrate the increasingly complex ways in which people who stammer try to conceal stammering in order to maintain an outward appearance of being fluent. Table 12.2 describes how Sheehan's areas of avoidance were applied to Carlos.

Therapy

Initially Carlos was introduced to the concept of his comfort zone, namely the space within which he currently feels comfortable operating. In order for this comfort zone to grow in size, Carlos

TABLE 12.1

Domains and types of therapies targeted in Phase 1 of Carlos's therapy

Enhancing communication	Identifying and dismantling barriers to social participation	Promoting autonomy and choice	Adaptation of identity	Promoting a healthy psychological state	Health promotion & illness prevention
Increasing self-knowledge (i.e., personal strengths, needs, communication strategies)	Avoidance reduction therapy	Developing competence and confidence in return to previous leisure and social activities (e.g., bowling, cinema)	Development of new means of expressing South American roots (e.g., teaching staff to salsa dance)	1:1 and group discussions regarding living with a communication disability, changes, needs	Accessible information about stroke and aphasia (e.g., leaflets, video materials)
Impairment-based therapies (e.g., word finding, syntax)	Graded community assignments (supported and unsupported)	Exploring new leisure interests (e.g., going to a gym)	Expressing opinions in conversation (e.g., Arsenal's performance, golf)	Expressing emotions, opinions re. life, pleasures, losses, hopes etc.	Relatives' group
Reading and writing activities	Conversation group	Developing self-advocacy skills to increase confidence in dealing with challenging situations	Enhanced communication skills and confidence enabling greater participation in family, social and leisure activities	Maintaining connections with previous network of friends	
Developing competence and confidence in conversational skills	Identifying acceptable strategies for explaining aphasia and practising using them across people and situations	Preparation and support re. Step Back to Study programme	Referral to London support group for younger people with aphasia Relatives' group	Accessing new and former interests/roles	
Developing competence and confidence in telephone, internet and email skills	Keyworker support in exploring and accessing "Step Back to Study" programme at the local adult education centre			Education and support for family	
Input to family members, girlfriend and friends through joint sessions, information and training					
Education and provision of accessible information to tutors at local adult education centre					

was introduced to the idea of risk-taking, that is stepping outside of his comfort zone in order to test out his fears. This can be done in a hierarchical way, which involves identifying people and speaking situations that are just outside the perimeter of the comfort zone as compared to those further away. Consideration of the differences between Carlos's pre- and post-injury lifestyles quickly enabled him to identify that there were many changes that needed to be made in

TABLE 12.2

Sheehan's areas of stuttering avoidance as applied to Carlos's difficulties with aphasia

Level of avoidance	Explanation in relation to stammering	Relevance in relation to Carlos
Word level avoidance	This is when someone anticipates stammering on a word and therefore changes it for another word (e.g., asking for "lager" instead of "bitter" or introducing themselves by another name, not their own)	Carlos would avoid saying any word he anticipated difficulty with, even if he was able to successfully achieve partial retrieval or total retrieval on rehearsal
Speech level avoidance	This is when a person is in a situation and chooses to stay quiet because they do not want their stammering to be apparent (e.g., staying quiet in a discussion or meeting)	In conversation Carlos kept all contributions to a minimum, avoiding saying anything where at all possible in all situations across all communication partners
Situation level avoidance	This is when someone avoids going into a situation at all because of their concerns about stammering (e.g., they do not go out for a meal or make a phone call)	Carlos avoided most speaking situations and had narrowed down those he was willing to enter into to either in the home or therapy settings
Relationship level avoidance	This occurs when an individual does not involve themselves in certain relationships because of feelings about stammering (e.g., intimate relationships, friendships in general, relationships with authority figures)	Carlos had narrowed down his conversational partners to his immediate family, therapists and a small group of close friends. All other friends, acquaintances and unfamiliar people were avoided
Feelings level avoidance	This might involve not letting other people know about what you feel about stammering or alternatively can relate to cutting yourself off from your own feelings as a way of protecting yourself	On admission Carlos had significant difficulty verbalising his emotions with anyone. His parents in particular were concerned by his frequent withdrawal to his bedroom in either anger or distress and absolute reluctance to discuss this with them at a later time
Role level avoidance	This relates to not wanting to take on the role of someone who stammers. It is about not wanting others to see or know about this aspect of yourself through trying to adopt the role of a fluent speaker. It is probably the most fundamental and pervasive aspect of avoidance	Carlos was struggling to conceal his aphasia from everyone and thereby present as "normal". A concrete example related to his refusal to take off his baseball cap for fear of people seeing his surgical scar

relation to his home situation, relationships with his family and friends and ability to participate in his former leisure and social activities before tackling return to study.

Goal planning became an integral part of Carlos's therapy and provided a means of actively engaging him in the therapy process, both in terms of driving the therapy, but also in terms of evaluating its success (McIntosh & Sparkes, 1997; McMillan & Sparkes, 1999). Initially, however, Carlos strongly equated a "therapist" with a "teacher". He expected that therapy/rehabilitation would involve being told what to do, doing it, being evaluated by the "teacher/therapist" and then being told how he had fared. Thus, engaging in a partnership model of therapy, being given responsibility for directing aspects of the therapy process himself and evaluating its usefulness were alien concepts for Carlos. Attention, therefore, needed to be given to this process in order to facilitate his development of the necessary skills.

Table 12.3 describes some of the different therapy tasks carried out with Carlos in relation to each of the levels of avoidance.

OUTCOME

The outcome of all speech and language therapy intervention will be described within the framework of Byng et al. (2000; and see Figure 12.1). Avoidance reduction therapy will then be focused on more specifically as it played such an integral part in Carlos's therapy.

Communication

Formal assessment
Formal assessments completed at the beginning of therapy were re-administered. A comparison of results can be found below in Table 12.4. At a single word level, Carlos now demonstrated increased semantic knowledge with more noticeable gains in concrete as opposed to abstract concepts. Significant gains were also apparent in both oral and written naming skills. At a sentence

level there was evidence of increased verbal comprehension skills, although the test completed was clearly insufficiently sensitive to reflect his true abilities. More noticeable gains were apparent in Carlos's written comprehension skills at a sentence level. On admission, the written version of the TROG was not carried out due to having to abandon written single word assessments (e.g. PALPA 49: Written Synonym Matching). Thus, successful completion of this assessment on discharge indicates changes in reading ability, as well as overall confidence. It is anticipated that these results reflect therapy-related gains (e.g. spoken and written word-finding) as well as spontaneous recovery.

Informal assessment
Informal assessment included analysis of spoken and written discharge self-report, language sample and discourse analysis (picture description, conversation about football), conversation skills rating scale, confidence rating scale and parents' spoken and written discharge self-reports. These assessments reflected gains in Carlos's understanding of aphasia in general and his own strengths/needs in particular; his actual language and conversational skills; overall self-confidence and openness with familiar people.

Social participation
By the end of therapy, Carlos had resumed all of his previous social and leisure activities. He frequently went out with groups of friends for meals, to bars or clubs, to go bowling or to the cinema. Whilst he still preferred being with people who he was more familiar with, he was beginning to enter into short exchanges with people he did not know (e.g., friends of friends). On discharge he only reported avoiding speaking situations involving extended exchanges with unfamiliar people or acquaintances he had not seen regularly since his injury.

Carlos had resumed playing golf with his father on a regular basis and, whilst still frustrated by the impact his visual-perceptual difficulties had on his game, was able to recognise steady improvements. He had beaten his father on a couple of occasions. He had also resumed playing

TABLE 12.3

Different therapy tasks for different levels of avoidance (after Sheehan, 1970–1975).

Levels of avoidance	Therapy tasks and activities
Avoidance reduction at the word level	*Go for the word* Carlos set himself the goal of attempting all words he anticipated difficulty with in the presence of the therapist in the first instance. Experience of success enabled him to transfer this hierarchically to conversations with his girlfriend, parents, close friends, etc. Joint sessions with Carlos and his girlfriend, parents and close friends enabled Carlos to explain to them what he was trying to do, why and how they could support him (e.g., through giving him time, feedback, etc.) in order to prepare them in advance. *What I can do when I get stuck for a word?* Carlos was given information about different compensatory strategies and identified those most acceptable to him. He was subsequently encouraged to problem solve which approach would be most useful when he experienced difficulty recalling a word in conversation. *Video analysis* When Carlos became more confident with the above he agreed to being videoed talking to the therapist in order to analyse the video and see how he came across to other people in conversation. This increased Carlos's awareness of the strategies he was skilfully employing to compensate for his word retrieval difficulties and also validated his many strengths as a communicator. *Impairment work* As Carlos became more willing to engage in extended conversations, he expressed a desire to work directly on his vocabulary knowledge and word retrieval skills. He therefore identified key topics of conversation relating to his principal communication partners and researched the vocabulary he wanted to target in subsequent impairment level therapy (e.g., father – football, golf; friends – music, cars, weight training, clubbing)
Avoidance reduction at the speech or "conversational" level	*Increasing speaking opportunities* Graded assignments were negotiated with Carlos to increase his opportunities for sharing his views and experiences. These included a regular "chat" slot at the beginning of each session, supported community assignments (e.g., lunch at Pizza Express, salsa lessons which Carlos gave to his SLT and physio), less supported assignments (e.g., meals out with his girlfriend and/or parents) and attendance to a conversation group. *Exploration of fears about speaking out* Carlos was asked to describe the extremes of his concerns about speaking out and to imagine the worst consequences. Evidence for this was sought in relation to Carlos's past experiences in order to challenge the probability of their occurring and practical strategies explored should they ever arise. For example, different ways of explaining his aphasia were initially discussed and then consolidated through worksheets and role play.
Avoidance reduction at the relationship level	*Drawing up a people and speaking situation hierarchy* As above

	Independent assignments As above. Examples included meeting up with friends he had not seen since his injury individually in the first instance, meeting up with a *small group* of *close friends* initially, phoning someone on his university course to wish them happy birthday, but giving himself permission to *keep the conversation short*, using public transport *on his own* to get to the WNRC, going shopping *on his own* for a CD, etc.
Avoidance reduction at the feelings level	*Creating opportunities to explore feelings as situations arose* Over time Carlos became more open to disclosing and discussing his feelings about his communication disability and the impact this had on his lifestyle and relationships. Space was always given to this when it occurred in addition to encouraging Carlos to access other means of emotional expression on a more regular basis (e.g., personal journal keeping, personal counselling). *PCP approaches* Self-characterisation was a method employed to assist Carlos's exploration of the impact of his aphasia. Comparison of successive self-characterisations over time also provided him with a means of plotting change. *Joint sessions with Carlos and his parents* Joint sessions gave Carlos and his parents a forum to discuss the impact of Carlos's aphasia on their relationships and the home situation. Reasons behind his mood swings and anger outbursts were therefore discussed and strategies to increase open lines of communication identified.
Avoidance reduction at the role level	*Conversation group* The conversation group provided Carlos with a peer group with which to discuss issues pertaining to living with a communication disability. It comprised a group of people of all ages with either aphasia, dysarthria and/or cognitive-communication difficulties. *Referral to the support group for young people with aphasia* As few people attending the WNRC at the time of Carlos's admission had aphasia and none were his age, he was referred to a support group for young people with aphasia based at the City Dysphasic Group (City University, London) and subsequently at Connect, the communication disability network. It was felt that this would provide him with access to other young people in the process of reconstructing their lives in the context of aphasia.

football with friends on a weekly basis and playing pool. In addition, he was planning a 2-week holiday abroad with a good friend in the summer. He had joined a local gym and was working out several times a week in addition to teaching some of his friends how to salsa.

Carlos was reading a newspaper regularly on discharge and had just started reading his first book. He had also re-established contact with a pen pal in Spain and had resumed letter writing to family members in South America. Finally, Carlos was very proud of the fact that an email he had sent in to a football programme had been shown on TV.

The Becker's Assessment Scales of Handicap Relative's Questionnaire (now the Brain Injury Community Rehabilitation Outcome Scales; BICRO), completed by his parents on discharge, showed a post-injury score after therapy of 90 as compared to a post-injury score of 126 on admission and a pre-injury score of 77. Positive changes from the beginning of therapy were noted in all areas (i.e., independence, activities, relationships and emotional behaviour).

TABLE 12.4

Comparison scores on formal tests

Instrument	Pre-assessment	Post-assessment
PALPA 47: Spoken Word–Picture Matching	36/40 (all errors close semantic)	39/40 (error was close semantic)
PALPA 50: Spoken Synonym Matching	40/60 (24/30 HI; 17/30 LI)	47/60 (28/30 HI; 19/30 LI)
Test of Reception of Grammar (Auditory)	75/80	80/80
PALPA 48: Written Word–Picture Matching	39/40 (error was close semantic)	40/40
Test of Reception of Grammar (Written)		80/80
PALPA 53: Spoken Naming	14/40 (semantic errors, phonological errors and approximations)	30/40 (semantic errors, phonological errors and approximations)
PALPA 53: Written Naming	20/40 (semantic errors and regularisations)	36/40 (one semantic error and three regularisation errors)

Adaptation of identity

Attending the WNRC had given Carlos access to other people with experience of brain injury, which he indicated had been helpful for him:

It wasn't meeting them, it was just seeing them 'cos . . . that's . . . you know, it was making me feel that I wasn't the only one 'cos I . . . I mean never in my life had I heard about strokes and aphasia and dysphasia and all this . . . words like that and then when you come to a place like this you see all these people that watching TV and being in wheel-chair and you listen to them talking and they can't talk properly, then it just makes me feel that it wasn't just me then. I'm not like the only . . . the only person who . . . who is like that . . . the only person who . . . who sounds different . . . and I think that's better. That makes me feel better.

On discharge Carlos had clearly gained a greater understanding of aphasia in general and his own aphasia in particular, thus enabling him to explain it to others more clearly. He was continuing to struggle with the hidden nature of his communication disability, however, and in some situations still preferred to conceal his aphasia.

Psychological state

Both Carlos and his parents reported a reduction in mood swings on discharge and a significant decrease in arguments at home. Carlos's increased community access and self-occupation was also identified as reducing instances of boredom. Emotionally, however, Carlos was still struggling to reconcile himself with a number of longer-term consequences of his injury. The first related to his aphasia and the second related to his visual perceptual difficulties and inability to drive. It was shortly before his discharge from the WNRC that Carlos had been informed of the unlikeli-hood of his ever being able to drive again due to the poor prognosis of his vision. This coincided with his younger sister passing her driving test and being given his car to drive. In addition, Carlos was beginning to face the reality of all of his friends finishing university a year ahead of him.

Autonomy and choice of lifestyle

Carlos had started using public transport during his admission to the WNRC, which significantly increased his community access. He also reported greater willingness to go shopping on his own or to access the gym independently, for example. Whereas initially he had wanted to be accompanied in order for someone to speak on his behalf, he was now comfortable entering into these situations on his own and did so on a regular basis.

Carlos had commenced a Step Back into Study programme at his local adult education centre as a stepping-stone back to university. This involved him attending mathematics, business and study skills classes three times a week. He had also tried out a couple of visits to his university in order to meet up with old friends and sit in on some lectures. He had found the latter more difficult than he was expecting, however. He was nevertheless consciously beginning to forge relationships with people in the year below him in order to prepare for his return in the September of 1999.

Evaluation of the avoidance reduction therapy

When asked about his therapy during this first admission to the WNRC during his in-depth interview, Carlos highlighted the significance of the avoidance reduction therapy for him, in particular the organisation of the bowling trip:

C: At the time it was really . . . I was like really, really scared . . . but after it . . . then you find it helpful . . . it is helpful, a lot helpful, yeah 'cos you have to get used to it . . . 'cos you have to do that every day . . . every time you go out you have to tell someone, even if . . . even if it's just buying the train card or you know buying little things or if you want to go to a shop, you have to buy something, you have to talk to someone who you don't know, so you have to get used to that . . .

Int: What do you think was the thing that helped you get used to that most . . . ?

C: That . . . having to . . . having to call them and speak to them on the . . . on the thing . . . and it was better doing it on the phone because then they don't see you, so I'm saying

you can just hang up, but I mean if you were talking to someone, what . . . what can you do just run? Of course you can't. So, it's better . . . I think the first time you're going to do that the best thing to do is on the phone . . . you feel better after . . .

Int: What do you think you've learnt from that looking back . . . ? What changed as a result?

C: Like I said that since that . . . now when I go to shops and I'm do . . . buying things and talk to people just to pay for something or . . . I can do that it's no . . . it's not a problem. I can do that, so I feel comfortable with that . . . I don't . . . I don't see anything wrong with that at all and if . . . if . . . there's something that I don't like say whatever I don't really . . . sometimes I don't really care . . . I don't really mind, it's just . . . 'cos now I'm used to that . . . whether I know or not I have to do things like this . . . little things like talking to people I don't know sort of thing. I don't get scared . . . as much . . .

This clearly demonstrates that the avoidance reduction therapy was effective in enabling Carlos to break the negative cycle of avoidance and fear. Through a carefully graded process of testing out his fears Carlos has significantly extended his comfort zone and the speaking situations he is willing to engage in, with positive consequences for his psychological state. It is also evident that Carlos has maintained and built upon these changes since the original block of therapy (July 1998 to February 1999). Importantly, he now has a greater understanding of his communication strengths and is less embarrassed by his aphasia, thus enabling him use his existing skills more readily to maximise his competence across speaking situations. In addition, the explicit hierarchical approach and responsibility given to Carlos to identify the steps in the therapy process have enabled him to make direct links between specific therapy tasks and their impact on other aspects of his life (i.e., how a supported telephone call with the therapist has paved the way to increased confidence in unsupported interactions with strangers). Thus, the relationship between therapy and real life has been made transparent to him.

The in-depth interview also highlighted that the practical, real-life focus had been an important aspect of the therapy for Carlos:

C: Well, 'cos like well you . . . you don't just . . . you don't just learn on your . . . in a rehabilitation centre . . . you can just actually . . . you feel like you're learning like doing normal stuff, like just going bowling . . . just going bowling and actually feeling like you're learning and enjoying it, so I found that . . . helpful . . .

Being able to work on increasing his communicative competence and enjoy himself at the same time is something he has made frequent reference to and, together with the practical real-life focus referred to above, is a common theme amongst other clients I have worked with of this age group. I only have to consider how I was spending my time at his age to appreciate the significance of this. Also, the fact that therapy was focusing on many of the activities he was carrying out before his injury made it easier for him to discuss what he was doing in therapy with his friends and family. The therapy process was, thus, rendered more tangible.

One other significant consequence of the avoidance reduction therapy is that Carlos has become increasingly willing to take risks in therapy and, more importantly, recognises the value of this for himself as risks have been rewarded by tangible evidence of change. This has had important consequences for his ability to engage in the therapy process and experiment with change.

Finally, Carlos made a comment about the importance of the therapeutic relationship and how this can be usefully employed in avoidance reduction therapy:

C: I don't know, it's like sometimes you're doing it with someone that you feel comfortable with . . . sometimes like . . . like . . . I don't know how to say that . . . basically you'll . . . you'll be doing . . . you'll be doing normal stuff . . . things that . . . that normal people do while at the same time learning from it . . .

the . . . the while at the time you're not like . . . really bothered about it . . . you're not really worrying about it, you know what I mean . . .

Int: And one of the reasons . . . you said something about being with someone you that feel comfortable with . . . ?

C: Yeah, someone you feel comfortable with . . . someone . . . it's like sometimes when you're with friends it's like . . . you're with friends and you go somewhere . . . someone who you've known like for years and stuff and you've gone somewhere . . . to this like . . . places like . . . normal places . . . well, places that everyone else goes, normal places, yeah . . . it's like if you don't want to say . . . if you're thinking of what to say, then you have to think about it first and if you can't say it then don't say . . . don't say it at all . . . whilst if you go with someone who teaches you and who you feel comfortable with . . . and you go to somewhere like a place like this like . . . you feel normal . . . you feel like you used to be and you don't mind what you say in front of them 'cos it's like . . . I'm saying it doesn't bother you, you know . . .

This illustrates how we developed an alliance that enabled Carlos to gain experience of feeling at one with his aphasia in a real-life setting. This gave him tangible evidence that his aphasia did not have to be a barrier to social participation.

My reflections on Carlos's first phase of therapy

Carlos had clearly made some significant changes at a lifestyle level during his first admission and on discharge was equipped with a structured plan to work towards his overall goal (i.e., to return to his university course) and an identified professional support network (i.e., referral back to his previous community speech and language therapy and access to a young person's support group). However, in spite of this, in my opinion, Carlos was still very vulnerable when he left the WNRC due to his ongoing belief in his overriding restitution narrative (Frank, 1995).

Referring him on had been a difficult process

for me. The fact that all the other team members had gradually withdrawn from his management during his admission had resulted in my becoming his sole advocate at that time. I was indeed very fired up about his case, which my supervisor often commented on when I brought him up in sessions. I had a strong belief in his potential, however felt that he would need ongoing, long-term support in order to realise this, which within the current UK National Health Service is all too frequently not available. When I look back, I can see that Carlos had brought out my own restitution narrative as a therapist at that time and a desire to ensure that he received the optimum service available over as long a time frame as possible. However, my anxiety and sense of urgency resulted in my not fully attending to issues pertaining to the timing of therapy in the context of Carlos's overall adjustment to living with aphasia.

As I was the only therapist involved in Carlos's case on discharge, this led to him only being referred on for further speech and language therapy. In retrospect this gave Carlos a clear message that it was his communication that presented the sole barrier to his return to study. It also left his community speech and language therapist working with him and his family in isolation. Whilst we regularly liaised on the telephone over subsequent months, it was apparent that she felt a tremendous sense of responsibility at having inherited this role of principal advocate, mirroring my feelings on Carlos's discharge. Interestingly, Carlos also appeared to be appealing to her restitution narrative.

CARLOS'S JOURNEY FOLLOWING THE WNRC

The young person's support group
Carlos commenced a young person's support group just prior to his discharge from the WNRC. It differed from the groups that Carlos took part in at the WNRC as only young people with aphasia attend. Whilst Carlos was initially reluctant to go along, this group has proved to be an invaluable source of support for him:

I really . . . I found . . . really . . . I found that really, really, really helpful . . . going there just to be with people who've had what you've had, so . . . you don't have to . . . you don't have to . . . hide . . . you don't have to fake . . . you don't have to show like there's nothing wrong with you and . . . places like this there's something wrong with you and "so what!" . . . people know and same thing has happened to them, worse things have happened to them and stuff, so it's . . . so I find that really eas . . . really helpful.

Carlos reported feeling very different in this group from the groups at the WNRC, where other group members had a variety of communication difficulties (e.g., dysarthria or cognitive-communication difficulties)

C: Everyone else could talk . . . they were like . . . I think there was a couple who were in a wheelchair, but like they sounded normal . . .
Int: Normal . . . ?
C: As in normal . . . as in how normal people talk . . . they talk . . . whatever they want to say they say and they know how to say it . . .
Int: So, it sounds like you didn't really feel like you fitted in . . . ?
C: Yeah . . . being the only one who can't talk properly . . .

The importance of a peer group with which you can clearly identify is well documented; however, its significance at the age of 20 is not to be underestimated. Clearly for Carlos the similarity of the communication disability was more important than similarity of age.

Community speech and language therapy
Carlos returned to his previous community speech and language therapist in order to continue working towards resuming his university course. Following his discharge from the WNRC, Carlos's attendance at the Step Back to Study programme at his local adult education college became increasingly erratic and he eventually chose to give it up. His reasons were as follows:

The maths I found it really, really, really easy 'cos it was all GCSEs and that was just numbers and I find that very, very easy . . . business I found that really difficult, but then again the thing is I never did business I was . . . always doing economics, so I wasn't sure if it they were completely different . . . the other one just all reading . . . and reading with people and in groups and stuff . . . that I don't know . . . I really found that . . . difficult and uncomfortable because being with normal people who go to college who know how to read and know how to explain things . . . so that I was sort of I was really scared doing stuff with them.

In hindsight he was able to reflect on the timing of this attempt to return to college and his readiness for it:

Int: Looking back on it now what do you think would have helped make that experience easier?

C: I don't know . . . I . . . I just don't . . . maybe I shouldn't have gone, so . . . so close to when I left the hospital. I should have waited bit longer before going to college straight away . . .

Int: Did you think that at the time or do you think that's something you realise looking back?

C: I think that now . . . not then, 'cos then all I was thinking was like well it doesn't matter, by next year it should be alright, when I go back to university it should be alright, I'm gonna be out of this, so don't worry about it.

Int: So, do you think anyone could have said anything to you at that time that would have put you off college?

C: Yeah, I was told . . . yeah, I was told many times (laughs) and . . . you see if, maybe I should just take a year out, don't go back to college not . . . not yet, but I was . . . just be me . . . wanted to do it and when I want to do things whether people tell me not to do it or not I still do it . . . and I . . . I should have done what they told me to do . . .

It is evident from the above, however, that Carlos was only able to achieve this insight retrospectively through experience of failure. Interestingly, in spite of abandoning his college course due to aspects of it being too challenging for him, Carlos remained determined to trial university in the autumn of that same year and firmly held on to the belief that this was within his capabilities. Thus, he returned to university in September 1999 and described the experience as follows:

I went back to university in the September and I found it so, so, so, so difficult . . . as soon as we went in there we had essays to do, assignments to do . . . and I had lots of it . . . to do with basically reading, reading books and writing and stuff like that, so I found it really, really difficult. We . . . when we were doing marketing in the groups, even like 2 weeks after we started, there was a presentation, which we had to give already . . . I did that and I felt so, so uncomfortable with it . . . and . . . and for that for marketing we had to do like every single week we have to read the whole chapter and summarise it and hand it in, so basically the . . . for the whole months that I stayed there all I was doing was marketing 'cos I couldn't . . . just reading the . . . the . . . chapters that would take me easily . . . each chapter used to be about 60 pages, so that used to take me ages to do it . . . first of all just by reading it first to understand what it actually meant and then write and summarising and stuff. I found it really, really difficult and I had all these assignments in groups or in pairs or . . . I just couldn't . . . I couldn't do it I couldn't really.

It is evident that in spite of ongoing preparation and liaison with Carlos's university on the part of his community therapist in order to establish links with the learning support service, Carlos had not accessed this identified support network when it was needed:

Int: What stopped you from going and asking for help . . . ? From going and saying to them that you were having difficulty?

C: Because ... there was no one else doing that ... no one else in my class was doing that I was ... was ... was the only one who doesn't understand everything. I mean people ... when people don't understand things they go home and study and they understand ... me I didn't understand in the lectures, I got home, tried to understand it, no still don't, try it again, no don't understand and again, no don't ... and then you just ... you just don't want to be the only one who doesn't understand this stupid little thing ...

Thus, Carlos's pride and overwhelming desire not to be seen to be different resulted in him battling the situation out alone and finally withdrawing from university altogether with his father's consent. Thus, aspects of Carlos's personality, his beliefs about disability and his overall independent coping style became barriers to the achievement of his overall goal.

Counselling

It was this decision to leave university that led Carlos to start a period of personal counselling with a trained counsellor at the aphasia centre. Carlos reports this to have been extremely beneficial, not only in terms of giving him a safe space to explore the implications of not having achieved his overall goal and the emotional impact of his injury, but also by providing him with a positive role model, as his counsellor has also had experience of stroke and aphasia:

It's helpful because just ... because I talk whatever I want to talk about ... I mean like sometimes ... some of the stuff that I've talked to him about it's like it's stuff that I ... that I ... that I haven't told people because I ... I haven't wanted to talk to people about it, but then him ... he's like someone who ... a person who ... who's had a stroke and who's ... moved on and been alright and been normal ... then it's ... and that's really, really helped me that's ... you see, look up ... look up to him like and you think ... "that's what I want to do. I want to be like him" ... and I think that's

what helps me ... it makes me ... you know what I mean ... hope that one day I'll be like that see ... that to me helps me ... when I think someone like that ... when I see someone like that then I think seeing as he's done that why can't I? I am going to do that. I can.

The timing of this is also significant. Carlos had been exposed to the idea of personal counselling on many occasions throughout therapy; however, the situation clearly needed to reach crisis point in order for him to make use of this kind of support. Validation from his friends was also important in increasing his receptiveness to counselling.

A new pathway

Having abandoned the idea of a career in business on leaving his business course, Carlos sought to identify a new direction in life. It is apparent from his in-depth interview that the positive role model his counsellor provided him with played an important part in this process, enabling him to entertain the possibility of starting again and recreating a new future. Carlos, therefore, reached a decision to start a different career in sports:

The thing is ... because as I said before the only reason I was doing business was for the money. I never found it interesting ... finance and operations ... I never found that interesting at all ... I want to do something which I like ... I like ... I love ... I love music and I love sports. Now music ... I don't ... don't really know what I could do because my dad was already telling me, "Think about ... I don't know what it's called ... music manager and stuff like that", but I'm thinking that comes back to business, so I'm not gonna ... it's not like I can sing and I can ... I can you know ... it's not like that ... by the way I'm learning to play the guitar now ... something else that I love is sports, so I'm thinking, "well, maybe I can do sports and that's something that whatever I'm gonna be learning that's stuff that I actually do want to learn" ... so, that's why I'm hoping to start in September I'll be doing sports ... something which I find interesting and would want to know about it.

He has gradually undergone a re-evaluation of his priorities in the context of his current capabilities and limitations with evidence of the beginnings of a quest narrative (Frank, 1995) coming to light:

Int: So, your plans then are to try and study sport ... how do you see the future now ... ?

C: I'm not sure, but I was ... was thinking that I ... either be a ... one of those personal fitness instructors or own a gym, don't know, don't know yet ... I think something like that ...

Int: OK, so working as a fitness instructor or owning a gym ... ?

C: Just doing sports stuff ... doing sports stuff ... and own a house ... own a flat ... that's all ...

Int: How do you feel about the fact that that dream has changed to something that's different ... it's no longer business and money, it's more about sport and something you enjoy ... ?

C: As I said it's ... I find that ... it's about the only good thing that I've found from this ... stroke ... the fact that ... I'm actually going to do something that I want to do ... something that I love. I'm definitely not gonna do business and I wanna do sports which is something that I like, so ... may be that's the good thing that's come out of this ... I'm gonna ... I'm gonna be doing something that I like ... and I enjoy.

Thus, through sport Carlos is beginning to make sense of his injury and re-align his past, present and future in order to reconstruct his life map and identify a way of living with his aphasia.

However, it is apparent that during this process Carlos had not fully taken into account the implications of his aphasia for full-time study at degree level. His high ambitions remained and it soon became apparent that Carlos had not entirely abandoned the idea of returning to university. However, instead of studying business, he was now considering a course in sports science. He was confident that this new goal would be attainable

and was having difficulty translating some of the difficulties he had experienced the first time round to this new course (e.g., in relation to the technical aspects of the course):

Int: How different do you think it will be studying business and studying sport at university?

C: I think it will be different definitely ... different ... I've been talking to people who have done sports and I've been hearing that it's so easy ... and it's been really ... not ... not just easy, it's been really ... interesting ... no, it's been a good laugh ... a good laugh.

Re-referral to the WNRC

Carlos's community speech and language therapist made contact to inform me that she was shortly going to be leaving her post. In relation to Carlos, she felt he was particularly vulnerable at that time and was, therefore, keen for him to be considered for re-referral back to the WNRC for ongoing support and intervention. Indeed, her anxieties at this time in many ways mirrored my own when discharging Carlos after his first admission to the WNRC. The same themes were apparent—a strong belief in Carlos's potential, but recognition of the ongoing input this would require over the longer term.

THE SECOND ADMISSION

There are many important differences in the intervention that has been offered to Carlos during this second admission. The first difference relates to the fact that he has attended as part of the Cognitive-Communication Group Programme. Thus, six young adults with mild to moderate cognitive and/or communication difficulties have attended together. Whilst they all have had access to individual therapy, a large focus is given to the group process and working together. Second, his therapy has not just involved speech and language therapy, as the group programme has a strong interdisciplinary emphasis involving primarily occupational therapy, speech and language therapy and clinical neuropsychology. Furthermore, the programme runs for a 24-week period, with clients attending 2 days a week for the first half of the programme and gradually reducing this to 1 day, then once a fortnight over the second half. Thus, dependency on the Centre is minimised and clients are able to increase their level of community participation whilst maintaining links with the staff and support from the group. From the outset this had many obvious advantages for Carlos. He was not going to be working solely with a speech and language therapist, but would have access to a larger team. Also, he would be able to receive the ongoing support, reinforcement and validation of a peer group over a longer period.

Problems on admission

The following are the key issues that Carlos and his family identified during the initial team goal-planning meeting.

Carlos

- "I'm not sure where I'm going with my life"
- "I find it difficult to ask for help"
- "I find it difficult to say when I don't understand"
- "I don't speak properly"
- "I read very slowly and don't understand the big words"
- "I have difficulty spelling words when I'm writing"
- "I'm not confident any more" (e.g., with acquaintances, girls and in groups)
- "I want to go to university to study sports science".

His parents

- "Carlos has no dream that he wants to work for"
- "Carlos has almost given up"
- "Carlos won't help himself"
- "Carlos is more argumentative again now".

The team

- High expectations of potential recovery on the part of Carlos and his parents
- Carlos's ability to identify realistic, future lifestyle goals in the light of past experience

- The potential risk to Carlos's psychological health of another experience of failure.

As a result, the following long-term goals were drawn up with Carlos:

- Carlos will have explored how realistic it is for him to study sports science at university and investigated other training options
- Carlos will have an established means of structuring his week to combine regular self-directed study time with exercise, leisure and social activities
- Carlos will feel more confident talking to his friends at university, acquaintances, girls and in group situations (as determined by a self-rating scale)

My concerns

In retrospect, I now recognise that for the first time I had an increasing number of concerns about Carlos's potential for change. Whilst it felt important to support Carlos's developing quest narrative and to facilitate his move into a career in sport, I was aware that there remained a strong restitution theme in my discussions with Carlos. He was still in search of the "miracle cure" that would render his attendance at the university possible:

> Well, I need help . . . I need help to be ready for university . . . and I need . . . I need more speech and writing and reading . . . and . . . and be with people who've had the same thing as me and . . . be more confident and feel more comfortable and . . . the whole thing . . .

It felt important that this should not get over-looked in our enthusiasm to foster Carlos's quest narrative.

INTERVENTION

Let us briefly reconsider Carlos's situation. Here we have a young man who has received a large amount of input over a 2-year period from a variety of different sources. He had made significant gains at both an impairment and disability level, but was still in a vulnerable position, struggling to achieve an autonomous lifestyle with aphasia. Whilst on the one hand we were confident he would benefit from the Cognitive-Communication Group Programme in particular, as compared with an individual admission, a number of barriers to change were now apparent with regard to Carlos's personality and coping skills and style. A completely different management approach would be needed to enable Carlos to make the necessary identity and lifestyle changes in the longer term—an approach that was not necessarily centred in speech and language therapy, aphasia therapy or even brain injury.

Theoretical background

Recently, as a team we have become increasingly interested in a model of change put forward by Prochaska and DiClemente (1986) and the motivational interviewing techniques described by Miller and Rollnick (1991) in their work with people with addictive behaviours. It is beyond the scope of this chapter to go into either of these approaches in any depth, so the reader is referred to the original texts. Briefly, Prochaska and DiClemente's wheel of change describes six specific stages of change that a person may go around several times before achieving stable, long-term change. Table 12.5 describes three of the stages that were pertinent to Carlos's therapy. The table also describes the therapist's role for the stages as laid out by Miller and Rollnick.

In relation to Carlos it was evident that he was oscillating between the stages of contemplation and determination on his second admission. His overall goal was to return to university to study sports science despite growing evidence that a full-time university degree course was unrealistic for him. This ambivalence became the target of therapy. This therapy was carried out by the full multidisciplinary team and involved the following kinds of activities:

- interdisciplinary assessment was done by each member of the team

- study skills group was co-facilitated by an OT and myself
- carlos attended a workshop in the physiotherapy department for physio assistants to gain insight into the content of his course and experience note taking
- a discussion was held with Carlos to reflect on ways that his aphasia impacted on his ability to resume his business course and the emotional consequences of this
- Carlos was asked to elaborate on the worst case scenario he could face, e.g., a further experience of failure
- he identified specific skills needed to successfully complete his course
- we devised ways with him to test out those skills at the rehabilitation centre
- he identified a goal entitled "Carlos will reach a decision about how realistic it is for him to go to university to study sports science"
- emphasis was placed on Carlos's roles and responsibility for participating fully in therapy sessions, scheduling of sessions and preparation for sessions
- he developed a menu for non-university training options and researched those options to make comparisons
- he developed strategies for managing his difficulties, e.g., maintaining the focus of his attention on reading for 15 minutes followed by a break enabled him to read for longer periods
- focus was on self-awareness and researching study options to draw up a profile of the advantages and disadvantages of each option in relation to his specific needs
- he attended a monthly peer support group to obtain access to positive role models.

In order to follow this process cohesively across the team, roles were at times blurred. This has, however, enabled us to consistently integrate the theoretical concepts in the different aspects of our work with Carlos. My dual roles as his chairperson and principal speech and language therapist have led to my moving beyond the traditional boundaries of a speech and language therapist.

TABLE 12.5

Six stages of change as depicted in Prochaska and DiClemente (1986) and associated tasks for the therapist from Miller and Rollnick (1991)

Prochaska and DiClemente stages	*Miller and Rollnick's outline of therapists' motivational tasks for the Prochaska and DiClemente stages*
Pre-contemplation: At this point a person is not yet considering the possibility of change. Before the first time round the wheel the person has not even contemplated having a problem or needing to make a change.	Raise doubt: Increase the client's perception of the risks and problems with their current behaviour. This is in part achieved through the feedback of assessment results.
Contemplation stage: Once some awareness of the problem arises, the person enters a period characterised by ambivalence: the contemplation stage. The contemplator both considers change and rejects it, alternating between reasons for concern and justifications for unconcern.	Tip the balance—evoke reasons to change, the risks of not changing and strengthen the client's self-efficacy for change of their current behaviour. A primary focus is on developing a discrepancy between the client's current behaviour and their broader goals.
Determination stage: From time to time the balance tips and the person begins to make statements indicating motivation for change, such as "I've got to do something about this problem". This stage denotes a window of opportunity.	Help the client determine the best course of action to take in seeking change. This involves drawing up a menu of all of the options available, exploring the pros and cons of each to identify the most desirable option, setting goals and delineating responsibilities.
Action stage: Here the person engages in the particular actions intended to bring about a change.	Help the client to take steps towards seeking change through an ongoing process of goal setting and evaluation, validating self-efficacy.
Maintenance stage: Making a change does not guarantee that the change will be maintained. During the "maintenance" stage, the challenge is to sustain the change accomplished by previous action and prevent relapse. Maintaining a change requires a different set of skills and strategies from those needed to achieve the change in the first place.	Help the client identify and use strategies to prevent relapse.
Relapse stage: If relapse occurs, the individual's task is to move around the wheel again. Slips and relapses are to be expected in any process of change and people need to develop the skills to avoid discouragement and demoralisation.	Help the client to renew the processes of contemplation, determination and action without becoming stuck or demoralised because of relapse.

PRELIMINARY EVALUATION

After 12 weeks of therapy, Carlos reached the action stage of the Prochaska and DiClemente model (1986), having gradually worked through contemplation and determination. Thus, discussions with Carlos and his contributions in the groups have shown a greater understanding of the implications of his aphasia and his cognitive difficulties for his return to study. He also now has a greater knowledge of practical compensatory strategies (e.g., pacing, note-taking, reading comprehension) and the type of support he would benefit from in relation to his return to study (e.g., requesting handouts in advance of the session in order to pre-read, sharing notes with his peers in order to identify any omissions or misinterpretations, specific learning support for reading and understanding more complex concepts). Carlos's increased insight, coupled with having definite study alternatives, has enabled him to reach the decision that a university-based course is now too challenging for him. He fully recognises his need for a part-time course in a centre with a clear commitment to supporting student learning and has found a suitable course on which he is currently enrolling.

This change, however, is not fully established and consistent. Although Carlos has taken action with regard to his decision not to return to university, in many ways he is now starting the cycle of change again in terms of dealing with the consequences of this decision. Thus, whilst his decision can be seen as a significant gain from the point of view of Carlos's journey towards healthy living with aphasia, it has not been without its losses. Carlos has expressed guilt at not fulfilling his parents' dreams of his having a university education and sadness at the loss of the singleton lifestyle he had hoped for at university now that he is no longer with his girlfriend. He is also currently questioning whether he will successfully manage to complete a non-university based training course and is more appreciative of the challenge that this represents. Access to different disciplines and a closed peer group has also enabled Carlos to spread his dependencies and access more varied support throughout this admission.

DISCUSSION

Carlos's case study raises a number of important issues with regard to working with younger people with aphasia. These can be categorised into three groups: issues pertaining to a longitudinal management approach, issues pertaining to an integrated therapy approach and finally issues pertaining to collaborative working across services and disciplines.

Longitudinal approach across the lifespan

The importance of taking a client's entire life history and experiences into consideration has been emphasised in this case study. In my work with Carlos it has been extremely important to have had an understanding of Carlos's pre-aphasic identity. By this I am referring to knowledge of his biography, his personal achievements, his aspirations and prospects pre-injury, an appreciation of his social status, personal attributes, attitudes and beliefs and coping style and strategies. I consider this to be of equal importance to my in-depth knowledge of the dimensions of his aphasia and cognitive-communication difficulties, as it is against these two variables that I have considered his post-aphasic identity, that is, the degree to which his aphasia has impacted upon his lifestyle and his sense of self and the personal significance of these changes. Therapy has, thus, tried to marry these different dimensions in parallel.

At the time of his stroke, Carlos was just beginning to firm up his sense of himself and his aspirations. It is not surprising that Carlos has hung on to his dream of a university education in order to maintain some sense of constancy in all of the chaos and uncertainty. His youth also brought with it advantages that allow him to adapt more flexibly to his new situation.

Attention to Carlos's narratives over time has been an integral part of the therapy. They have been relevant to the assessment process. Carlos's pre-admission assessment for the Cognitive-Communication Group Programme took the form of an in-depth interview, enabling therapy goals to be framed entirely within his reality. Listening to his personal story enabled me to identify the predominant narrative type being used at any given moment, which in turn assisted in determining the most appropriate therapy approach for Carlos. Thus, for example, at times Carlos needed his chaos narrative to be witnessed in order to move forward; alternatively, roles and responsibilities needed to be carefully negotiated in the presence of his restitution narrative and, finally, a broader focus on coping and healthy living with aphasia was employed to facilitate his emerging quest narrative. The ongoing monitoring of Carlos's narratives has also allowed for changes in his predominant narrative type to be observed, variations according to different contexts to be identified and peaks and troughs along the journey to be tracked.

The narrative concept has also been of relevance to me, as Carlos's therapist, and to Carlos's own family. By listening to recurring plots in these story lines, other considerations have been brought to light. Analysing and attending to narratives of all those involved in the therapy process created a more sensitive way of planning and carrying out therapy.

Integrated therapy approach

Carlos's management has upheld the importance of an integrated therapy approach. Speech and language therapy has not only combined impairment and disability approaches to aphasia therapy, but has also used ideas from different fields of thought (e.g. stammering therapy, work with addictive behaviours, the concept of narrative). These approaches have not been employed in a sequential manner (i.e., one after the other). Instead they have been fully integrated simultaneously. Similarly, therapy has integrated task and process work. Specific attention has been given to fostering a productive therapeutic relationship with Carlos with an explicit focus on the balance of power. As highlighted above, this is of particular relevance to Carlos given his age

and limited experience of different models of learning.

Goal planning has also been upheld as a useful way of directly linking therapy with real life. It provides a tangible way of working hierarchically towards broader goals and, in the case of Carlos, was a useful means of making steps in therapy more explicit and giving him greater control in addition to providing a framework for measuring outcome. Similarly, the narrative approach adopted has allowed attention to be given to the different plots and themes over time in order to influence therapy and in turn be influenced by therapy, thus integrating the two. Finally, this case study has also shown the importance of integrating "work" and "play" in the therapy process, not simply in terms of making learning fun, but in terms of incorporating the more diversional aspects of life into therapy (e.g., bowling in Carlos's case). The significance of this for Carlos's age group cannot be overstated.

Collaboration

Carlos's management has illustrated the importance of collaboration across disciplines (i.e., SLT, Psychology, OT, PT) and settings (i.e., acute, community, rehabilitation centre and aphasia centre) over the long term when working with younger people with aphasia. The complementarity of the different services has been apparent, with one or two coming to the fore at any one point in time. Integral to this have been strong lines of communication across the different settings and a clear understanding of each other's services, strengths, roles and boundaries. Carlos's case also brings to light issues to do with the timing of therapy. It has shown the need to consider when intensive rehabilitation is more appropriate as compared to a more graded, gradual approach. It has also shown the importance of collaboration in terms of giving clients access to a broader range of services, such as group therapy and counselling. Carlos, for example, was attending the WNRC and the young person's support group concurrently for a period of time, followed by community therapy, the support group and counselling thereafter.

In addition, this case has shown the importance

of collaborative working with clients, their families and friends. Regular joint and individual sessions with Carlos's family and friends have enabled knowledge to be shared, their active participation in the therapy process to be facilitated and support to be provided. Their influence on the client and the rehabilitation process again cannot be underestimated. Finally, Carlos's case illustrates the importance of an interdisciplinary management approach to young people with brain injury. The shortcomings of his first admission are only too apparent when I consider the valuable contribution of occupational therapy, clinical neuropsychology and physiotherapy at a later date. Examples of this are comprehensive assessment of his cognitive function, information about his psychological state and intervention in relation to the development of sports science study skills and strategies. It would have been only too easy for Carlos's needs to have been identified as solely language-based and for him to have received uni-disciplinary intervention.

FINAL COMMENT

As stated in the Introduction, this case study represents a typical case in a busy clinical setting and I am only too aware that methodologically it is not tight in research terms. Therapy is messy in real life. In many ways Carlos has been an influential client for me and I have learnt many things from working with him. It has reinforced the need to be respectful of a client's life choices and how it is possible to work within these. I have been made aware of the value of being prepared to look to other disciplines and approaches outside of my field to identify the most effective way of facilitating change with clients. Similarly, of the value of being quick to admit when therapy is not working and obtaining support to change direction. Finally, it has confirmed my belief in the value of the narrative concept, not only as a means of listening to clients' life stories and obtaining a fuller understanding of their perspective, but also as a means of becoming more

self-aware of my own narratives as a therapist. For example, I have identified how strong a restitution narrative I have at times, enabling me to become more insightful as to when it is helpful to bring this into the therapy room and when it is not.

REFERENCES

Barrow, R. (2000). Hearing the story. *Royal College Speech Language Therapy Bulletin*, April, 8–10.

Byng, S., Pound, C., & Parr, S. (2000). Living with aphasia: A framework for therapy interventions. In I. Papathanasiou (Ed.), *Acquired neurological communication disorders: A clinical perspective*. London: Whurr.

Clarkson, P. (1995). *The therapeutic relationship*. London: Whurr.

Damico, J., & Simmons-Mackie, N. (1996). *Maintaining impairment in aphasia therapy: The co-construction of deficit via talk-in-interaction*. Paper presented at the International Pragmatics Association Meeting, Mexico City, Mexico, July 1996.

Elwyn, G., & Gwyn, R. (1998). Stories we hear and stories we tell . . . analysing talk in clinical practice. In T. Greenhalgh & B. Hurwitz (Eds.), *Narrative based medicine: Dialogue and discourse in clinical practice*. London: BMJ Books.

Frank, A. (1995). *The wounded storyteller: Body, illness and ethics*. Chicago: The University of Chicago Press

Greenhalgh, T., & Hurwitz, B. (1998). Why study narratives? In T. Greenhalgh & B. Hurwitz (Eds.), *Narrative based medicine: Dialogue and discourse in clinical practice*. London: BMJ Books.

Kay, J., Lesser, R., & Coltheart, M. (1991). *Psycholinguistic assessment of language processing abilities*. Hillsdale, NJ: Lawrence Erlbaum Associates Inc.

Kleinman, A. (1988). *The illness narratives: Suffering, healing and the human condition*. New York: Basic Books Harper Collins.

McIntosh, J., & Sparkes, C. (1997). Goal-setting: Can the process be empowering? *Royal College Speech Language Therapy Bulletin*, December, 9–10.

McMillan, T.M., & Sparkes, C. (1999). Goal planning and neurorehabilitation: The Wolfson Neurorehabilitation Centre approach. In S. Fleminger & J. Powell (Eds.), *Evaluation of outcomes in brain injury rehabilitation*. London: Taylor & Francis.

Miller, W.R., & Rollnick, S. (1991). *Motivational interviewing: Preparing people to change addictive behaviours.* New York: Guilford Press.

Nettleton, S. (1995). *The sociology of health and illness.* New York: Blackwell.

Parr, S., Byng, S., Gilpin, S., & Ireland, C. (1997). *Talking about aphasia.* Buckingham, UK: Open University Press.

Pound, C. (1999). Learning to listen and helping to tell. *Speech Therapy in Practice*, Autumn, 20–21.

Pound, C., Parr, S., Lindsay, J., & Woolf, C. (2000). *Beyond aphasia: Therapies for living with communication disability.* Bicester, UK: Winslow Press.

Prochaska, J.O., & DiClemente, C.C. (1986). Toward a comprehensive model of change. In W.R. Miller & N. Heather (Eds.), *Treating addictive behaviours: Processes of change.* New York: Plenum Press.

Sheehan, J.G. (1970). *Stuttering: Research and therapy.* New York: Harper & Row.

Sheehan, J.G. (1975). Conflict theory and avoidance-reduction therapy. In J. Eisenson (Ed.), *Stuttering: A second symposium.* New York: Harper & Row.

Simmons-Mackie, N., & Damico, J. (2001). Social role negotiation in aphasia therapy: Competence, incompetence and conflict. In D. Kovarsky, J. Duchan, & M. Maxwell (Eds.), *Constructing (in)competence.* Hillsdale, NJ: Lawrence Erlbaum Associates Inc.

Simpson, S. (2000). *Making sense of aphasia and disability: The impact of aphasia on sense of self and identity and factors influencing the reconstruction process.* Unpublished MSc project.

Somers, M.R. (1994). The narrative constitution of identity: A relational and network approach. *Theory and Society, 23*, 605–649.

Stainton Rogers, W. (1991). *Explaining health and illness: An exploration of diversity.* Hemel Hempstead, UK: Harvester Wheatsheaf.

Van Riper, C. (1973). *A treatment of stuttering.* Englewood Cliffs, NJ: Prentice Hall.

13

A case study of a client with mild language problems

Alex Stirling

INTRODUCTION

The chapter describes a client whose aphasia may be considered "mild" in terms of impairment. This type of client may raise issues for the therapist in terms of prioritisation. Perhaps the client with mild impairment is at risk of being neglected within a context of scarce therapy resources for people with acquired communication disability. What factors determine prioritisation? How have prioritisation decisions been affected by the increased recognition of our role in terms of addressing with the person the real-life consequences of aphasia, regardless of severity of impairment?

Two types of therapy are discussed: work on organising discourse, and work on identity. These therapies occurred simultaneously, led by the client. Questions and dilemmas are then raised for readers to consider.

BACKGROUND

B was 23 when I met him, and was half-way through a PhD in the performance arts. He was already a successful performer, having won competitions. He was a friendly, humorous, talkative person, with a wide circle of friends and interests. He seemed to have a great deal of confidence, particularly about his physical appearance, and enjoyed socialising and partying. He was passionately interested in all aspects of the arts, understandably proud of his achievements and (by his own description) very ambitious. He had parents and two siblings. He lived with friends while at university.

B was a very determined person and not afraid of confrontation if he felt it would help him achieve his goals. His mood could alter quickly from despair to elation and he had strong likes and dislikes (with no grey areas in between!).

B was diagnosed with epilepsy at the age of 7. It was caused by a left, benign fronto-temporal brain tumour. The epilepsy became increasingly intractable, so that despite extremely large doses of medication, he was having severe fits every day, with long periods of drowsiness afterwards.

Even though the epilepsy was severe, B appeared to have let it interfere with his life very little. He was fulfilling all his goals, and seemed to be very philosophical about the (few) restrictions placed on his independence. It was a very difficult decision to have the surgery to remove the tumour, but he finally felt that the fits were having an impact on his life that could no longer be tolerated.

B was dyslexic and left-handed. The WADA test, named after its originator, was administered pre-operatively. The test involves injection of intracarotid sodium amobarbitol, which temporarily suspends function of one cerebral hemisphere at a time. The results showed that his language was lateralised to the left side of the brain.

FIRST MEETING

Initial assessment of B's language was on the hospital ward 3 weeks post-surgery. (He was transferred to the Younger Rehabilitation Unit shortly afterwards.)

B was a talkative, lively communicator with a good sense of humour. There was no evidence of receptive difficulties, or delay in processing conversation. His expressive language appeared slightly hesitant, with reduced speed, apparently due to occasional slowness in accessing a word. He was able to access the word without assistance, and with no evidence of circumlocution. He had a wide vocabulary, accessing words like "feasible". Speech quality was normal and prosody was unaffected by the reduced speed.

He immediately expressed his perceived problems with his speech:

I can talk but I can't use difficult sentences

with complicated words in them. I find it hard to think of those difficult words.

In addition, he commented that the thoughts in his brain were "*jumbled*" and that "*my brain feels like cotton wool*". He told me in detail about the nature of his PhD, and his worries that he would now be unable to do some of the tasks.

I can't imagine being able to get up and give a talk at the moment, the thought of it makes me feel sick.

He reported no difficulty reading. Indeed, he felt that his concentration was actually better now than before the operation. He said that he was premorbidly dyslexic, but felt that it had no impact on his ability to process written information, other than his needing more time to do so.

B felt that it was much easier to write the complicated sentences that he needed, rather than speak them. He said that he had some spelling difficulties with the dyslexia, but that he managed very well using the spell check on his computer. He showed me the letter he had been writing, which was very well-formed syntactically. The few spelling errors were phonological in nature.

ASSESSMENT

B expressed a great deal of anxiety regarding formal assessment. He had found the pre-operative psychometric assessment very threatening, and was concerned that his anxiety would prevent him doing justice to himself. I attempted to reassure him that the purpose of the assessment was to help us both "pin down" the things to work on together that would be relevant for him. We agreed that the aims of the assessment would be to have a more detailed look at his occasional difficulty in finding words, and attempt to discover the reasons why he was finding it difficult to express himself verbally. While reassurance was partially successful, it was nevertheless preferable to limit the formal assessment as much as

TABLE 13.1

Results of formal tests administered to B prior to therapy

Test	Score	Comments
Palpa Naming Test	39/40	1 semantic paraphasia (screw for nail). He was slow to access lower frequency items.
Graded Naming Test	16/30 (average)	B rated his own vocabulary pre-test as "average". While his level of education and spontaneous speech might have suggested an above-average vocabulary, it is possible that the dyslexia could have had a mildly negative effect on his vocabulary acquisition. He was slow to access the items, and showed evidence of word-finding difficulty, including one of the early items, "thimble". He generally provided semantic substitutions, but in one case appeared to have some phonological (as well as semantic) information (for "blinkers" he said "blinds", then "shutters").
Palpa Written Sentence To Picture Match	100%	
Jones Sentence Order Test	100%	

possible. Table 13.1 displays the results of the formal tests given.

B was also asked to tell the Cinderella Story (see Appendix 13.1). Here B showed no real difficulty with verb access, or with complex sentence structure. He was slow to access some of the appropriate items (e.g., pumpkin, coach). He seemed to have mild problems ordering and organising the material and there was a long pause at the beginning, where he seemed to be attempting to marshal his thoughts. However, once he started, it seemed that the familiar story and structure assisted him. He needed to seek reassurance about his performance.

The following conclusions were drawn from the results of the assessment of B:

- he was an excellent and lively communicator
- he had mild word-finding difficulties and slowness in access, apparently resulting from high level semantic problems
- he had no apparent difficulties processing at the sentence level
- there were reported (and mildly evident) difficulties organising his thoughts to translate into verbal output

- he expressed anxiety and lack of confidence about his communication.

THERAPY

B was eager to start some work related to his academic studies, and therefore I felt that it was appropriate to explore his abilities more through this route, which was meaningful to him. I asked him to list the tasks that he would need to perform in a typical week at university, so that we would ensure that we were working on relevant goals. He was able to list these as follows:

- using the telephone to talk to supervisor, colleagues, other staff
- sending and replying to emails
- taking a tutorial for a small group of undergraduates
- talking to his supervisor
- giving lectures (once a fortnight) to a bigger group of students
- presenting to a small group of colleagues

- taking part in a department discussion (small group)
- preparing lectures
- writing long essays for his PhD
- writing letters (rarely)
- reading textbooks.

I began therapy by giving B very short snippets of academic articles, and asking him to tell me what they were about. This was the kind of task that he would need to do when reviewing a journal article for his colleagues or to instruct students.

It was evident that he had no problem comprehending the passages. He was able to answer complex questions and showed he had no difficulty inferring meaning.

However, B did have some difficulty conveying the sense verbally without prompts. Again, he used appropriate syntactic structure but the presentation was somewhat muddled. He often said; *"I don't know where to start"*. And indeed, he would sometimes start with a piece of information that was peripheral, rather than central, to the meaning of the passage. Sometimes he would start with the correct initial idea, and then skip to a point later in the passage, without making a clear link between the segments of discourse.

B would sometimes go back over the sentence he had just said, and attempt to rephrase it, even when it was entirely well constructed the first time. This backtracking interfered with his fluency and communicative effectiveness.

I decided to go back and impose some structure, to see if that aided his performance. A very short passage was selected, which contained only one key idea; he was asked to read it, and use one sentence only (without backtracking) to convey the key idea.

B had no difficulty with this, and we built up to a newspaper article with one key idea, and three or four other points contained within that. Again, he was asked only to verbalise the key idea of the article. Then he was asked to write the other points down in note form, and use those points as a plan to verbalise the whole. I felt that the written points would make it more tangible. With this structure provided B improved very quickly, and he was encouraged to capitalise on his written

ability to help him plan and organise his oral output.

In a task with less structure, he was asked to explain a term or concept that was unfamiliar to me, for example "dat recording", "modal" (working with him on his academic articles gave me endless opportunities for this kind of practice!). He was asked to be as concise as possible. A measure of success was whether I was able to demonstrate that I had comprehended the term correctly. B was always good at tailoring his explanation at the appropriate level.

B began to tackle small amounts of material from textbooks. He was eager to try to plan some lectures for the next year. We agreed that he should start by preparing a short presentation for us on the theme of "current art exhibitions".

B's difficulty in organising his thoughts became apparent in his approach to study. It was immediately obvious that he was unable to work out how to extract the salient information from textbooks; the volume of material overwhelmed him. He seemed to have little idea of how to go about planning or organising the content of the presentation. He also seemed unable to spontaneously generate strategies that might help, for example, taking notes as he read.

We therefore spent a lot of time on work that might be labelled "study skills", and which included:

- brainstorming on paper the key points of the talk
- organising the key points into a logical structure (so for this talk, a chronological order made sense)
- using the index of the book, the chapter headings, and the chapter subdivisions, to identify relevant information
- taking brief notes as he read, rather than trying to remember it later
- generating his own strategies, e.g., brainstorming on paper, with arrows radiating from a central idea (it was important for me to recognise that he needed to use his own strategies, not mine, to be successful)
- deciding the relative importance of the key

points and estimating timing for different parts of the talk

- practising the talk using the outline, and timing it
- practising sending and receiving emails and using the Internet.

OUTCOMES

Language and discourse

B left our unit after 4 months. At that time:

- He was still experiencing the occasional word-finding problem. While usually able to access even the most obscure word, he would occasionally now make a phonemic error, e.g., "*phemonemal* (not corrected); *is it archal type? no, archetype*".
- He felt more able to "organise" his thoughts and his speech, and this was noted spontaneously by his parents.
- He was returning to his academic work with enthusiasm, planning a series of short lectures from books and articles, and using his self-generated strategies as well.
- After one false start, where anxiety made him freeze, he successfully gave a short talk in the unit (using the plan for the talk to be given at his university).
- While his planning had improved, he still had a tendency to backtrack, and had some difficulty with timing.

Identity

There were several aspects of B's former identity that had changed. The first was that he no longer had epilepsy. B had had epilepsy almost all of his life, and it had become an increasingly dominant part of his life.

He also now perceived that another identity, that of "disabled", was being forced upon him. He was in a wheelchair (temporarily) with an unusable right hand (almost certain permanently). B was very aware that the wheelchair and the weak right hand caused society to label him—to impose an identity on him. He constantly

related his amazement at how, for example, people would now ignore him and speak to the person pushing the chair. It seemed the attitude he experienced from others was internalised, causing him to lose confidence and feel self-conscious.

> I feel when I go into a room that everyone is looking at my hand.

While B's new image of himself as disabled was negative, he took a great deal of care in his appearance, and seemed confident in his appeal to the opposite sex.

As B improved physically, he was able to abandon the wheelchair, and thus abandon the label. Indeed, as he recognised this, it was evident that he increasingly set himself apart from the other people in the unit, preferring not to mix with them. His dissociation was evident in a comment he made at a point when he was only using the chair for long distances:

> I feel confident: it doesn't bother me in a chair. Because I feel confident, I go out looking confident, and it doesn't fit with the stereotype of disabled people looking hunched up and sorry for themselves.

Now B was able to relate, with some pride, that he used the wheelchair to jump the queue at a disco, and then to get out of it briefly to dance. He did experience conflicting feelings, however, expressing guilt both at his desire not to be disabled, and at his rapid improvement.

In addition to his awareness of identity change, B also expressed a great deal of anger at the consequences of the operation, the right-sided weakness. There appeared to be a need to assign blame. He angrily claimed on several occasions that he had not been made aware of the possible consequences of the surgery before the operation, and that had he known, he would have refused the surgery. He also said that the reason he was not recovering hand function was that the therapy provided was not enough, or was sub-standard.

There was an apparent idealisation of B's past life, with a temporary denial that this had become so poor in quality (which he was able to recognise at times). It may be that anger arose partly from guilt; it was possibly hard to accept that he chose to have the operation, and perhaps this explained his need to find someone to blame.

A third aspect of his changed identity had to do with his perceived communication difficulties. Communication is obviously a fundamental part of a person's identity. It may be that B's perceived change in communication could not be separated from his perceived identity in general.

Initially, B felt that his speech was "different" and for this reason he avoided certain people and situations. He was also reluctant to confront his perceived difficulties, refusing to be videoed or audio-taped, and finding assessment a threat. He was particularly apprehensive about speaking to people whom he hadn't seen since before the operation. He felt different, and thus he expected them to feel he was different as well.

B was very aware of how his communicative confidence varied dramatically depending on how he felt about a certain communication situation. "I'm fine in here with you." Less structured, and therefore less predictable situations seemed particularly problematic. I observed him confidently ask a librarian to check the email address he had been allocated, but he was unable to say a word to a very chatty taxi driver 10 minutes later.

He often sought reassurance about his output, and "backtracking" was a big feature initially. While it would have been difficult to detect any difficulty in conversational output, B appeared to feel like an "impostor" in conversation; as if he had "got away with it" if he completed a successful interaction.

IDENTITY THERAPY

The following aims for the clinician governed the aspect of therapy concerned with B's identity:

- to encourage him to express his feelings and to acknowledge these feelings
- to identify difficult situations and, most

importantly, the reasons why he found them difficult.

In order to achieve these aims, we had B identify difficult situations. These included:

- speaking to a stranger, face to face
- negotiating with a stranger on the phone (e.g., use of the library)
- seeing a friend whom he had not seen since before the operation
- phoning a friend whom he had not seen since before the operation
- phoning a colleague (who was a rival in the field of composition)
- giving a presentation.

Our therapies involved working on the above goals in situations where he would experience success. B was able to teach me to use the Internet, and I was able to demonstrate to him that he had instructed me clearly.

Much of the therapy involved direct discussion about his difficulties. We explored the beliefs he held about himself and about the attitudes of other people towards him. He was confronted with the contradictions. For example, he was terribly worried about his speech, yet we showed him that one of his friends was amazed that he was having speech therapy.

We also worked directly with B to confront the situations he found difficult, starting with the easiest. We suggested, for example, that he telephone a friend. We discussed it in detail with him before hand, and attempted role play, though this was not very successful, as B felt that it did not relate to the situation. With situations where there was a specific role, he was encouraged to plan this.

Outcomes of identity therapy

As a result of our discussions and activities, B became more able to recognise that other people may not be perceiving him in a negative way. He developed confidence, as evidenced by his ability to successfully negotiate a range of situations.

Following the therapies, B was able to think more positively about long-term strategies. For example, he started collaborating with a set designer to modify a set to make it more accessible for people with disabilities. He was also able to see that he could use his experience in a positive and creative way; for example, he was asked to contribute to an exhibition on arts and disability.

The biggest problem we experienced together was not resolved when he left. We felt that it was very important for him to talk about how he was feeling. However, because we were listening unconditionally, it sometimes felt as if we were being asked to collude with his wish to find someone to blame, including expressing negative feelings about other professionals in the Unit. When we refused to agree with these comments, the resultant confrontation led to the anger being directed at us, which was still the case when he left.

DISCUSSION

B was not a typical client of mine, nor probably of any other speech therapist. It could be argued that he did not have a great need for speech therapy (particularly, perhaps, compared to other clients on our caseload.) He was able to communicate very well, in comparison.

The difficulties he experienced, although mild, had huge impact on his life in terms of impairment, however. First, his ability to resume his chosen career depended on an extremely high level of language functioning. Furthermore, his attitude to his communication would be an obstacle to his real-life communication in terms of work, forming new social relationships, etc.

In this case the speech therapist and the client both recognised the need and the client was highly motivated to work on his language.

We were in the very unusual position with B, in being able to see him as long and intensively as we liked. My colleague and I at the Younger Rehabilitation Unit are in the situation of having a number of sessions that must be allocated to a certain (small) client group, allowing those clients to be seen intensively (even daily), if required. Most services to people with communication disability, as we all know, are hopelessly under-resourced, and there is not this comparative luxury.

So what would have happened if B had been in a different setting? What if we were forced to prioritise him in the context of a caseload of two hundred? Might the client's perception of need then have to become a very different thing? It may be that the prioritisation criteria differ between districts, and even between therapists. For example, a person with very severe aphasia may be perceived as high priority because of the magnitude of their problems, or low priority because they are judged unlikely to make a big improvement. And on what criteria are we judging "improvement"? Is it in terms of impairment, or in terms of re-engaging with real life? Or both?

In this case, the client and I both perceived a need that we were able to act on. But what happens when the client's and therapist's perception of need do not correspond? How might this mismatch be addressed?

Another important issue regarding service delivery is the timing of our intervention. B was in the acute phase and still experiencing spontaneous recovery in terms of his impairment when we saw him. Had we waited, he would have received no speech therapy at all. But what are we doing in the acute phase? Can we only prove our efficacy if we are working with someone who is no longer spontaneously improving? This may be so if we are looking solely at the impairment, but increasingly we are aware that we are able to offer something important for the client at every stage of therapy.

We discharged B naturally when he was transferred to another unit, and, therefore, to another speech therapist. During the 4 months we worked with him I felt he was beginning to approach the end of his need for speech therapy. While still needing to practise skills, he was becoming (as intended) far more confident and self-directed. But what would he have felt? Would it have been more difficult to end speech therapy if he had remained in the Unit? Would that have meant that we could not have seen the person in the next bed? Here, then, are the broader questions that working with someone with a mild impairment raised for us:

- What determines who gets therapy?
- How do we prioritise who to work with?
- How does the setting influence prioritisation?
- How do we resolve differences in perception of need between client and therapist?
- When is the right time for therapy?
- What determines how long people get therapy for?

(See Hersch, 1998 and 2003, for more discussion of these issues.)

Working with B also raised issues about a speech therapist's role with regard to the psychological side of communication difficulties. The nature of the role of the speech therapist in terms of psychological support is still controversial. The view has been expressed that speech therapists are not trained in counselling, and that these issues need to be addressed by a psychologist. However, it seems to me that psychological issues are a part of speech therapy. First, as we see with B, the person's communication is a part of them and influenced by how they feel. If we address the language difficulty but not how the person feels about it, our goals of communicative effectiveness and confidence surely are not met. The person with good language function (like B) offers us particularly fascinating insights into the emotional response to language difficulty, which may help us in our therapy with clients who are less able to articulate their emotions verbally.

Moreover, as we all have experienced, the environment of the speech therapy session may be the most conducive for the client to express their feelings. Speech therapists are trained to listen, to interpret meaning, and to facilitate communication. Initially B was hostile to clinical psychology, because his first experience of it was psychometric testing, which he found threatening.

This is not to deny the importance of psychologists, nor the role they played in B's rehabilitation. Perhaps the important thing is to recognise the issues that we do not feel capable of addressing with the client, and then to seek advice and make sure the client has the possibility of addressing these elsewhere.

With B, I felt that we were in a position to listen to him and acknowledge his feelings. However, the situation of possible collusion was, for me, an example of where I needed to stand back, and indeed seek advice from a psychologist.

REFERENCES

Hersch, D. (1998). Beyond the "plateau": Discharge dilemmas in chronic aphasia. *Aphasiology*, *12*, 207–243.

Hersch, D. (2003). "Weaning" clients from aphasia therapy: Speech pathologists' strategies for discharge. *Aphasiology*, *17*, 1007–1031.

APPENDIX

APPENDIX 13.1: The Cinderella story

Oh god yes, that story, where do you start? Um. (long pause) There was a girl called Cinderella, well let's start with the mother, there was a wicked woman who married Cinderella's father, I think, yeah, and she had two ugly daughters so Cinderella was the step daughter and these two . . . oh, it's getting the bits right, . . . um, yes, . . . they were invited to go to a ball, but Cinderella couldn't go, she was treated like a slave, . . . she was always in the kitchen.

So the rest of them went off to the ball. But while she was doing the washing up, or whatever, the . . . fairy godmother appeared, I can't remember how, did she rub something? (laughs) . . . and told her that she could go to the ball. But she didn't have . . . wait a minute have I missed, . . . no, she said that she didn't have any clothes and stuff, so the fairy godmother, I can't remember how she got it, but she turned something into a beautiful dress, it was magic anyway! And, oh yes she turned a . . . um a . . . a . . . pumpkin into a . . . coach to take her to the ball, and she used the mice for people who . . . no, I can't remember how she got the horses; was that the mice maybe?

So anyway she went to the ball, and when she got there no one recognised her, and she looked really beautiful but . . . the Prince was there, and they danced together . . . oh and there was the thing about . . . the woman, th . . . er, fairy godmother had told her to be home by midnight, because the um all the things, like the dress, would turn back into . . . what, you know, what they really were . . . back into mice and everything. Is this OK so far, I'm not sure if I've got it all the right way round?

So, she was dancing, and she looked very beautiful and suddenly it was . . ., well the clock started striking and she realised it was midnight and that . . . she would have to run away.

And the Prince came looking for her . . . Oh it was the shoe! The glass shoe, Cinderella dropped it . . . it fell off her foot when she ran away. And he knew it would only fit one woman, and he found her, and I think that's it!

AL: Accessing the predicate argument structure

Janet Webster and Anne Whitworth

INTRODUCTION AND OVERVIEW

AL was a 68-year-old gentleman who had a left CVA resulting in a severe receptive and expressive aphasia. Ten years post-onset his speech was non-fluent and characterised by word-finding difficulties and abandoned, incomplete sentences. An analysis of his narrative speech identified a deficit in the production of thematic structure at the functional level representation (Garrett, 1980). Detailed assessment showed that AL's difficulties included a verb retrieval deficit, a deficit in the creation of the predicate argument structure and thematic role and/or mapping difficulties. The aim of therapy was to improve access to predicate argument structure information, with a view to enabling AL to use more complex and a wider range of argument structures and to reduce the number of verbs used in an inappropriate argument structure.

Therapy was based on a programme designed by Whitworth (1994) to improve thematic role assignment. The programme involved the explicit identification of thematic roles in a wide range of sentence types with canonical word order. Feedback focused on predicate argument structure information and the optional or obligatory nature of verb arguments. Two subsequent stages of therapy involved the identification of thematic roles in sentences with the same verb in different predicate argument structure arrangements and in non-canonical, passive sentences.

Therapy consisted of 10 weekly sessions supplemented by self-study exercises. In order to monitor efficacy, multiple baselines of AL's narrative production were taken prior to therapy and performance on a control task was assessed pre- and post-therapy.

AL's comprehension and production of reversible sentences improved as a result of therapy.

Within constrained tasks, he was able to produce more sentences with an appropriate predicate argument structure and began to produce more complex, three-argument structures. Improvement was also evident in his production of narrative speech, with a reduction in the number of sentences with an undetermined thematic structure. Performance, however, remained below normal limits. No improvement was seen in his performance on the control task and in other aspects of sentence production.

Therapy targeting predicate argument structure information and thematic role assignment resulted in significant gains in sentence production. It is suggested that predicate argument structure deficits may be frequent contributors to sentence production deficits in aphasia and that treatment for deficits affecting the production of thematic structure should be preceded by detailed assessment of the sub-processes involved.

BACKGROUND

Garrett's (1980) model of normal sentence production has been used to describe the deficits seen in individuals with aphasia (Schwartz, 1987). This model conceives sentence production as a series of independent processing levels each corresponding to a level of representation. The message level representation corresponds to a non-linguistic, conceptual level. The functional level representation is a thematic representation that specifies the verb and its arguments. The positional level representation specifies the syntactic and phrasal structure of the sentence in phonological form. Phonetic and motor planning information is specified at more peripheral levels of processing. The processes that produce these levels of representation can be selectively impaired with differential effects for sentence production (Webster, 1999).

Schwartz (1987) elaborated Garrett's model by suggesting a set of processes that operate to produce each level of structure. She hypothesised that three discrete processes are involved in the production of thematic structure at the functional

level representation. First, a lexical search based on the semantic form and the grammatical category of the word is performed. Second, the predicate argument structure is specified; this is a conceptual representation that determines the number and type of arguments associated with a verb. The predicate refers to the concept that specifies the action or relation; the arguments refer to the concepts identifying the participants in the event (Byng & Black, 1989). The semantic role played by each of the participants in the sentence is described as its thematic role. Third, and finally, the lexical items are assigned to each of the thematic roles. Thematic role assignment precedes the specification of word order; the same functional level representation can be translated into sentences with different syntactic forms— for example, active and passive sentences. The association of sentence meaning (thematic structure) and sentence form (syntactic structure) has been described as mapping (Saffran, Schwartz, & Marin 1980; Schwartz, Saffran, & Marin, 1980). Mapping involves the association of the functional level representation with the syntactic frame produced at the positional level. Mapping is thought to involve a combination of lexically specified information and general rules and procedures (Byng, Nickels, & Black, 1994).

Studies investigating the production of thematic structure in aphasia have focused predominantly on access to semantic information for nouns and verbs and on the process of mapping. These studies have identified parallel deficits in production and comprehension, suggesting that the processes are central. Semantic deficits have been reported to result in semantic paraphasias in production, confusion of semantically related items in comprehension (Berndt, Mitchum, Haendiges, & Sandson, 1997b) and an excessive reliance on pronouns instead of specific nouns (Gleason et al., 1980) and "light" verbs instead of specific verbs (Berndt et al., 1997b; Breedin & Martin, 1996).

Word retrieval difficulties may result in the omission of a noun and, thus, the omission of an obligatory argument from the sentence. The omission of a verb may result in a more fundamental breakdown in the production of the thematic structure of the sentence as it is the verb that specifies the semantic character of the sentence as a whole (Shapiro, Brookins, Gofdon, & Nagal, 1991).

Mapping deficits have been reported to result in difficulties in the production and comprehension of reversible sentences (Byng, 1988; Saffran et al., 1980; Schwartz et al., 1980). Mapping in non-reversible sentences may be aided by real-world information that specifies the relationship between sentence participants. This information is not available in the processing of reversible sentences, so reverse role errors may result. Mapping difficulties increase in sentences where there is no transparent relationship between thematic structure and the word order specified within the syntactic frame (Schwartz, Linebarger, Saffran, & Pate, 1987). The centrality of the mapping mechanism has been confirmed by the parallel gains seen in production following therapy targeted at comprehension (Byng, 1988; Jones, 1986).

Few studies have considered the impact of predicate argument structure and thematic role assignment difficulties on sentence production. Thompson, Lange, Schneider, and Shapiro (1997) investigated the production of the predicate argument structure by people with aphasia in a conversational task. They concluded that, compared to non-aphasic speakers, people with aphasia produced argument structures with fewer predicate argument arrangements and sentences with fewer arguments. It is proposed, therefore, that predicate argument structure difficulties may result in a reliance on simple one- and two-argument structures. Poor access to predicate argument structure information for particular verbs may also result in the omission of obligatory arguments or the addition of arguments, as the participants may be unaware of the arguments that are required alongside the verb.

It is difficult to assess thematic role assignment independently of its subsequent mapping onto word order. Thematic role difficulties will also result in reverse role errors in the production and comprehension of reversible sentences, but as thematic role assignment is independent of syntactic form, all sentence types should be equally affected, i.e. there should be no marked effect of syntactic transparency. Thematic role assignment

difficulties have also been reported to result in the omission of verbs and verb arguments (Schwartz, Fink, & Saffran, 1995). The omission of obligatory arguments, as a consequence of thematic role assignment difficulties, is thought to increase in sentences with an increased number of arguments (Whitworth, 1994). It can be seen from the description of the deficits resulting from semantic, predicate argument structure, thematic role assignment and mapping deficits, that there is some overlap in the surface symptoms resulting from impairment to each of the processes. Detailed psycholinguistic assessment is thus required to identify the impaired processes responsible for the observed pattern of symptoms.

METHOD

Participant
AL was a 68-year-old gentleman who had a left CVA in 1988. He was a retired electrical safety officer who had worked in the mines. He lived with his wife and had two children and four grandchildren who lived locally. Following his CVA, AL presented with severe receptive and expressive aphasia and a right hemiparesis. When seen 10 years post-onset, AL had made significant progress physically but remained aphasic. He had received some speech and language therapy following his stroke and was still attending a special club for people with speech difficulties after stroke, although the activities offered by this group were socially oriented. AL led a very active social life but felt his limited ability to communicate affected his participation in conversation. On initial impression, he had good functional comprehension. His speech was non-fluent and was characterised by apparent word-finding difficulties and abandoned sentences and his verbal communication was supplemented by pointing, gesture and intonational changes.

Analysis of narrative speech
A narrative sample was obtained using the procedure suggested by Saffran, Berndt, and Schwartz

(1989). The sample was analysed for its thematic, phrasal and morphological structure, using an analysis developed by Webster (1999). A transcript of the narrative can be found in Appendix 14.1.

AL's production of the narrative was also compared to that of non-aphasic speakers. His performance was considered to differ from normal speech if it fell outside two standard deviations of the non-aphasic mean. AL was able to convey the main events of the story, suggesting that his message level representation was intact. In the production of the functional level representation, he produced a high percentage of utterances with an undetermined thematic structure. These utterances consisted of single phrases or strings of phrases not including a verb. Sentences with a definite argument structure consisted of predominantly two-argument structures around the copula verb. Obligatory arguments were sometimes omitted from two-argument structures and no three-argument structures were produced. His production of the syntactic frame at the positional level representation was characterised by some substitution errors in the production of determiners, pronouns, verb auxiliaries and morphology. AL was, however, capable of producing elaborated phrasal structure.

AL had a combination of thematic and syntactic difficulties. The impaired thematic structure had a significant impact on his ability to convey information. More detailed assessment was carried out to determine which of the processes involved in the production of thematic structure was impaired.

Differential diagnosis

AL's language was tested to determine his access to semantic information and word retrieval, access to predicate argument structure information, thematic role assignment and mapping in sentence production and comprehension. The results of these tests can be seen in Table 14.1. The retrieval of nouns and verbs was assessed using the Verb and Noun Test (VAN; Webster & Bird, 2000). AL showed good retrieval of nouns (54/54) but his verb retrieval (42/54) was significantly impaired compared to non-aphasic speakers (independent sample t-test, $t = 2.546$, $df = 29$,

$p = .016$). This revealed a significant difference between noun and verb retrieval ($\chi^2 = 65.3$, $df = 1$, $p = .00$). Verb retrieval was very slow and was characterised by the production of semantically related verbs and nouns.

Verb comprehension was assessed using the verb comprehension video (described in Byng, 1988). AL's verb comprehension was relatively intact, with only three errors on reverse role verbs. Access to predicate argument structure information and the creation of an appropriate predicate argument structure for verbs with different argument structures was assessed using a sentence generation task. This involved giving AL the verb and asking him to produce a sentence containing that verb. It was hoped that giving him the verb might bypass his verb retrieval deficit. AL was able to produce a sentence containing the target verb; in 16% of the sentences, however, the verb was used in a sentence with an inappropriate argument structure. These errors were predominantly the omission of obligatory arguments in two arguments in two-argument structures, for example, "build a new house" and "I ensured . . .". When given 45 of the verbs in a sentence anagram task, where AL had to select and then order sentence components from a choice of distracters, only 26 of the sentences were produced correctly on his first attempt.

AL also differed significantly from non-aphasic speakers in his ability to identify appropriate and inappropriate predicate argument structure in a grammaticality judgement task, scoring 102/120 (independent sample t-test, $t = 3.392$, $df = 13$, $p = .002$). His errors were predominantly the acceptance of an inappropriate predicate argument structure as correct.

Thematic role assignment was assessed via the production and comprehension of reversible sentences. His production of reversible two-argument sentences involved the production of a reverse role error and two sentences in which an obligatory argument was omitted. A similar mix of reverse role errors and omitted arguments was seen in AL's production of three-argument structures.

Sentence comprehension was assessed using the reversible sentence comprehension test

TABLE 14.1

Results of pre-therapy tests

Test	n	Non-aphasic mean	Non-aphasic range	AL's score
Semantic information				
VAN: Noun retrieval	54	53	49–54	54
VAN: Verb retrieval	54	50	44–53	42*
Verb comprehension	46	NA	NA	43
Predicate argument structure information				
Sentence generation: % inappropriate predicate argument structure		0.90	0–4.11	16*
Grammaticality Judgement Test	120	113.4	108–117	102*
Sentence Anagram Test	45	NA	NA	26
Thematic role assignment				
Production of 2-argument reversible sentences	20	NA	NA	17
Production of 3-argument reversible sentences	10	NA	NA	7
Reversible Sentence Comprehension Test: spoken version	70	NA	NA	55
Reversible Sentence Comprehension Test: written version	70	NA	NA	54

NA = normal data not available. VAN = Verb and Noun test (Webster & Bird, 2000).
* Performance differed from non-aphasic speakers.

(described in Black, Nickels, & Byng, 1991). AL's written and spoken comprehension was characterised by the selection of reverse role errors, particularly in the comprehension of passive sentences.

Thematic Roles in Production (TRIP; Whitworth, 1994) was used to contrast the production of one-, two- and three-argument structures. This tests noun and verb retrieval and the production of predicate argument structure as well as thematic role assignment. AL's performance on the TRIP is detailed in Figure 14.1. There was a significant difference in AL's noun retrieval, verb retrieval and the thematic completeness of sentences across the one-, two- and three-argument structures (chi square tests,

FIGURE 14.1

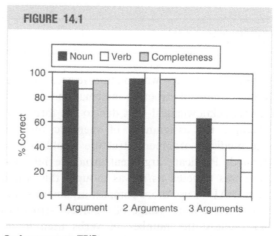

Performance on TRIP.

p < .001). This seemed to be a consequence of his severe difficulties with three-argument structures. His production of three-argument structures was characterised by the omission of arguments and the omission of verbs. For example, for the picture "the woman is giving the shell to the baby", he produced "the woman is . . . the shell".

From the results of the assessments, it was concluded that AL's difficulties in the production of thematic structure did not have a single origin. First, a verb retrieval deficit was evident resulting in the production of semantic paraphasias, a reliance on "light" verbs (for example, "have", "do" and "be") and the omission of verbs in sentences. Second, AL had significant difficulty in accessing predicate argument structure information and using it to create an appropriate sentence frame. This resulted in the omission of arguments and a reliance on simple one- and two-argument structures. Finally, AL's difficulties with reverse role verbs and the presence of reverse role errors in the production and comprehension of reversible sentences suggested a deficit in thematic role assignment or mapping. The prominence of this deficit in the comprehension of passive sentences may implicate a mapping deficit. These difficulties in the assignment of thematic roles and mapping may also account for some of AL's difficulties in the production of complex argument structures.

THERAPY

The aim of therapy was to improve access to predicate argument structure information, although it was acknowledged that due to the format of therapy, the assignment of thematic roles in the predicate argument structure would also be treated. Predicate argument structure information was targeted as it was thought this would enable AL to use more complex argument structures, use a wider range of argument structures and reduce the number of verbs used in an inappropriate structure. Therapy was based on

a programme designed by Whitworth (1994) to improve thematic role assignment; this focused on the explicit identification of thematic roles in a wide variety of written one-, two- and three-argument structures. A brief description of the therapy and the sentence types used can be found in Appendix 14.2.

Thematic roles were given easy labels and associated with specific "wh" questions and cue words. Colour coding was used initially to introduce each sentence type. AL was initially given the questions and cues by the therapist. He was then encouraged to generate the cues himself and then to identify the thematic roles without explicit cues. If thematic roles were not correctly assigned to lexical items, the task was repeated with cues from the therapist. An explicit comparison between correct and incorrect thematic role assignment was then made. Following the correct assignment of thematic roles, feedback concentrated on predicate argument structure information; the optional or obligatory nature of the arguments in the context of that sentence and other sentences was discussed. Each argument was covered up in turn and AL was asked to judge whether the sentence was still appropriate. The semantic selection restrictions of the verb were discussed and AL was sometimes asked to generate another lexical item that could fulfil a particular role. Therapy sessions were used to introduce a particular sentence type or types, with subsequent home practice during the week. These home exercises were checked in the subsequent session and AL was asked to complete some unseen examples without cues. Therapy consisted of 10 weekly session and the associated home exercises.

As therapy progressed, two subsequent stages of therapy were considered necessary. AL was able to identify the thematic roles and judge the optional or obligatory nature of arguments within a particular given context but it was clear he couldn't envisage the use of the verb in a different context. For example, when given the sentence "the boy gave the present to the girl", he was able to identify the thematic roles and knew that they were all obligatory arguments. He was, however, unable to see that in a different context "the

professor gave the lecture on Egypt", the third benefactive argument was not always necessary. It was, therefore, considered important to focus on the different predicate argument structure arrangements associated with the verbs. Originally, it was hoped that AL might be able to generate sentences containing the verb in a different predicate argument structure context but he was unable to do this. He generally just produced a sentence in which one of the lexical items fulfilling an argument had changed. For example, after identifying the thematic roles in "the man ate his breakfast", he produced "the woman ate her breakfast" or "the man ate his dinner". AL was, therefore, given examples of sentences with different predicate argument structure, e.g., "the man sailed to the island" and "the man sailed the boat" and was asked to identify the thematic roles. Treatment of thematic role assignment in active sentences resulted in no improvement in the comprehension of passive sentences. Thematic role assignment and mapping in passive sentences was thus introduced as a separate stage of therapy with subsequent comparison of the active and passive forms.

RESULTS

A comparison of the results on the test of predicate argument structure and thematic role assignment pre- and post-therapy can be found in Table 14.2. It can be seen that following therapy, AL was able to produce sentences with an appropriate argument structure. This resulted in an improvement in his performance on the sentence generation task and an improvement in his ability to produce three-argument structures in the TRIP. Post-therapy, no significant difference was identified in the production of one-, two- and three-argument structures in noun retrieval, verb retrieval or thematic completeness (chi square tests, $p > .05$) and his performance was now within the non-aphasic range. His production of reversible two- and three-argument structures also became error free.

In the comprehension of reversible sentences, both his spoken and written performance improved significantly (McNemar's test, spoken version $p = .002$, written version $p = .001$). This improvement was a consequence of the reduction in reverse role errors. There was no change in AL's performance on the task involving writing words to dictation.

AL's improvements suggest that targeting predicate argument structure was an appropriate choice of therapy. But if therapy is considered to be effective, improvement must also be seen in the production of more spontaneous speech.

A transcript of post-therapy narrative is presented in Appendix 14.3. Figure 14.2 shows the distribution of argument structures in the production of narrative speech pre- and post-therapy. Improvements were indicated by the lower proportion of utterances with an undetermined thematic structure (UTS) (single phrases) and an increase in the percentage of one- and three-argument structures in the post-therapy sample. Although the percentage of two-argument structures remained constant across the two samples, the second sample was characterised by a shift to the more prominent use of lexical verbs. AL still produced no utterances with thematic embedding. Therapy thus resulted in some improvements in less constrained tasks of sentence production but performance remained outside normal limits. As therapy progressed, AL's wife used the "wh" questions to prompt him if obligatory information had been omitted during conversation. This increased AL's awareness of the adequacy of his sentences and towards the end of the block of therapy, he showed evidence of self-monitoring. AL reported that he felt that this awareness had helped him improve his conversation.

Following therapy, therefore, AL's sentence production improved with more accurate production of non-reversible and reversible two- and three-argument structures in constrained tasks. In spontaneous speech, he relied less on single phrases and produced more sentences, thus allowing him to convey more information. His comprehension of reversible sentences also improved.

TABLE 14.2

Comparison of pre- and post—therapy performance

Test	n	Pre-therapy performance	Post-therapy performance
PAS information			
Sentence generation: % inappropriate PAS		16	0
Thematic role assignment			
Production of 2-argument reversible sentences	20	17	20
Production of 3-argument reversible sentences	10	7	10
Reversible Sentence Comprehension Test: spoken version	70	55	68
Reversible Sentence Comprehension Test: written version	70	54	68
TRIP			
Word retrieval (nouns)			
Single words	35	34	34
1-argument structures	15	14	15
2-argument structures	40	38	38
3-argument structures	30	19	28
Word retrieval (verbs)			
1-argument structures	15	13	15
2-argument structures	20	20	18
3-argument structures	10	4	10
Thematic completeness			
1-argument structures	15	14	15
2-argument structures	20	19	20
3-argument structures	10	3	10
Control task			
Writing words to dictation	40	20	19

DISCUSSION

AL, a client with aphasia, had difficulties with verb retrieval, predicate argument structure, thematic role assignment or mapping. Therapy aimed to improve AL's access to predicate argument structure information for a wide variety of verbs in different sentence types. In addition, therapy targeted thematic role assignment in sentences with canonical word order. A subsequent stage of therapy focused on thematic role assignment in passive sentences. In these non-canonical sentences, there is no transparent relationship between thematic and syntactic structure.

Therapy resulted in improved production of thematic structure in constrained tasks with a reduction in the proportion of sentences with an inappropriate argument structure and an increase in the use of three-argument structures. In narrative speech, there was some decrease in the proportion of sentences with an undetermined thematic structure. It is suggested that this improvement

FIGURE 14.2

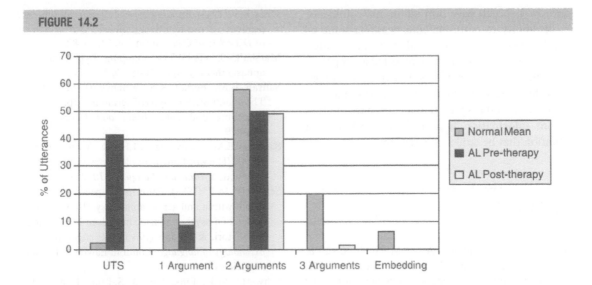

Distribution of argument structures in narrative speech: Comparison of pre- and post-therapy performance.

in sentence production was a consequence of improved access to predicate argument structure information associated with a wide range of sentence types. The remaining difficulties in the production of thematic structure may be a consequence of his impaired verb retrieval; this was an aspect not targeted in this phase of therapy. Alternatively, it may be that the strategies learnt in therapy were not yet so automatic that they could be used in more complex tasks. AL's improved comprehension appears to be a consequence of improved mapping between thematic and syntactic structure. The lack of initial improvement in the comprehension of passives following therapy targeted at thematic role assignment suggests that it was the mapping process that was impaired initially.

During therapy, it was clear that AL had difficulty appreciating that verbs could have multiple predicate argument structure arrangements and could thus be used in a variety of different sentence types. This is an important aspect to consider when planning therapy for predicate argument structure deficits and may be treated more successfully via production tasks. It is suggested that predicate argument structure difficulties may be frequent contributors to sentence

production deficits in aphasia and that the presence of these difficulties may account for some of the discrepancies seen in the outcome of mapping therapy studies, for example, the varying degrees of generalisation seen in untreated sentence types (Byng, 1988; Marshall, 1995). When considering the treatment of deficits affecting the production of thematic structure, it is suggested that the sub-processes producing that level of structure need to be considered and that treatment should be directed as specifically as possible to the process that is impaired. It is, therefore, important not to plan treatment on the basis of the observed symptoms but on detailed assessment of those sub-processes. The nature of the relationship between the processes involved in verb retrieval, the creation of the predicate argument structure, thematic role assignment and mapping need to be considered further if the assessment and treatment of sentence processing disorders in aphasia is to be refined in the future.

On a more functional level, AL's improved expressive language had two consequences. He had been leading an active social life before the intervention. However, he reported frequently feeling left out of group conversations. His improved speech gave him additional confidence in his ability to communicate, negating some of the feelings of isolation within group settings. Second, both he and his wife reported an improvement in their conversations. Frustration between them had reduced when talking, partly due to a realisation on AL's part that he may have omitted salient information within the conversation—a situation that he could now remedy.

REFERENCES

Berndt, R.S., Haendiges, A.N., Mitchum, C.C., & Sandson, J. (1997a). Verb retrieval in aphasia: II. Relationship to sentences processing. *Brain and Language, 56*, 107–137.

Berndt, R.S., Mitchum, C.C., Haendiges, A.N., & Sandson, J. (1997b). Verb retrieval in aphasia: I. Characterizing single word impairments. *Brain and Language, 56*, 68–106.

Black, M., Nickels, L., & Byng, S. (1991). Patterns of sentence processing deficit: Sentences can be a complex matter. *Journal of Neurolinguistics, 2*, 79–101.

Breedin, S.D., & Martin, R.C. (1996). Patterns of verb impairment in aphasia: An analysis of four cases. *Cognitive Neuropsychology, 13*, 51–91.

Byng, S. (1988). Sentence processing deficits: Theory and therapy. *Cognitive Neuropsychology, 5*, 629–676.

Byng, S., & Black, M. (1989). Some aspects of sentence production in aphasia. *Aphasiology, 3*, 241–263.

Byng, S., Nickels, L., & Black, M. (1994). Replicating therapy for mapping deficits in agrammatism: Remapping the deficit? *Aphasiology, 8*, 315–341.

Garrett, M.F. (1980). Levels of processing in sentence production. In B. Butterworth (Ed.), *Language production I*. New York: Academic Press.

Gleason, J., Goodglass, H., Obler, L., Green, E., Hyde, M., & Weintraub, S. (1980). Narrative strategies of aphasic and normal speaking subjects. *Journal of Speech and Hearing Research, 23*, 370–383.

Jones, E.V. (1986). Building the foundations for sentence production in a non-fluent aphasic. *British Journal of Disorders of Communication, 21*, 63–82.

Marshall, J. (1995).The mapping hypothesis and aphasia therapy. *Aphasiology, 9*, 517–539.

Saffran, E.M., Berndt, R.S., & Schwartz, M.F. (1989). The quantitative analysis of agrammatic production; Procedure and data. *Brain and Language, 37*, 440–479.

Saffran, E.M., Schwartz, M.F., & Marin, O.S.M. (1980). The word order problem in agrammatism II: Production. *Brain and Language, 10*, 263–280.

Schwartz, M.F. (1987). Patterns of speech production deficit within and across aphasia syndromes: Application of a psycholinguistic model. In M. Coltheart, G. Sartori, & R. Job (Eds.), *The cognitive neuropsychology of language*. London: Lawrence Erlbaum Associates Ltd.

Schwartz, M.F., Fink, F.B., & Saffran, E.M. (1995). The modular treatment of agrammatism. *Neuropsychological Rehabilitation, 5*, 93–127.

Schwartz, M.F., Linebarger, M.C., Saffran, E.M., & Pate, D.S. (1987). Syntactic transparency and sentence interpretation in aphasia. *Language and Cognitive Processes, 2*, 85–113.

Schwartz, M.F., Saffran, E.M., & Marin, O.S.M. (1980). The word order problem in agrammatism: I. Comprehension. *Brain and Language, 10*, 249–262.

Shapiro, L.P., Brookins, B., Gofdon, B., & Nagal, H. (1991). Verb effects during sentence processing. *Journal of Experimental Psychology: Learning, Memory and Cognition, 17*, 219–246.

Thompson, C.K., Lange, K.L., Schneider, S.L., & Shapiro, L.P. (1997). Agrammatic and non-brain damaged subjects' verb and verb argument structure production. *Aphasiology, 11*, 473–490.

Webster, J., & Bird, H. (2000). *The verb and noun test (VAN)*. Ponteland, UK: STASS Publications.

Webster, J.M. (1999). *A semantic and syntactic analysis of aphasic speech*. Unpublished PhD thesis, University of Newcastle upon Tyne.

Whitworth, A.B. (1994). *Thematic role assignment in word retrieval deficits in aphasia*. Unpublished PhD thesis, University of Newcastle upon Tyne.

APPENDICES

APPENDIX 14.1: Cinderella narrative (pre-therapy)

Once upon a time there lived a . . . Cinderella . . . the sisters . . . er . . . fat the Cinderella working all the time . . . cleaning cooking and erm . . . so the the sisters went to the ball . . . erm . . . Cinderella is crying . . . but the magic genie he says you shall be the best erm . . . ball so she the pumpkin changed into coach . . . the rats comes into erm the coachmen and . . . Cinderella lovely gown erm well she went to the ball and they danced with her . . . erm . . . can't say the words erm she went to the ball danced her and the . . . prince he said . . . erm I know her . . . can't know her so he ran twelve o'clock he ran the Cinderella ran then . . . he erm the prince depressed but the slipper was on the stairs then ah who the fat one that's mine . . . try it on . . . no the . . . try it on . . . no . . . I I I can't I just . . . all around . . . the city try it on then . . . the prince is . . . Cinderella . . . try it on the it fit . . . then happy ever after

APPENDIX 14.2: Details of the therapy programme

Mapping thematic roles onto syntactic frames: A therapy resource (Whitworth, 1994)

Therapeutic aims
The therapy programme aims to increase the person with aphasia's (the participant) awareness of the thematic roles (or meaning relations) of individual words within sentences and develop an understanding of how meaning is mapped onto the predicate argument structure.

Sentence types targeted within the programme
Verb
Agent + Verb
Experiencer + Verb
Agent + Verb + Patient (non-motion verb/pragmatic bias)
Agent + Verb + Patient (non-motion verb/ no pragmatic bias)
Agent + Verb + Patient (non-directional motion verb/pragmatic bias)
Agent + Verb + Patient (directional motion verb/ pragmatic and non-pragmatic bias)
Agent + Verb + Locative
Experiencer + Verb + Attribution
Possessor + Verb + Patient
Agent + Verb + Patient + Benefactive (pragmatic bias)
Agent + Verb + Patient + Benefactive (no pragmatic bias)
Agent + Verb + Patient + Instrument

APPENDIX 14.3: Cinderella narrative (post-therapy)

The story of Cinderella . . . Cinderella lived with her . . . er the mother and the two daughters . . . then she cleans cooks erm all sorts washes clothes and makes the beds but the two sisters swans you know the er . . . the meals served by Cinderella then . . . she's er fed up sits down crying and nobody loved me you know but er then the godmother erm . . . appeared what you're crying for I've got no clothes and I haven't got money and well . . . the ball is next week so . . . the sisters dress up and they go in the carriage then OK . . . Cinderella beautiful gown the rats the er . . . the coach then the mouse the coachmen then go to the ball and dance so she looked lovely gown and the coaches and the horses then she went to the ball then she didn't know anybody but she's so lovely and the prince thought oh that's that's a lovely girl dancing with me and they all danced and danced and then the sisters er mad so . . . erm . . . one twelve o'clock she go in the coach and go home but er twelve o'clock she run and her slipper dislodged then the coach went the prince he says lovely girl where are they nobody knows . her slippers her slippers oh I'm going try all the town all over so she tried it she tried it then Cinderella goes . . . house and just the rags and the mouse and the rats erm so the daughters two two daughters we'll try this on and she tried and then she tried and the other one tried and they tried and no good then the prince saw tried it and she tried it and she went the slipper lovely fit then the prince married the girl and lived happily ever after.

A framework for describing therapies and discovering their whys and wherefores

Sally Byng and Judy Duchan

In this final chapter we will introduce a framework for highlighting common issues and differences raised in the previous chapters. When examining the similarities and differences between what authors in this volume have to say, we have been struck by the diverse ways of undertaking therapy with people with aphasia. Of course, different individuals need different therapies at different times, but these differences seemed to go beyond what would be expected. We were also noticing that authors in this book had different ways of describing the people they were working with, and seemed to be justifying what went on in their therapies in different ways. In order to show how all of the chapters compare with one another we have applied the framework to all of them.

Readers who are less interested in such a comparison and more interested in how the framework functions might want to skip over the details offered in the individual tables.

These discrepant ways of writing about therapy can make it hard to compare different therapies and to compare the beliefs and assumptions of the authors that were explicit or implicit in their writings. In recent years much has been written about different types of implicit beliefs, and how they influence therapies in the field of communication disabilities. Some have talked about influences of conceptual frameworks (Byng & Duchan, 2005; Duchan, 2001, 2004); others have talked about different philosophical approaches (Petheram & Parr, 1998; Weniger & Taylor Sarno, 1990). One question that we are asking is whether the thinking underpinning authors' therapies described in this book could be uncovered by laying out how they describe the people with aphasia they work with and their therapies.

THE THERAPY DESCRIPTION FRAMEWORK

We have developed a framework for describing therapy and applied it to each of the studies in this volume; thus, different therapies could be more easily compared with one another and the different sorts of thinking underpinning each study could be made more transparent. The framework provides a means of capturing, in descriptive non-theoretical language, a portrait of the significant issues about the person or people involved in the therapy, and a catalogue of the therapy tasks.

We found that each of the chapters offered therapy information that fitted the framework, even though the therapies varied considerably. They ranged from highly structured sentence processing tasks through to loosely structured discussions, from individualised therapy to group therapy, and from impairment-focused to socially focused therapy designs.

The therapy framework has three main parts, one involving details about *the person or people with aphasia*, the second involving details about *the therapy* and the third representing the *rationale* of therapy. Each of the first two parts has three subsections.

Part One: The "facilitators and barriers facing the *person* with the communication disability" contains details about:

- (A) the *facilitators*—what this person can do communicatively, or the resources they can draw and build on
- (B) the *barriers*—what this person has difficulty doing, or the complications and barriers they have to overcome
- (C) the *checks*—what further issues need to be explored.

Part Two: The "description of the *therapy*" contains details about:

- (A) the *content* of therapy (the what of therapy)
- (B) the *process* (the how of therapy)
- (C) the *context* of therapy (the who, when, where, and with what of therapy).

Part Three: The *rationale* of therapy captures the relationship between the person and what was done in the therapy described in Part Two:

- the factors from Part One that are taken into account in designing the therapy tasks in Part Two are identified
- for example, therapy involving visual support described in Part Two of the protocol might have arisen from the knowledge that the person is benefited by visual presentation of material, information that is found in the facilitators section of Part One
- this comparison of items in the two parts of the protocol can help explicate the relationship between factors about the person and features of therapy and reveal some of the thinking that goes into decisions about what actually happens in therapy.

What follows is a brief yet detailed explanation of the framework and representation of the components. Then we apply the framework to each of the 13 chapters of this volume that describe therapies. By explicating the various elements and issues comprising a person and his or her therapy, the reader can better see the similarities and differences between different therapies and compare these with their own practices. We will also make the case at the end of the chapter that the framework has the potential for revealing some of the thinking that went into the therapy descriptions.

Part One of the therapy framework—the person

This part focuses on what it is about the person that might aid or hinder the design or progress of therapy and what more needs to be found out. The three subsections of Part One are facilitators, barriers, and checks (see Table 15.1).

TABLE 15.1

A framework for describing therapies and their relationship to the issues confronting the person with aphasia

Part One: The facilitators and barriers facing the person with aphasia

A: Facilitators—e.g., what can this person/these people do communicatively, or what resources can they draw and build on?

1.
2.
3.
4.
5.
6.
7.
8. Etc.

B: Barriers—e.g., what does this person have difficulty doing, or what are the complications & barriers to overcome?

1.
2.
3.
4.
5.
6.
7.
8. Etc.

C: Checks—e.g., what else do I need to find out about/think about/explore?

1.
2.
3.
4.
5. Etc.

Part Two: A description of the therapy

WHAT: The content of therapy—what were the tasks/events of therapy?	*HOW: The processes of therapy—how was the therapy carried out by the therapist?*	*WHO, WHEN, WHERE, WITH WHAT RESOURCES: The context of therapy—how was the environment/context set up to enable the therapy to happen?*
Activity 1:		

Rationale

Facilitators:
Barriers:
Checks:

Activity 2:

Rationale
Facilitators:
Barriers:
Checks:

Facilitators are any factors to do with the person with aphasia that seem to be working well for them and that could be used to advantage in supporting them in therapy. A facilitating factor may be something specific to the individual, like a good sense of humour, relatively strong written naming ability, ability to write the first letters of some words, a supportive family, a positive outlook on life, a creative employer, good understanding of single words, and so on.

Barriers, on the other hand, are the factors working against someone, the barriers they face, or the factors causing a problem or difficulty. They may range from depression, lack of initiative, frustration, difficulty finding the phonological form of a word, impairment to the orthographic output lexicon, an unsympathetic family member, lack of local support networks, and so on.

Sometimes an issue can act both for and against someone: the supportive family member can also be over-protective of their relative. Frustration can also be part of a strong motivational force for an individual. The framework does not, of course, preclude placing an issue in both the facilitators and barriers lists. There is no pre-determined weighting of any of these issues, because the significance of an issue will depend on an individual's reaction to it. Rather these two categories represent simply a list of the issues.

Facilitators and barriers will differ depending upon the points of view of the evaluator. In this chapter, we will be describing the therapies from our own point of view as readers of the authors'

therapy descriptions. We have, however, checked these interpretations with the authors of each of the studies, but not with the people with aphasia or their families, for obvious reasons. Readers interested in employing these frameworks in their own practices might want to use them as a vehicle for discussion and corroboration with the people with whom they are working.

Checks are what the therapist is also trying to explore when they undertake a specific therapy. Very often we describe therapy as an investigative process—assessment as therapy—through which we try to understand more about the person's language and communication skills, and their reaction to their aphasia. The "checks" are intended to find out about those as yet unknown aspects of the person's aphasia, or their response to them.

Part Two of the therapy framework—the therapy

This second part of the framework (see Part Two of Table 15.1), focuses on the "activities" of therapy. It is divided into three categories that separate out the tasks of therapy from what the therapist does within those tasks and the environment within which the therapy task take place.

The content of therapy involves a description of the tasks used. It can be anything from structured worksheets, to discussion groups, to talking with potential employers. The content of therapies described by Montagu and Marshall (Chapter 7), Perkins and Hinshelwood (Chapter 8) and Webster and Whitworth (Chapter 14) includes a step-by-step description of the task and the materials used.

The process of therapy has to do with how the therapist carries out his/her therapy. How the therapist reacts and responds in the therapy event may vary across therapists, even with the same task or activity. Some therapies, such as those that are based in interaction and discussion, focus more on process than on content.

The last component in the therapy section of the framework has to do with what might be termed broadly environmental factors. It includes how the environment or context for the therapy is set up in order to enable it to happen; that is, who is involved, where, with what resources and how often therapy takes place.

Part Three of the therapy framework—the rationale

Together, the two parts of the framework can reveal relationships between what is done in therapy and the issues facing the person with aphasia. We have done this by devising a coding system to compare the two parts. Each of the factors working for (the facilitators) or against (the barriers) the person with aphasia, and each of the checks the therapist wishes to make, is assigned a number. The numbers assigned in Part One of the framework are inserted under each of the tasks in Part Two of the framework so that one can see how aspects of the person relate to specific aspects of the "activities of therapy" in Part Two. This relationship between relevant factors and activities make up the "*rationale*" for each therapy activity analysed in Part Two of the model. This makes it easier for the reader to see and evaluate a possible rationale for a therapy. It also makes it easier to see at a glance a therapist's perceptions of the issues associated with each therapy for an individual.

Our position as readers is comparable to any reader of this volume. That is to say, we positioned ourselves as naïve readers, who must depend upon the details of the case in order to understand and evaluate what was done. A big part of such an understanding is to draw inferences from the case description about why certain therapies were chosen in the first place. One can safely infer, for example, that a person receiving therapy for word finding has word-finding difficulties.

Some rationales such as this are obvious. Either they are provided explicitly by the authors of the report, or they can be logically inferred. That is what we have done, using the framework to guide our thinking. We are well aware, however, that our rationales are being applied as outsiders. We presume that were the therapists themselves asked to provide rationales, they might offer justifications that go beyond their descriptions or that draw upon a logic in the descriptions that is different from ours.

APPLYING THE THERAPY FRAMEWORK TO EACH OF THE THERAPIES IN THIS VOLUME

We have applied the framework to some or all of the therapies carried out by the authors of the studies in this volume. We have done this in Part One of the framework by simply listing all the characteristics of the person or people described by the authors in each chapter. Part Two of the framework was constructed by taking each author's descriptions of the content of therapy, the processes used in the therapy event and contextual factors.

As far as possible the authors' own language and description has been used to complete the framework, and as little extrapolation or interpretation as possible has been applied. Each author has approved the framework that was constructed for their therapy study. We have not commented on the application of the framework to the individual studies: to do so would be to negate the purpose of the framework as a purely descriptive, value-free, means of describing person and task. We do, however, raise some issues at the end of this chapter about how to use the framework for making certain observations and comparisons about implicit assumptions of therapy.

Chapter 2: Deborah Cairns
Part One of the framework (Table 15.2) applied to Deborah Cairns' therapy summarises the key

TABLE 15.2

Chapter 2: Cairns' therapy for communication and identity

Part One: The facilitators and barriers facing Tony at the point this therapy began, 18 months after his stroke

A: Facilitators

1. Tony was previously confident as a speaker
2. Tony was supported by his wife
3. He had long experience of being bilingual/multilingual
4. He wanted a communication book and to communicate through any means possible
5. He was assertive about his use of alternative means of communication
6. Tony wanted to join a group, to discuss what aphasia meant with others with the same experience
7. Tony could work as a model alternative communicator for other group members and as an explicit commentator on other group members' skills
8. He was prepared to get involved in a discussion, even if it was on the wrong tack
9. He made good use of contextual supports to compensate for difficulties in expressing himself
10. He used non-verbal communication, especially intonation and facial expression, effectively
11. He used writing of single words and short phrases in English and Portuguese to communicate, even if he could not spell them accurately
12. He was aware of his speech difficulties
13. He had a small repertoire of clear gestures
14. He had a reasonably reliable clear nod and shake of his head for conveying yes and no, which could be verified
15. Tony indicated when he thought he had not understood
16. Tony drew arrows to indicate relationships between ideas/ people etc. to clarify communication

B: Barriers

1. Tony's speech was largely absent and what there was, was unintelligible and effortful
2. The words he could write were often hard to interpret because of misspellings or being written in a language his interlocutors didn't speak
3. Tony's wife was very anxious
4. His less specific gestures could sometimes be hard to interpret
5. Questions aimed to clarify could cause confusion
6. Tony was sometimes puzzled by the need to clarify
7. His comprehension sometimes broke down, leading to misunderstanding
8. Written sentence comprehension was more difficult than spoken
9. His enthusiasm for communication and frustration when not understood could overwhelm others
10. His Portuguese/English language switching could cause him distress when he realised it was making it difficult for others to understand him
11. He was sometimes unaware that he had switched between languages
12. His non-aphasic communication partners could get anxious about not understanding him and were worried about over-interpreting/misinterpreting his meaning

Part Two: Cairns: Describing the therapy initially aimed at addressing developing a means of communication with Tony

WHAT: The content of therapy	HOW: The processes of therapy	WHO, WHEN, WHERE, WITH WHAT RESOURCES: The context of therapy
Activity 1: Developing a communication book • Review of other people's communication books • Selection of formats/media for the book • Taking supplementary photographs • Selecting ready-made "communication ramps" • Set goals and deadlines for completing the compilation work on the book *Rationale* Faciitators: A2, A3, A8, A11 Barriers: B1, B2 Checks:	• Discussed Tony's ideas for a new communication book • Discussed formats, styles, size, use of icons to facilitate discussion on certain topics • Discussed how to represent the forms of communication to encourage and how to represent his communication strengths in the book • Identified responsibilities for different parts of the work • Identified the therapeutic rationale for each step of the process • Developed an idea of how Tony wanted to use therapy time for developing the book	• Provided other people's communication books for Tony to look at as examples • Organised opportunities to take photos to put in the book
Activity 2: Using the communication book *Rationale* Facilitators: A2, A3, A6, A7 Barriers: Checks:	• Listened to Tony carefully and reflected on how he wanted to use the book • Changed the therapist's own assumptions about how to use a communication book • Enabled Tony to become clear about how he wanted to use the communication book	

strengths and opportunities that are supporting Tony and the key factors that are causing him difficulty. The therapy described in Part Two of the framework represents only the second "project" carried out with Tony, for reasons of length.

Chapter 3: Gatehouse and Clark

Part One of the framework (Table 15.3) applied to Claire Gatehouse and Liz Clark's therapy summarises the key strengths and opportunities that are supporting WL and the key factors that are causing him difficulty. Parts of both phases of the therapy carried out with WL are included in Part Two of the framework in order to illustrate how the framework can capture any kind of therapy and also to illustrate how the description provided in Part One of the framework also serves as a description to underpin any kind of therapy.

TABLE 15.3

Chapter 3: Gatehouse and Clark's reassembly therapy

Part One: The facilitators and barriers facing WL in his journey for the first year after his stroke

A: Facilitators

1. WL's comprehension in conversation appeared good
2. Could choose between semantic alternatives in spoken and written languages
3. Used his communicative resources extremely well—acting, gesturing, and circumlocuting effectively
4. Able to preserve the broad meaning of phrases in phrase repetition
5. Relatively better written naming than spoken naming
6. Initially supportive partner
7. Monitored accurately whether listeners' guesses were correct
8. Independently mobile in the community due to absence of physical disabilities
9. Workplace colleagues open to involvement in supporting WL
10. Good ability to make lexical decisions
11. Good monitoring own errors

B: Barriers

1. WL had frequent pauses and attempts at repair
2. Fluent spoken language was relatively empty and displayed neologisms
3. Unable to name or be cued to find names
4. Difficulty with repetition
5. Difficulty writing although errors bore some relationship to the target
6. Graphemic and phonological assembly difficulties with phonological assembly being more severely impaired
7. Longer words more difficult to write to dictation or repeat
8. Loss of contact with family and frustration with their apparent lack of interest
9. Facing loss of job, income and career prospects
10. Loss of role as father and authority figure, causing anger and humiliation
11. Loss of social status and peer group and social withdrawal
12. Loss of attractiveness to women
13. Occasional outbursts of anger

14. No local community-based speech and language therapy available

15. Familiar social life communicatively inaccessible—noisy and language based

16. Work was largely communication based

17. Inaccessible communication from service providers explaining lack of services

18. Impenetrable financial benefits systems to work out WL's entitlement to benefits

19. Lack of understanding of aphasia and its impact by family, friends and benefits agencies

20. Difficulties in selecting information relevant to potential advocates

21. Communicatively inaccessible information from information sources

22. Partner, J, bore the brunt of WL's anger and their relationship deteriorated

C: Checks

1. What should the role of the speech and language therapist be in facilitating complaints?

2. Are there potential cultural reasons for differences in reactions to "the system" failing people?

3. Are there other treatment studies of people with similar problems?

4. Are there any theoretical models that might aid hypothesising about the nature of the impairment and help to guide therapy?

Part Two: Describing the therapy aimed at WL's language impairments and social and psychological situation

WHAT: The content of therapy	HOW: The processes of therapy	WHO, WHEN, WHERE, WITH WHAT RESOURCES: The context of therapy
Activity 1: Establish reliable auditory discrimination		
• WL's partner says two words that differ initially or finally • WL identifies whether the difference is at the beginning or end	• Constructed a task that could be given as homework, based on interpretation that listening for auditory differences would facilitate self-correction of errors	• Programme developed to be given as homework involving WL's partner • Provided list of single-syllable real-word pairs differing by one phoneme
Rationale Facilitators: A6, A7, A10 Barriers: B2, B3 Checks:		
Activity 2: Written anagram sorting, memorising of correct form of word, writing word from memory and checking of answer against the target		
• Written words and non-words presented, which were anagrams of the real words • WL makes lexical decision • View correctly ordered words and memorise	• Designed task and developed set of resources for WL to use • Monitored use of task and modified instructions for the task and task requirements • Monitored compliance with task	• Set of words taken from PALPA 39, turned into anagrams and set out on paper to allow covering of correct version • Task designed to be used as homework and for use with student

- Write the correctly ordered word next to the misordered word without copying
- If difficult, multiple check-backs to correct word allowed
- When reordering complete, check back against correct
- 3- then 4- then 5-letter words used

Rationale
Facilitators: A10
Barriers: B2, B3
Checks:

- Decided when to introduce reassessment
- Ensured maximal success in therapy tasks
- Kept tasks as similar as possible to enable WL to "overlearn"

- Identified time for follow-up on outcome of language therapy
- Student speech and language therapist assigned to WL to increase the level of input

Activity 3: Action on lack of services available to WL locally

- Asked other professionals to complain to the healthcare facility on his behalf
- Advised family to complain to Trust, GP, Member of Parliament
- Contacted patient organisation to ask them to complain on WL's behalf
- Patient organisation drew up standard letters of complaint for family
- Contacted professional body for advice
- Wrote a letter with WL outlining his predicament

Rationale
Facilitators:
Barriers: B2. B17, B18, B19
Checks: C1

- Advised family to make complaints to hospital, doctor and local politicians
- Requested support from a not-for-profit campaigning organisation for people with aphasia
- Asked advice from professional body about how to lobby for local resources for WL
- Helped WL write a letter to a range of agencies about his predicament

- Wrote letters and contacted advisory organisations
- Assigned a student to work with WL to provide extra resource
- Referred WL to a specialist agency

Activity 4: Negotiation and investigation around return to work

- Visit to employer
- Identification of components of WL's role
- Development of therapy tasks mimicking WL's role at work

Rationale
Facilitators:
Barriers: B9, B16
Checks:

- Clarification of potential role in assisting WL's return to work with WL's former employer
- Researched the nature of WL's job and identified the tasks WL was still likely to be able to do
- Engaged in simulated tasks with WL

- Visits to WL's employment
- Design of therapy tasks to simulate tasks at work
- Involved staff from WL's place of employment

Activity 5: Supporting WL to be a self-advocate about his aphasia

- Development of accessible training session for all primary care practice staff in WL's workplace
- Development of a video of WL talking about his specific needs
- Opportunity for open discussion with practice staff about how to support WL
- Opportunity for WL to describe his predicament to his colleagues

- Designed a means of WL being able to contribute to the training of staff in his place of employment
- Prepared the training with WL
- Set up training with all types of staff
- With WL, explained the nature of aphasia to these staff
- Facilitated discussion between WL and other staff about ways to reduce barriers for him at work
- Followed up to identify effectiveness of training with one key member of staff

- Identified sessions to prepare the training
- Secured co-operation of employers
- Assembled ready-made training materials to combine with specific information from WL
- Supplied the videos for WL to use with his family

Rationale
Facilitators: A1, A3, A4, A7
Barriers: B19

Activity 6: Promoting a positive identity with aphasia .

- Identified an appropriate counsellor to refer WL to
- Identified potential of a personal portfolio

- Referred WL to a counsellor
- Showed WL sample portfolios
- Began discussion with WL about possibility of developing his own portfolio
- Used judgement about when to give up the idea of trying to implement a portfolio and the conditions that might be more conducive to portfolio development

- Managed referral to counselling
- Assembled sample portfolios for WL to see

Rationale
Facilitators:
Barriers: B10, B11, B12
Checks:

Chapter 4: Debbie Graham

Part One of the framework (Table 15.4) as applied to Debbie Graham's therapy summarises the facilitators that supported KB's therapy and the things that got in the way. Part Two of the framework summarises the three activities that she carried out during the second of her three phases of therapy programme.

Chapter 5: Julie Hickin et al.

Part One of the framework (Table 15.5) applied to Julie Hickin et al.'s therapy summarises the key strengths and opportunities that supported HM and PH, and the key factors that caused them difficulty. Part Two of the framework summarises all of the activities that are described in this therapy study.

TABLE 15.4

Chapter 4: Graham's therapies with KB, a person with mild aphasia

Part One: The facilitators and barriers facing KB in Debbie Graham's phase two therapy: online processing, complex sentences, low frequency verbs

A: Facilitators

1. Highly motivated
2. High expectations of himself
3. Good access to high frequency nouns
4. Good sense of humour
5. Enjoyed conversation
6. Fluent oral reading
7. Less struggle in output than previously
8. Some self-monitoring and self-correction
9. Coping with functional demands of everyday conversation
10. With planning time KB produced some clear sentence structures.

B: Barriers

1. Frustrated and subject to fatigue
2. High expectations of himself—sophisticated use of language a major part of both work and social life
3. Hesitant effortful output
4. Made some sound substitutions, repetitions and false starts, difficulty with polysyllabic words
5. Difficulty finding verbs
6. Word accessing difficulties affecting his planning of sentence structure and ultimately fluency
7. Vulnerable to language breakdown in "on-line processing"—processing overload, fatigue and word-finding difficulties for low frequency words affect his overall fluency
8. Difficulty recognising that ideas could be combined using more sophisticated structures or using connectives

C: Checks

1. Assess types of discourse that would highlight KB's ability to use complex and varied structures
2. Determine KB's ability to cope with the increasing cognitive demands of more complex tasks

Part Two: A description of KB's therapy in phase two of Debbie Graham's therapy study

WHAT: The content of therapy	HOW: The processes of therapy	WHO, WHEN, WHERE, WITH WHAT RESOURCES: The context of therapy
Activity 1: Mapping task for low frequency verbs such as "examine", "incinerate", moving on to verbs that lead to a more complex clause structure: for example "feel", "believe", "perceive", "think"	• Therapist asked KB questions to help determine the number of thematic roles that need to go with each type of verb, e.g., who, what, why, where? • Discussed optional versus obligatory thematic roles • Material used in examples was built into a separate spoken task for KB to do and then to evaluate for himself • This was then developed into another modality for practice outside of the session	• In-patient rehabilitation to facilitate frequent sessions • Tasks developed to facilitate independent practice
Rationale: Facilitators: Barriers: B5, B6, B7 Checks:		
Activity 2: Writing a letter of complaint	• Therapist checking out types of discourse that would reveal planning difficulties and how to make that apparent to KB • Also checking out what actions by KB would facilitate greater control over the task	
Rationale Facilitators: Barriers: Checks: C1, C2		
Activity 3: Developing complex syntactic structures		
Procedural discourse: e.g., "Describe how to sharpen a pencil" Narrative discourse: Story telling centred around events and characters Complex sentences: • combine two given sentences into one by identifying redundant information and using embedding	• Therapists asked KB to compile description as a range of simple syntactic structures temporally and hierarchically related • Therapist gave KB characters and a basic setting to build a story around. He produced stories in written format using a word processor	• Use of word processor for writing tasks facilitated writing and reduced fatigue • Picture-based material enabled therapy to focus on impact of taking different perspectives

- join short sentences using appropriate connectives
- use sequential and composite pictures to generate coordinating or subordinating sentence structures
- formulate a short story from a set of short simple sentences.
- generate a series of short sentences about an activity that happened over the weekend and then link into cohesive narrative text

- Increasing complexity of pictures increased demands on perspective of events in picture

Rationale
Facilitators:
Barriers: B8
Checks:

TABLE 15.5

Chapter 5: Hickin, Herbert, Best, Howard, Osborne. Therapy for word retrieval and conversation

Part One: The factors affecting therapy for HM and PH

A: Facilitators

1. PH has a large and supportive family, with some of whom she has regular contact
2. PH is involved in many activities available at her sheltered accommodation
3. PH is able to read single words aloud
4. HM and PH both have little or no difficulty understanding single words
5. HM and PH are both phonemically cueable
6. HM and PH are both able to concentrate for at least one hour
7. HM and PH are part of a larger research study of therapy
8. HM and PH are both aware of their problems and understood how therapy might help them

B: Barriers

1. HM's marriage has ended since his stroke and he has limited contact with his children—presumably affecting opportunities for communication
2. HM lives alone and goes to a day centre where he is building a model railway—presumably both factors provide little opportunity for communication
3. HM has difficulties reading aloud via both the lexical and non-lexical routes
4. HM and PH make semantic errors in naming
5. PH and HM both have short-term phonological memory problems so long lists of distractors potentially difficult
6. Neither HM nor PH have anyone to support daily use of file in Phase 2

Part Two. Describing the therapy for HM and PH aimed at improving word finding in picture naming, connected speech and conversation

WHAT: The content of therapy	HOW: The processes of therapy	WHO, WHEN, WHERE, WITH WHAT RESOURCES: The context of therapy
Activity 1: Cueing picture naming through providing the word sound or the written word form		
• A hierarchical procedure (see chapter) giving progressive cues of either more of the target word's sound form or the target word's written form • The cues also included distracter items that did not provide the correct cue	• Presented the task and explained how to do it with examples • Made individualised adjustments within the hierarchy to suit individual differences between people	• Developed sets of target and distracter words and pictures to use in the task • Asked HM and PH to select their own words to include • Designed the therapy task and its progressive procedure • One-to-one with a research speech and language therapist
Rationale Facilitators: A1, A2, A3, A4, A5, A6, A8 Barriers: B1, B2, B3, B5, B6 Checks: Determine the 20 personally relevant words Determine what therapy tasks would be interesting for Phase 2 Evaluate client's views of therapy		
Activity 2: Use of target words in everyday speech		
• Naming to definition • Making lists • Reminiscing • Telling anecdotes • Conversations about chosen subjects	• Set up the communication situations to be used • Therapist and client agreed useful topics for file, making lists and for reminiscing etc., in conversation during Phase 2	• Ensured pictures and written name cues for target words were available for use if required • Creation of a file of pictures sorted into conversational categories
Rationale Facilitators: A1, A2, A3, A4 A5, A6. A8 Barriers: B1, B2, B3, B4, B6 Checks: Evaluate client's views of therapy		

Chapter 6: McVicker and Winstanley

Part One of the framework (Table 15.6) applied to Sally McVicker and Leonie Winstanley's therapy summarises the key strengths and opportunities that supported members of the group of people with cognitive communication difficulties with whom they worked, and the key factors that caused them difficulty. Part Two of the framework summarises the three modules that comprised the therapy programme implemented in this therapy study.

Chapter 7: Montagu and Marshall

Part One of the framework (Table 15.7) applied to Ann Montagu and Jane Marshall's therapy summarises the key strengths and opportunities that supported SH and the key factors that caused her difficulty. Part Two of the framework describes all of the activities that are described in this therapy study.

TABLE 15.6

Chapter 6: McVicker and Winstanley's group therapy

Part One: The facilitators and barriers facing the people with acquired brain-injury in a community-based group

A: Facilitators

1. Some members with little or no difficulty following conversational speech

B: Barriers

1. Difficulty coping in the community

2. Poor attention and listening skills for five out of seven group members

3. Some people with considerable comprehension difficulties

4. All had memory difficulties

5. Six out of seven people had expressive language characterised by verbosity and marked problems with planning and maintaining the focus of conversation and occasional disinhibition

6. Three group members had specific difficulties with language, including semantic errors, overuse of non-specific terms and some word-finding difficulties

7. One group member had more marked language difficulties—more word-finding difficulties, slow speech and hesitant, and difficulty with sentence planning

8. All group members profoundly affected by loss of role and lack of confidence, resulting in avoidance and isolation

Part Two: Describing the therapy aimed at addressing long-term life issues associated with brain injury

WHAT: The content of therapy	*HOW: The processes of therapy*	*WHO, WHEN, WHERE, WITH WHAT RESOURCES: The context of therapy*
Activity 1—Module 1—Getting to know one another		
• Non-verbal and verbal tasks	• Maintain balance between verbal and non-verbal tasks	• Group environment in a "Healthy Living Centre", a local recreation centre open for use by the public
• Memory task		
• Descriptive task	• Reinforce value of non-verbal as well as verbal communication	
• Establishing ground rules		

- Completion of grids about pre-morbid and current activities
- Discussion about the negative and positive aspects of living with brain injury
- Brainstorming about issues faced by the group

- Ensure respect across the group for the cultural and social diversity of members
- Manage group dynamics to create foundation for future discussions of difficult topics

Rationale
Facilitators:
Barriers: B1, B4, B8
Checks:

Activity 2: Module 2—Education, information & self-perception of strengths and weaknesses

- Education and information about the concepts of attention and memory
- Completion of self-rating scales
- Peer evaluation
- Implementation of "personal logs"
- Personalised strategy identification   .
- Homework tasks to bring feedback to next session

- Identification of group's own priorities for group therapy with a group like this—how the group wanted to use the time
- Negotiation about goals
- Provided educational and informational content
- Supported group members to identify appropriate strategies for individual group members
- Varied complexity of information to accommodate varying levels of comprehension difficulty across the group
- Encouraged use of strategies outside the group

- Provided handouts to explain attention and memory
- Setting up of video in order to give feedback
- Development of rating scale for use by group

Rationale
Facilitators:
Barriers: B2, B3, B4, B8
Checks:

Activity 3: Module 3—Stress management

- Identification of personal interpretation of stress
- Personal stress awareness exercises
- Stress rating scales
- Discussion of stress-inducing situations
- Problem-solving role-play scenarios

- Facilitated brainstorming session
- Managed group dynamic for discussions about difficult and emotional issues
- Introduced rating scales for personal stress
- Supported the dynamic for group feedback

- Adaptation of published materials on handling stress
- Devised tasks to provoke stress
- Prepared body diagrams to illustrate effects of stress
- Booked a physiotherapist to demonstrate relaxation techniques

- Identifying adaptive strategies
- Undertook illustrative role-playing to model different scenarios
- Identified local community resources available
- Assisted group members to write individual goals for using their own strategies
- Observed and reinforced practice of individual strategies throughout the module
- Supported self-evaluation of achievement of goals

Rationale
Facilitators:
Barriers: B1, B8
Checks: Rating scale assessing personal stress

TABLE 15.7

Chapter 7: Montagu and Marshall's errorless therapy

Part One: Factors about SH that represented strengths or difficulties identified

A: Facilitators

1. SH asserts her independence
2. Her children and grandchildren visit regularly
3. SH has normal hearing
4. In normal conversation she copes with understanding with little or no facilitation
5. She picks up on humour easily
6. She reads single words and short sentences aloud well
7. She can capture the meaning of short newspaper articles
8. She can repeat single words well but has more difficulty with words of three or more syllables
9. She can write her name and copy words and write some short words accurately
10. SH uses finger spelling as a self-cueing medium
11. SH is a very communicative person, using intonation, humour and sarcasm, gesture and facial expression to convey meaning
12. She has intact face recognition
13. She understands proper and common nouns equally well
14. The production of personally familiar names is significantly better than for names that are not personally familiar
15. Phonemic cues help more than semantic cues
16. She provides rich circumlocutions, indicating good semantic knowledge of the target, leading to correct naming on some occasions

17. Place names are slightly easier than famous people's names
18. SH benefits from a high level of success and encouragement
19. SH wanted to work on writing

B: Barriers

1.   She has few opportunities to mix with others
2.   She is depressed and takes medication
3.   She has word-finding difficulties that affect and frustrate her in conversations
4.   She has difficulty with proper names, which causes her particular distress
5.   She is dependent on her communication partner to help repair conversations
6.   She has transport and mobility difficulties
7.   She has difficulty introducing herself or greeting others
8.   She has high level comprehension difficulties at a complex sequential ideational level
9.   She has difficulties with increased auditory load
10. She has more difficulty communicating with more than one person
11. She does not feel confident in reading and says she can't read
12. She makes phonological errors in speech leading to real and non-word substitutions
13. She circumlocutes, is hesitant and groping and uses conduit d'approche in naming
14. She reverses pronouns
15. She make morphemic errors
16. She is not confident about writing and finds it effortful
17. She does not use writing spontaneously in everyday communication
18. She is considerably frustrated by her communication difficulties
19. She walks with great difficulty and uses a wheelchair when she goes out
20. Proper nouns and common nouns are equally difficult

Part Two: Describing the therapy aimed at enabling SH to say proper names for a set of people and places

WHAT: The content of therapy	*HOW: The processes of therapy*	*WHO, WHEN, WHERE, WITH WHAT RESOURCES: The context of therapy*
Activity 1: Naming given a cue		
• Given a picture of a famous person or place • Given the spoken name and the written name simultaneously • Told the initial letter of the person's name • SH repeats the name and copies it • Each week distracter names added to the card with the written name on it	• Organised and presented the items to SH in a carefully controlled sequence • Gave SH the instructions about what she had to do • Ensured that the task, although repetitive, maintained some interest for SH by progressively demanding more from her • Provided feedback and encouragement	• Set up the task in a careful way to include equally items that she could or couldn't name in the pre-therapy assessment, and created a treatment set and a control set • Task devised sensitively in such a way that SH could not make any errors, as the task corresponded exactly to strengths in language skills that SH had shown in pre-therapy assessment

- The distracters were distantly related in meaning, sound or spelling to begin with and then became closer in meaning, sound or spelling
- In those cases SH had to read all the names and pick the right one first
- Finally she had to write the first letter of the word before being given any other cues

Rationale
Facilitators: A8, A15, A18
Barriers: B3, B4
Checks:

- Discussed the nature of the words that were the focus of the therapy, especially those that SH found more difficult
- Allowed conversation about the people whose names SH was learning
- Allowed SH to attempt to self-cue

Activity 2: Naming pictures without cues

- Naming of the same pictures without a cue
- If picture could not be named, SH read aloud her own written version of the name
- SH introduced naming of the word after she had copied it

Rationale
Facilitators: A8, A15, A18

Checks:

- As above
- Also SH to introduce her own modification to the sequence of events in the task as the therapy gradually developed over time

- As above

Activity 3: Homework

- Each week given half of the set of items being worked on
- Picture was accompanied by 4 names—correct, 2 distracters close in meaning, 1 distracter from an unrelated proper name category
- SH had to select the correct name and record her choice on a chart
- Chart set up to allow SH to do the task 5 times during the week

- Task devised that SH could do on her own, at home, using same errorless learning conditions
- Modified the chart that SH was using in the homework at SH's request

- SH started to copy the words as well
- She also introduced finger-writing the name to cue herself

Rationale
Facilitators: A8, A15, A18
Barriers: B3, B4, B6
Checks:

Chapter 8: Perkins and Hinshelwood

Part One of the framework (Table 15.8) applied to Lisa Perkins and Fiona Hinshelwood's therapy summarises the key strengths and opportunities that supported FR, and the key factors that caused him difficulty. Part Two of the framework summarises the therapy programme that was implemented in this therapy study.

Chapter 9: Carole Pound

Part One of the framework (Table 15.9) applied to Carole Pound's therapy summarises the key strengths and opportunities that supported Tony and the key factors that caused him difficulty. For reasons of length, Part Two of the framework describes the activities only in Phase 2 of Tony's therapy—activities that were designed to increase his confidence.

TABLE 15.8

Chapter 8: Perkins and Hinshelwood's therapy to retrieve words in connected speech

Part One: Factors affecting FR's ability to communicate in conversational situations and exercises

A: Facilitators

1. FR had no physical disability

2. FR and his wife had a high level of commitment to work on exercises together at home

3. Prepared to persevere with and work at a therapy task that he did not like initially

4. Confidence grew as he persevered with the therapy, felt a sense of achievement working through the different levels of the therapy

B: Barriers

1. FR's speech was hesitant

2. He had difficulty expressing complex sequences of ideas—he can't explain things to his wife

3. FR had lost his confidence in his ability to communicate and avoided situations where he needed to speak

4. FR relied on his wife to speak for him and she initiated most talk at home

5. Difficulty with naming pictures in both speech and writing, and made semantic errors—hypothesised central semantic impairment

6. Difficulty understanding low imageability words

7. The more complex the argument structure of a verb, the more difficulty FR had with retrieval of nouns and verbs in a sentence

8. Difficulty with processing thematic roles for both speech and understanding of language led to structurally incomplete utterances

9. FR relied on questions from his interlocutor to elicit conversation

10. FR repeated back words and structures from his interlocutor in conversation

11. FR relied on listing lexical items and used a limited range of verbs in conversational speech

12. FR relied on the copula in conversational speech

13. FR relied on phrases with low clausal embedding

14. FR equated the therapy with school work initially, for which he felt he did not have an aptitude

15. FR did not understand why he should be working on input tasks in therapy when his difficulty was with speech

16. Use of metalinguistic task prevented FR from having to produce sentences in therapy, which he found difficult.

Part Two: Describing the therapy aimed at enabling FR to retrieve words in connected speech

WHAT: The content of therapy	HOW: The processes of therapy	WHO, WHEN, WHERE, WITH WHAT RESOURCES: The context of therapy
Activity 1: TRIP programme—developing the underpinning knowledge of language processing for production of thematic roles		
• 13 graded stages	• Introduced each stage	• One-to-one therapy
• Colour-coded cards represent the verb and different thematic roles	• Worked through the practice sentences	• Therapy took place in FR's home
• Verb is introduced in relation to concept of "what is happening?" within a sentence	• Discussed meaning of each role	• Systematic published therapy programme introduced, with pre-prepared materials
• 1-, 2- and 3-argument structures worked through progressively	• Drew attention to the obligatory nature of each role in the sentence	• Wife observed all the therapy sessions and worked with FR between therapy sessions using "the therapist's model"
• Different types of thematic role are introduced	• Identified the locus of the error when a mistake is made and used sentence cues to help FR to correct himself	• 16 hours of direct therapy from the therapist in total
• Each thematic role is assigned 3 explanatory terms—(i) a technical term—the thematic role, (ii) a question and (iii) a question word prompt	• Provided feedback and support	
• Each word type is identified in a written target sentence, by placing underneath it the card with the relevant technical term on it	• Introduced evaluation set at the appropriate time	
• Two sets of sentences for each stage	• Determined when FR ready to move to next stage on basis of evaluation	
• When accuracy is consistent across the two sets, an evaluation set is introduced		

- Practice sets are repeated until target level of accuracy on evaluation set is reached and move to next stage can take place

Rationale
Facilitators: A2, A3
Barriers: B4, B5, B7, B8
Checks: Evaluation for when can move on to next stage

TABLE 15.9

Chapter 9: Carole Pound's therapy for life

Part One: The facilitators and barriers facing Tony at the point the second therapy began, 3 years after his stroke

A: Facilitators

1. Sociable, cheerful and friendly
2. Supportive mother and sister, keen to assist
3. Highly motivated to work on his impairments and change his ability to use and understand words
4. Very mild weakness and altered sensation on his right side
5. Hearing and vision unimpaired
6. Good non-verbal problem solving and reasoning, orientation and memory
7. Insight into the presence and impact of his language difficulties
8. Made full use of his social speech and non-verbal skills
9. Used effective strategies to conceal the severity of his difficulties with receptive and expressive language
10. Able to follow simple, everyday conversation in context
11. Relatively well-preserved single word meaning, more so with written than spoken language
12. Comprehension facilitated by repetition, slower presentation, lip reading and context
13. Repeated attempts led to closer phonological approximation to the word
14. More access to orthographic than phonological knowledge
15. Therapy focusing on self-cueing and self-monitoring resulted in some ability to use a self-cueing strategy in conversations and some increase in fluency, increased understanding of his comprehension difficulties and use of listening strategies

B: Barriers

1. High degree of anxiety, embarrassment and bewilderment about the extent and nature of his communication disability
2. Unwilling to involve his relatives in therapy, discussions or facilitating him in any way
3. Very mild weakness and altered sensation on his right side—profoundly affecting ability to resume sporting interests
4. Required frequent repetitions and clarification to understand any conversation which lacked context or some form of visual support

5. Fast communication, background noise, fatigue or anxiety increased comprehension difficulties

6. Impaired comprehension of written language

7. Severe word-finding difficulties—conversations beyond social exchanges tended to be empty and lacking content

8. Rarely attempted extended conversation

9. Unable to self-correct despite sub-vocal rehearsal to try to avoid phonological errors, which caused acute embarrassment

10. Therapy for cueing strategies and self-monitoring strategies increased Tony's panic and lack of confidence

11. Loss of friends, interests, work and a growing sense of isolation

12. Feels likes a loser, a boring man, loss of personal pride

Part Two: Describing the therapy aimed at enabling Tony to develop confidence in living with and accommodating his aphasia, and identifying life and work skills, with options for returning to work

WHAT: The content of therapy	*HOW: The processes of therapy*	*WHO, WHEN, WHERE, WITH WHAT RESOURCES: The context of therapy*
Activity 1: Group challenging negative self-images • Generating a vocabulary for describing personal characteristics through identifying qualities in other people • Completing self- and peer-ratings on given and group-generated personality traits • Recording list of own qualities and reflecting on mismatches with peer observations	• Facilitated group dynamic to enable discussion about personal issues and discussions that contained elements of personal challenge	• Set up group therapy context with members wanting to address similar issues • Development of communication support materials e.g., pictures of celebrities to prompt discussion of personality traits • Accessing personality trait questionnaires to use as examples
Rationale Facilitators: A1, A5, A6, A7, A8, A9 Barriers: B1, B10 Checks: Explored personality traits using questionnaires		

Activity 2: Compiling a CV and developing interviewing skills
 • Reviewing Tony's life history
 • Creating a written record of all Tony's strengths and skills
	• Discussed one-to-one with Tony to enable him to:
	   – identify explicit work strengths and skills and less obvious skills and strengths
	   – link past and present skills
	   – identify new skills and experiences
		• Set up one-to-one sessions
		 • Set up role plays
		 • Set up mock interview

- Elaborated on Tony's identified personal strengths
- Monitored and discussed Tony's emotional response to activities
- Identified and fed back concrete examples of abstract issues

Rationale
Facilitators: A1, A5, A6, A7, A8, A9
Barriers: B1, B10
Checks: Worked with clients to identify own skills and strengths

---

Activity 3: Confidence hierarchies

- Group brainstorm to identify communicatively difficult or easy situations
- Rating situations or people on communicative ease or difficulty
- Using specific examples from these situations to tell the complete story of these experiences
- Brainstorming strategies for dealing with situations or people
- Role play of different situations using a prepared script or cue card
- Review progress towards achieving goal plans

- Established and managed group dynamic to be able to raise challenging issues
- Facilitated group dynamic to enable all members to participate
- Identified experiences that could act as a springboard for all group members to promote key issues
- Gave feedback/reflected with the group on what happened in role-play situations
- Shaped and extended role-play situations
- Broke down large goals into achievable steps
- Facilitated identifying the achievement of steps towards achieving goals
- Supported perception of therapy as a journey carried out in partnership with others

- Set up group therapy context
- Developed communication support materials for role plays (scripts, cue cards)
- Developed visual analogue scales
- Developed assignments for dealing with communicatively difficult situations/people outside the therapy context
- Used questionnaires to rate self-perceptions of confidence

Rationale
Facilitators: A1, A5, A6, A7, A8,
Barriers: B2, B8, B10
Checks: Clients rated situations and own confidence and progress

---

Activity 4: Assertiveness skills

- Group discussion about assertiveness
- Role play
- Observation of role play

- Established and managed group dynamic to be able to experiment with their communication styles

- Identified resources for activities
- Set up group therapy context

- Opportunity to experiment with new communication styles
- Identifying barriers created by others
- Developing a video about living and coping with aphasia—participating on equal terms and feeling OK about yourself
- Preparing for a visit
- Assisting in training volunteers and students to be better conversation partners
- Talking to non-aphasic people about the nature of stroke and aphasia

- Supported group members in giving each other feedback
- Identified internal and external barriers
- Challenged assumptions about their aphasia
- Prepared group members to deal with visitors

- Identified opportunities in the centre for Tony to participate as a volunteer rather than a recipient of services

Rationale
Facilitators: A1, A5, A6, A7, A8, A9
Barriers: B1, B2, B8, B10
Checks:

Activity 5: Establishing life goals

- Setting goals which reflected getting engaged with life rather than working on trying to "fix" specific aspects of language
- Sharing responsibility for finding ways to solve problems and find ways of moving on

- Therapist engaged in careful listening
- Therapist engaged in negotiation
- Therapist avoided tendency to fall back on concrete, tangible solutions to Tony's quest for recovery
- Worked on assertive bargaining
- Worked on asking questions
- Balanced respect for Tony's insider experience and expertise and Carole's experience and expertise as a provider of therapy services

- Set up one-to-one sessions with an experienced therapist
- Careful reflection by therapist about appropriateness of challenging Tony's assumptions about recovery

Rationale
Facilitators: A6, A7, A8
Barriers: A3, B1
Checks:

Chapter 10: Robson and Horton

Part One of the framework (Table 15.10) applied to Jo Robson and Simon Horton's therapy study summarises the key strengths and opportunities that supported the group of people with aphasia with whom they worked, and the key factors that caused them difficulty. Part Two of the framework summarises the two main stages of the therapy programme that was implemented in this therapy study.

TABLE 15.10

Chapter 10: Robson and Horton on replicating therapy for people with jargon aphasia

Part One: The facilitators and barriers facing the people with jargon aphasia in a group therapy study

A: Facilitators

1. All clients had some evidence of ability to access covert written word knowledge, either being able to sort anagrams of picture names or carry out delayed copying, i.e., they can access some orthographic information without written production

2. Comprehension skills were sufficient to be able to participate in formal assessment and therapy

3. Clients who were offered the second stage of therapy also had a carer available to support therapy and had maintained gains made in the first stage of therapy

B: Barriers

1. All clients had speech that was made unintelligible by the presence of non-words

2. All clients had difficulty with written picture naming

C: Checks—e.g., what else do I need to find out about/think about/explore?

1. Could the second stage of therapy successfully facilitate the transfer of skills for functional use?

Part Two: Describing the therapy aimed at enabling the establishment of a vocabulary of written words that could be used in everyday situations for people with jargon aphasia

WHAT: The content of therapy	*HOW: The processes of therapy*	*WHO, WHEN, WHERE, WITH WHAT RESOURCES: The context of therapy*
Activity 1: Picture Naming Therapy		
Specific tasks selected according to needs and abilities of each participant but could be any of the following: Decide tasks • written word to picture matching (with semantic distracters) • associated word to picture matching • categorisation judgements • odd-one-out judgements • generating semantic information about the target • matching pictures to their first letters • identifying initial letters from an alphabet chart	• Selected and implemented tasks flexibly from the menu of potential tasks according to the individual's needs and abilities	• Developed a personal vocabulary of 40 items for each person with aphasia • Developed pre- and post-therapy assessment tasks using the selected vocabulary • Created a "decide and produce" format as a basis for all the therapy tasks to be consistent with the underpinning *processing goal* of therapy: this involved maintaining a consistent format of accessing stored semantic and orthographic information about the target prior to priming or supporting its production

- categorising words according to length

Produce tasks
- writing the first letter of the word
- insert missing letters into the target word form
- complete anagrams
- delayed copying
- cued written naming
- uncued written picture naming

Rationale
Facilitators: A1, A2, A3
Barriers: B1, B2
Checks: Pre- and post-assessment tasks

- Developed therapy tasks using each individual's personal vocabulary

Activity 2: Message therapy

Decide tasks
- select a target word from a choice of semantically related words to match to a word, phase or message (or more than one of these) related to the target word
- select a picture from a choice of semantically related pictures to match to a word, phase or message (or more than one of these) related to the target word

Produce tasks
- delayed copying of the target name
- writing the name of the picture
- writing the target name from memory

Rationale
Facilitators: A1, A2, A3
Barriers: B1, B2
Checks: C1

- Selected and implemented tasks flexibly from the menu of potential tasks according to the individual's needs and abilities

- Created a "decide and produce" format as a basis for all the therapy tasks to be consistent with the underpinning *processing goal* of therapy: this involved maintaining a consistent format of accessing stored semantic and orthographic information about the target prior to priming or supporting its production

Chapter 11: Sacchett and Lindsay

Part One of the framework (Table 15.11) applied to Carol Sacchett and Jayne Lindsay's therapy summarises the key strengths and opportunities that are supporting FM and the key factors that are causing him difficulty. The therapy described in Part Two of the framework represents the tasks used to develop a communication book with FM and his wife, and was selected in order to facilitate comparison with the therapy described by Deborah Cairns in Table 15.2.

TABLE 15.11

Chapter 11: Sacchett and Lindsay's drawing and communication book for a person with severe aphasia

Part One: The facilitators and barriers facing FM in communicating with people around him

A: Facilitators

1. Keen to interact with people around him
2. Musician with international career prior to stroke
3. Keen football supporter
4. Understood pictured information reliably
5. Could point to pictured items on request
6. Able to indicate preferences
7. Able to select from a semantically grouped array
8. Able to read some single words for meaning
9. Uses an electric wheelchair independently
10. Minimal impairment of word meaning for highly imageable single words
11. Could use wife's name reliably
12. Able to follow simple conversation
13. Appropriate use of facial expression
14. Able to copy simple drawings
15. Drawing produced by FM moderately recognisable in context
16. After first part of therapy, FM using strategies in the use of drawing as a means of communication such as allowing the interlocutor time, listening to and responding to questions and providing additional information by modifying the drawing or gesturing
17. After therapy, FM's wife uses more interpretation strategies for FM's drawings
18. After therapy, FM using drawing spontaneously and successfully in real-life conversations
19. After therapy, able to separate a complex situation into a number of single events and to convey these in a "cartoon-strip" format

B: Barriers

1. Frustrated when people unable to understand his non-verbal communication
2. FM's wife sceptical about the usefulness of a communication book, because of experience of previous, unsuccessful non-verbal communication aids
3. Dense right hemiplegia and reduced sensation in his right arm—unable to use his arm or hand functionally
4. Apraxia in left arm
5. Spoken and written naming abilities severely restricted: output restricted mainly to string of unintelligible phonemes
6. Writing restricted to occasional first letters of words
7. Restricted ability to gesture, which improved to some extent after therapy

Part Two: Describing the therapy aimed at enabling FM to develop a communication book

WHAT: The content of therapy	HOW: The processes of therapy	WHO, WHEN, WHERE, WITH WHAT RESOURCES: The context of therapy
Activity 1: Negotiating the therapeutic relationship • Emphasis on FM setting his own goals for therapy in collaboration with AM, to share responsibility for change • Pictographs of the therapy "menu" on offer provided • Development of "ownership" of decisions about contents for the communication book • Development of "ownership" of the production of items for the communication book *Rationale* Facilitators: A1, A4, A5, A6, A10 Barriers: B2 Checks: Identified barriers	• Use of total communication (drawing, writing single words in "on-line" discussion) to: ⇒ facilitate FM's comprehension ⇒ confirm her interpretation of FM's meaning ⇒ summarise decisions reached • Identified the barriers to FM's developing the items himself to go in the book • Supported the student therapist to be flexible around alternative methods of achieving the goals of developing and selecting content and layout	• Prepared pictograph menu of therapy activities available for FM to choose from
Activity 2: Developing the content and layout of the communication book • Discussion of relevant sections and topics for the communication book • Discussion of relevant, personalised information to include • Discussion about format for representation of information (pictures and words) • Discussion about nature of the pictures—FM's drawings or clipart *Rationale* Facilitators: A1, A4, A5, A6, A10 Barriers: B1, B5, B6, B7 Checks:	• Negotiated and sometimes challenged FM's selection for his communication book • Continued attention to uncovering items and categories that were relevant and desirable for FM • Negotiated with AM around the addition of items • Developed communication support mechanisms to enable FM to engage in the process of selection and negotiation	• Assembled models of other people's communication books • Assembled materials to provide for FM's selection

Activity 3: Refining the content of
the communication book

- Increasing the specification of
  previously generic items
- Increasing the range of
  information within categories
  to provide more relevant
  options
- Addition of new resources (e.g.,
  maps and photographs to
  enable sharing of personal
  information)
- Addition of "category
  headings" and specific content
  within those category headings
  to speed up process of accessing
  content within topics specific
  to FM's career
- Addition of pages to tell whole
  "stories" from FM's past

Rationale
Facilitators: A1, A4, A5, A6, A10
Barriers: B1, B5, B6, B7
Checks: Therapist shifted idea about use of book

- Therapist shifted idea of use of
  the book as a means of
  transmitting information to a
  means of increasing social
  affiliation
- Therapist developed sensitivity
  about appropriate
  communication support
  mechanisms to enable FM to
  be engaged in the process of
  selection and negotiation

- Assembled materials to provide
  for FM's selection

Chapter 12: Sam Simpson

Part One of the framework (Table 15.12) applied
to Sam Simpson's therapy summarises the key
strengths and opportunities that are supporting
Carlos and the key factors that are causing him
difficulty. The therapy is described in Part Two of
the framework. Sam Simpson's chapter describes
two phases of therapy, but for reasons of length
Part Two of the framework describes only the
first phase.

TABLE 15.12

Chapter 12: Simpson's longitudinal study of life-based therapies

Part One: The facilitators and barriers Carlos faced at the point of the first intervention

A: Facilitators

1. Carlos's family (and friends) are very supportive

2. Carlos's family have a very strong ethos of "effort always brings success" and "positive thinking"

3. His university course has been held open for a year

4. Carlos found previous speech therapy helpful for revealing the extent of his difficulties and therefore his need for help

5. Wide variety of social interests prior to stroke

B: Barriers

1. Carlos feels stigmatised by his current state, feels like a weirdo, has a negative perception of himself and lacks confidence
2. Carlos feels his life is on hold
3. Carlos finds the hidden nature of his aphasia difficult to manage
4. Carlos's family have a very strong ethos of "effort always brings success" and "positive thinking"
5. Carlos can't play golf, drive his car, can't speak Spanish
6. Carlos finds that he gets angry and cries a lot
7. Carlos feels that work on his impairment is like going back to school, relates therapists to teachers and therefore gives the "teacher" the responsibility for telling him what to do and evaluating him
8. Carlos has perceptual difficulties
9. Carlos's friends and family are all moving on and achieving
10. Carlos has a reduced social network now and avoids conversations
11. Carlos has word-finding difficulties
12. Carlos has difficulty with reading and writing
13. Carlos has some difficulty with understanding
14. Carlos has some agrammatism

C: Checks—e.g., what else do I need to find out about / think about / explore?

1. Carlos's capacity to enter into a partnership in therapy, taking responsibility for his part in setting goals and evaluating his progress

---

Part Two: Describing the therapy aimed at addressing Carlos's avoidance tendencies

WHAT: The content of therapy	HOW: The processes of therapy	WHO, WHEN, WHERE, WITH WHAT RESOURCES: The context of therapy
Activity 1: Go for the word • Attempt all "difficult" words	• Supported Carlos to identify and attempt difficult words • Mediated between Carlos and his family to interpret what Carlos was trying to do • Explained how they could support him	• Initially one-to-one session with therapist, then joint sessions with Carlos and his family and close friends
Rationale Facilitators: A1, A4; Barriers: B1, B4, B11; Checks: C1		

Activity 2: What can I do when I get stuck for a word?

• Use a range of strategies for word finding	• Provided information about a range of compensatory strategies to assist word finding • Identified strategies acceptable to Carlos • Encouraged Carlos to develop problem-solving ability to find most useful strategy to use in a conversation	• Provided information materials to use in the therapy

Rationale
Facilitators: A4;
Barriers: B11;
Checks: C1

Activity 3: Video analysis

• Analyse own communication on video	• Facilitated Carlos's ability to identify his own communication and word-finding strategies • Enabled Carlos to identify communication strengths	• Included video as a therapy tool

Rationale
Facilitators:
Barriers: B11, B1
Checks: C1

Activity 4: Impairment work

• Research vocabulary for selected conversation partners	• Listened to Carlos's priorities • Identified a task Carlos can engage in to meet his priorities	• Provided sources for vocabulary search

Rationale
Facilitators:
Barriers: B10, B11
Checks:

Activity 5: Exploring feelings

• Active discussion of feelings about communication disability	• Listened to Carlos talking about his feelings and responding appropriately • Encouraged Carlos to use a range of methods of expressing his feelings	• Checked alternative opportunities available for Carlos's expression of feelings, e.g., counselling

Rationale
Facilitators:
Barriers: B1, B2, B4
Checks:

Activity 6: PCP approaches

• Use of "self-characterisation"	• Enabled Carlos to engage in self-characterisation through providing the concept and a way to do it • Set up method of charting changes in self-characterisations over time	• Regular use of the activity to enable Carlos to chart change over time

Rationale
Facilitators:
Barriers: B1, B2, B6
Checks:

Activity 7: Joint sessions

• Joint forum for discussion with Carlos and his parents	• Facilitated an exchange of perceptions between Carlos and his parents • Enabled discussion of strategies to support open expression of feelings within the family • Clarified possible reasons for mood swings	• Invited parents in for joint sessions

Rationale
Facilitators: A1, A2
Barriers: B1, B4, B6
Checks:

Activity 8: Conversation group

• Discussion of issues about living with a communication disability	• Created the conditions within the group for discussion of personal issues • Supported communication within the group to enable people to get their message out and understood	• Set up group of people with mixed aetiology of acquired communication disability

Rationale
Facilitators:
Barriers: B1, B3
Checks:

Activity 9: Referral to a support group for young people with aphasia

• Onward referral to another agency	• Considered constraints Carlos was experiencing within existing opportunities • Discussed possible referral with Carlos and implications for him • Made contact with new agency • Organised referral	• Identified an appropriate opportunity for Carlos in another agency

Rationale
Facilitators:
Barriers: B1, B3
Checks:

Activity 10: Increasing speaking opportunities

• Increase the range of communication situations Carlos takes part in	• Identified the need for Carlos to develop confidence in a range of communication situations • Facilitated Carlos to identify and set up potential communication situations • Discussed the demands of those situations • Debriefed after each assignment to review the experience	• Created some of the opportunities for Carlos to take part in

Rationale
Facilitators:
Barriers: B10, B11
Checks:

Activity 11: Exploration of fears about speaking out

• Facing the worst communication situations • Facing the worst things that could happen in those situations	• Discussed the likely situations • Challenged Carlos's perception of the probability of these situations arising • Developed with Carlos strategies to use in difficult situations • Enabled Carlos to identify the strategies to use for himself • Engaged in role playing the situations	• Prepared worksheets for Carlos to use to support him thinking through these situations

Rationale
Facilitators:
Barriers: B1, B3, B10
Checks:

Activity 12: Independent assignments

• Undertake the most difficult communication-related activities	• Focused Carlos on identifying difficult situations and setting them up • Prepared him to undertake them • Debriefed after the assignments	• Awareness of Carlos's life and lifestyle to see likely potential situations and their impact on Carlos

- Provided background support and confidence for Carlos to be able to consider undertaking them

Rationale
Facilitators: A1;
Barriers: B10
Checks:

Chapter 13: Alex Stirling

Part One of the framework (Table 15.13) applied to Alex Stirling's therapy summarises the key strengths and opportunities that supported B and the key factors that caused his difficulty. Part Two of the framework describes the range of activities and tasks carried out in the first part of B's therapy.

Chapter 14: Webster and Whitworth

Part One of the framework (Table 15.14) applied to Janet Webster and Anne Whitworth's therapy summarises the key strengths and opportunities that supported AL, and the key factors that caused him difficulty. Part Two of the framework summarises the therapy programme that was implemented in this therapy study.

TABLE 15.13

Chapter 13: Stirling's case study with a client with "high level" problems

Part One: The facilitators and barriers facing B in recovering from surgery for epilepsy, which affected his language and his self-perception

A: Facilitators

1. Friendly, humorous, sociable person with wide circle of friends and interests

2. Excellent communication skills

3. Successful young composer, passionate about music, engaged in postgraduate study

4. No apparent difficulties in processing sentences

B: Barriers

1. Mild word-finding difficulties, slowness in retrieving words apparently resulting from high level semantic problems

2. Mildly evident difficulties organising his thoughts to translate into verbal output

3. Anxiety and lack of confidence about his communication

4. High level of awareness of his right-sided hemiparesis

5. Experienced marginalisation as a disabled person by other people, causing him to lose confidence and feel self-conscious

6. Anger about the consequences of his surgery for epilepsy and wanting to assign blame for the outcome

7. Idealisation of his past (pre-operative) life

8. Felt his speech to be different post-operatively and therefore avoided certain situations or people, assuming they would find him different too

9. Felt an "impostor" in conversation

10. Less structured and less predictable situations particularly problematic

Part Two: Describing the therapy aimed at enabling B to cope with the changes to his language and communication post-operatively

WHAT: The content of therapy	*HOW: The processes of therapy*	*WHO, WHEN, WHERE, WITH WHAT RESOURCES: The context of therapy*
Activity 1: Working through tasks required during a typical week of B's work • Summarising part of an academic article • Identifying the key idea in a short passage with one key idea • Identifying the key idea in a short passage with one key idea plus other sub-points • Noting down in writing the sub-points • Using written sub-points and key idea to plan and organise spoken summary • Explaining concisely technical terms and concepts to naïve audience [*] * • Preparing a short presentation from textbook material *Rationale* Facilitators: A2, A3, A4 Barriers: B2, B3, Checks:	• Interpreted B's difficulties in completing a piece of work and devised an alternative task to address the difficulty that had arisen • Acted as a naïve audience	• One-to-one therapy in an in-patient rehabilitation unit • Preparation of articles controlled for complexity of number of ideas expressed
Activity 2: Study skills to prepare a presentation • Brainstorming on paper the key points of a talk • Organising the key points into a logical structure • Using the index, chapter headings and chapter subdivisions to identify relevant information • Taking brief notes as he read • Generating and identifying his own strategies • Deciding the relative importance of the key points and estimating timing for different parts of the talk	• Enabled B to identify and use strategies he generated himself rather than those imposed by the therapist, since these seemed more successful	• Identified and planned the appropriate sequence of tasks

- Practising the talk using the outline
- Practising use of the Internet and email

Rationale
Facilitators: A2, A3, A4
Barriers: B2, B3, B10
Checks:

Activity 3: Communicating in personally challenging situations

- Speaking to a stranger face to face
- Negotiating with a stranger on the phone
- Seeing a friend whom he had not seen since his surgery
- Phoning a friend as above
- Phoning a colleague
- Giving a presentation

- Direct discussion about B's difficulties
- Explored his beliefs about himself and the attitudes of others
- Confronted B with his contradictory responses
- Encouraged B to confront situations he found difficult
- Modified methods employed, e.g., abandoned role play
- Refused to collude in apportioning blame to other members of the rehabilitation team for the extent of B's physical disabilities

- Identified and planned the appropriate sequence of tasks
- Sought advice from a clinical psychologist

Rationale
Facilitators: A1, A2, A3, A4
Barriers: B1, B2, B3, B4, B5, B6, B8, B9, B10
Checks:

TABLE 15.14

Chapter 14: Webster and Whitworth's therapy on the predicate argument structure

Part One: The facilitators and barriers facing AL in understanding and producing sentences

A: Facilitators

1. Good functional comprehension

2. Verbal communication supplemented by pointing, gesture and intonational change

3. Able to convey the main events of a story (suggesting message level of representation intact)

4. Capable of producing elaborated phrasal structure

5. Good retrieval of nouns

6. Verb comprehension relatively intact

B: Barriers

1. Limited ability to communicate affected AL's participation in conversation

2. In spontaneous speech, abandoned, incomplete sentences—single phrases or strings of phrases without a verb

3. Deficit in the production of thematic structure at the functional level of representation

4. Impaired thematic structure impacted his ability to convey information

5. Verb retrieval deficit, slow retrieval with the production of semantically related verbs and nouns

6. Difficulty accessing predicate argument structure information and using it to create a sentence frame, resulting in a high percentage of utterances with an undetermined thematic structure, the omission of obligatory arguments, difficulty with three-argument structures and difficulty identifying incorrect predicate argument structures

7. Impaired thematic role assignment/mapping resulting in reverse role errors in production and difficulty with passive sentences in both spoken and written comprehension

Part Two: Describing the therapy aimed at enabling AL to improve access to predicate argument structure information

WHAT: The content of therapy	HOW: The processes of therapy	WHO, WHEN, WHERE, WITH WHAT RESOURCES: The context of therapy

Activity 1: Explicit identification of thematic roles in a wide variety of one-, two- and three-argument structures
 	
• Thematic roles given labels and associated with specific "wh" questions and cue words
• Progression of sentence types
• Colour codes included to introduce each sentence type
• Matching of thematic role labels, "wh" questions and cue words to verb arguments within sentences
• "Wh" questions and cue words given by therapist
• AL generates cue words
• AL identifies correct thematic role label without cue
• If assignment incorrect, task repeated with cue words from the therapist and an explicit comparison between correct and incorrect assignment made
• When assignment correct feedback provided
	• Therapist ensured systematic flow of task through the predetermined sequence of activities
	• Therapist's action was contingent on correct or incorrect response by AL
	• Discussion during the task focused on
	  – the optional or obligatory nature of the arguments in that sentence or other sentences, following correct assignment of the thematic roles
	  – semantic selection restrictions of the verb
		• Items illustrating critical issues were prepared and used in therapy sessions and for home assignments

- Arguments in sentences covered over for AL to judge whether sentence still correct (i.e. whether arguments were obligatory or not)
- AL asked to generate alternative lexical items to fulfil specific thematic roles
- Exercises to complete at home set and checked in subsequent session
- Task extended to include sentences with same verb but different types of argument and also to include passive sentences

Rationale
Facilitators: A5, A6
Barriers: B3, B4, B5, B6, B7
Checks:

SUMMARY OF DATA FROM THE TABLES GENERATED FROM THE THERAPY DESCRIPTION FRAMEWORK

The tables summarising each of the chapters offer a thumbnail sketch of the therapies described in this book. They also offer opportunities for comparing the therapies with one another and for reflecting on the content and processes that the therapists are using. Below are some observations and reflections associated with each component of the framework, the factors, activities and rationale.

The facilitators and barriers
We found that the facilitators and barriers highlighted by the authors of the chapters in this volume revealed interesting differences in their descriptions. First, there were differences in the detail that authors gave on their clients, with some providing lengthy descriptions and others short ones. The total factors used ranged from 39 by Montagu and Marshall to 5 by Robson and Horton.

There was also a difference among authors in this book in the relative emphasis they gave to facilitators vs. barriers. Some emphasise facilitators (e.g. Sacchett and Lindsay in Chapter 11 with 19 facilitators and 7 barriers), others emphasize barriers (e.g. McVicker and Winstanley in Chapter 6 with 1 facilitator and 8 barriers), and still others emphasised both (e.g. Montagu and Marshall in Chapter 7 with 19 facilitators and 20 barriers).

While these differences are tantalising, and point to different ways of thinking about what sorts of things bear on therapy decisions made by different therapists, we do not yet know how to interpret them. For example, some of the differences might be an artefact of writing vs. talking about therapy—perhaps therapists choose different issues to bring to the fore when they write. One might, for example, want to say that therapists differ in whether they focus on competencies or deficits in their clients. But facilitators and barriers are not the same as competencies and deficits. For one thing, they are not always about the client: some are about the situation, some about the spouse.

Also of concern when classifying factors into facilitators or barriers was that the same factor could be a facilitator in one activity and a barrier in another. For example, a factor that would logically be classified as a facilitator, such as a client's clarity on a therapy goal, could be a barrier for therapy that does not progress toward that goal. Evidence for the role of context in classifying factors is found when the same factors appear in the list of facilitators as well as barriers.

The section of the framework having to do with personal factors (Part One), felt a bit stretched when applied to therapies for groups such as those described in Chapter 5 by Hickin et al., Chapter 6 by McVicker and Winstanley and Chapter 10 by Robson and Horton. How does one go about reporting the characteristics of a group in group therapy? Do you describe those characteristics that are common to all members of the group—the ones that lead to the selection of the activities? Or do you describe the differences among group members to show how the activities allow for individual differences? Authors in this book did both.

The activities

The wide variety of activities are displayed in Part Two of the tables above. Further examination of those entries points to the differences in focus for different activities. For some activities, the focus was on involving users in their own decision making. Table 15.15 is a listing of what many of these authors did to obtain user involvement.

For other activities, listed in Table 15.16, the focus was on skill building, with a particular emphasis on skills that would serve to improve word-finding difficulties and linguistic problems.

The checks

Part One of the framework provides a category called "checks", where descriptions of therapists' "wonderings" can be placed. This section would be the one to use when carrying out investigative therapies to see what works, or diagnostic therapies to find out more about factors that bear on the

therapy enterprise. There are relatively few entries in this category of checks. Why aren't they more plentiful?

We suggest that these reports, as is likely for most reports written at the end of a period of therapy intervention, are not ones of therapy exploration, but rather are ones of therapy efficacy. In these descriptions, the authors were reporting on therapy done, not wondering about what might have been done.

The rationales

Many of the factors used in the descriptions by the authors did not bear directly on the choices of therapy. That is, they were not used to develop a rationale. This would suggest that the information is provided by authors in this book not only to justify their therapies but also to develop a picture of their client and their situation, as one would for a narrative.

The factors in Part One that served to provide a rationale for therapy did so in different ways. Some were tightly related to the therapy; others were more distantly related. For purposes of illustration, we classify the degrees of relationship ranging from tight to distant as level 1, 2 and 3 rationales.

Level 1 rationales, the ones whose Part One factors and Part Two therapy were most closely related, were exemplified by those in which the activity was designed to remediate a factor listed as a barrier. This type of tightly reasoned rationale is typical of those falling within a "symptom-focused" strategy, where a problem is regarded as a symptom that is then either eliminated or minimised. For example, Montagu and Marshall describe the word-finding difficulties of their client (Table 15.7, B3), which serves as a direct rationale for their cueing therapy (activity 1), and Robson and Horton's clients with jargon aphasia inserted non-words in their speech (Table 15.10, B1), which led to picture naming therapies (activity 1). This level 1 rationale could also be manifest as a facilitating factor, such as when a client identifies a goal and the therapy is designed to achieve that goal. This was illustrated in a rationale underlying Cairns' work on a communication book with Tony (Table 15.2, A4).

TABLE 15.15

Elements of activities emphasising user involvement

Location of activity description	*User involvement elements in the activity*
Chapter 2: Cairns Activity 2: Using the communication book	Listened to Tony carefully, reflecting on how he wanted to use the book. Challenged therapist's own assumptions about how to use the book and enabled Tony to clarify his own ideas.
Chapter 3: Gatehouse & Clark Activity 5: Supporting LW to be a self-advocate about his aphasia	Prepared the training with LW. With LW, explained the nature of aphasia to these staff. Facilitated discussion between LW and other staff about ways to reduce barriers for him at work.
Chapter 6: McVicker & Winstanley Activity 2: Education, information and self-perception of strengths and weaknesses	Identification of group's own priorities for group therapy—how the group wanted to use the time. Negotiation about goals. Supported group members to identify appropriate strategies for individual group members.
Chapter 6: McVicker & Winstanley Activity 3: Stress management	Facilitated brainstorming session. Assisted group members to write individual goals for using their own strategies.
Chapter 7: Montagu & Marshall Activity 3: Naming pictures without cues	Task devised that SH could do on her own, at home, using same errorless learning conditions. Modified the chart that SH was using in the homework at SH's request.
Chapter 9: Pound Activity 1: Group challenging negative self-images	Completing self- and peer ratings on given and group-generated personality traits. Facilitated group dynamic to enable discussion about personal issues and discussions that contained elements of personal challenge.
Chapter 9: Pound Activity 3: Confidence hierarchies	Group brainstorm to identify communicatively difficult or easy situations. Brainstorming strategies for dealing with situations or people. Established and managed group dynamic to be able to raise challenging issues. Facilitated group dynamic to enable all members to participate.
Chapter 11: Sacchett & Lindsay Activity 1: Negotiating the therapeutic relationship	Emphasis on FM setting his own goals for therapy in collaboration with AM, to share responsibility for change Pictographs of the therapy "menu" on offer provided for making therapy choices. Development of "ownership" of decisions about contents for the communication book. Development of "ownership" of the production of items for the communication book.
Chapter 11: Sacchett & Lindsay Activity 2: Developing the content and layout of the communication book	Negotiated FM's selection for his communication book. Developed communication support mechanisms to enable FM to engage in the process of selection and negotiation.

Chapter 12: Simpson Activity 3: Video analysis	Facilitated Carlos's ability to identify his own communication and word-finding strategies. Enabled CR to identify communication strengths.
Chapter 12: Simpson Activity 4: Impairment work	Listened to Carlos's priorities.
Chapter 12: Simpson Activity 5: Exploring feelings	Listened to Carlos talking about his feelings and responding appropriately.
Chapter 12: Simpson Activity 6: PCP approaches	Enabled Carlos to engage in self-characterisation through providing the concept and a way to do it. Set up method of charting changes in self-characterisations over time. Regular use of the activity to enable Carlos to chart change over time.
Chapter 12: Simpson Activity 7: Joint sessions	Facilitated an exchange of perceptions between Carlos and his parents. Enabled discussion of strategies to support open expression of feelings within the family.
Chapter 12: Simpson Activity 8: Conversation group	Created the conditions within the group for discussion of personal issues. Supported communication within the group to enable people to get their message out and understood.
Chapter 12: Simpson Activity 10: Increasing speaking opportunities	Facilitated Carlos to identify and set up potential communication situations.
Chapter 12: Simpson Activity 11: Exploration of fears about speaking out	Developed with Carlos strategies to use in difficult situations. Enabled Carlos to identify the strategies to use for himself.
Chapter 12: Simpson Activity 12: Independent assignments	Focused Carlos on identifying difficult situations and setting them up.
Chapter 13: Stirling Activity 2: Study skills to prepare a presentation	Brainstorming on paper the key points of a talk. Generating and identifying his own strategies Enabled B to identify and use strategies he generated himself rather than those imposed by the therapist, since these seemed more successful.
Chapter 13: Stirling Activity 3: Communicating in personally challenging situations	Explored his beliefs about himself and the attitudes of others. Encouraged B to confront situations he found difficult.

A level 2 rationale was one where factors in Part One were less closely related to the activity in Part Two. For example, a barrier such as abandoning sentences (Webster and Whitworth, Table 15.14, B2) was dealt with by using activities that focused on something else, such as therapy involving the teaching of thematic roles (activity 1). Level 2 examples also occurred for facilitating factors, such as when the presence of a supportive partner provided a rationale for assigning

TABLE 15.16	
Activities that focus on clients' skills and knowledge	
The skill / knowledge focused on	*Where the specific activity is described in this chapter*
Thematic roles	Table 15.8, Activity 1
	Table 15.14, Activity 1
Auditory discrimination	Table 15.3, Activity 1
Sound blending/ anagrams	Table 15.3, Activity 2
Verbs	Table 15.4, Activity 1
Complex sentences	Table 15.4, Activity 3
Naming	Table 15.5, Activity 1
	Table 15.7, Activity 1
	Table 15.10, Activities 1 & 2
Word-finding strategies	Table 15.12, Activities 1, 2, 3 & 4
Study skills	Table 15.13, Activity 2

homework with that partner (e.g. Gatehouse and Clark, Table 15.3, A6).

Level 3 rationales were ones that were based on a general or more abstract relationship between factors and activities. For example, Graham described KB as being highly motivated and subject to fatigue, both factors that were likely to affect KB's performance on any of the therapy tasks (Table 15.4, A1) and therefore influenced the design of the therapy tasks.

The framework's ability to uncover underlying conceptual models

We developed our framework with the hope that by displaying and analysing the descriptions of this book's authors, we might be able to uncover their beliefs. We are persuaded that the rationales, which were devised from finding factors in the descriptions that justify a choice of activities, are indeed a way into the thinking of the therapists who wrote these chapters.

We are not persuaded, however, that these rationales offer a way to uncover all of the beliefs about therapy held by our therapists. Among the beliefs that remain hidden in our data are those that derive from overarching models that have received attention of late—the social and medical models. We do not know, from the descriptions in this book, where the authors stand on the principles of these more philosophical underpinnings of therapy. For example, when examining facilitators and barriers, we cannot see whether the therapists subscribe to the principles of a social model, such as the ones listed in Table 15.17. This is because it is perfectly possible to undertake any kind of therapy activity using either a social model or a medical model philosophy—the philosophy does not determine the type of therapy conducted (see Byng & Duchan, 2005)

Besides not being able to determine an overall model from their descriptions, we are not able to see in their writings other justifications for therapy choices. For example, a therapist might offer a client a therapy because it fared well in evidence-based research studies. Or a therapist might favour certain therapies that they are familiar with or that a supervisor has asked them to try. In some cases, therapy decisions may be based on the preferences of an institution or the availability of materials. Understandably, these factors did not get talked about in the reports. Nonetheless, therapists who are dealing with the practicalities of their situations need to consider such influences. Neither did the authors discuss what ideas for therapy they had rejected, for example, why developing a communication book

TABLE 15.17
Princiiples associated with the social model of therapy practice (from Byng & Duchan, 2005)
1. Equalising the social relations of service delivery
2. Creating authentic involvement
3. Creating engaging experiences
4. Establishing user control
5. Becoming accountable users

was chosen rather than a word-finding therapy, or vice versa.

It would be helpful for therapists to explore other reasons that motivate their therapy choices. They might ask themselves questions about why they do what they do in order to be maximally self-aware of whether they are making the best choices. For example, they might ask whether their choices are designed to:

- keep within time constraints
- make use of limited resources
- satisfy a senior colleague
- conform to a research goal
- fit within a research paradigm
- conform to the demands of presentation to colleagues
- raise the profile of a department in a hospital
- fit with a perception of what therapy "should" be
- fit with the therapist's perception of the priorities of the client.

In summary, this instrument on describing therapy frameworks has served its purpose—to allow us to display an overview of the very different types of therapies of authors in this volume. It has also allowed us to infer rationales, or some of the thinking that went into therapy decision making and has revealed how authors approach an issue that someone with aphasia is facing. But it is not a vehicle for examining the philosophical beliefs of our authors, such as those are associated with social and medical models.

In these chapters the therapists described what they did after their therapies were over. This post-facto use of the framework helped us see the thinking that went into the preceding therapies and in so doing to compare the therapies and their descriptions with one another. So, for example, Cairns (Table 15.2) and Sacchett and Lindsay (Table 15.11) both wrote about their work with clients to develop a communication book. Their descriptions contain many similarities: both were working with severely disabled clients; both used more facilitators to justify their rationales than barriers; both emphasized negotiation with clients as a therapy method for designing communication books. Where they differ is in

their emphases. Cairns focuses on the function of the book (Activity 2) and discovers that her client was using the book differently from the way that she had anticipated. Sacchett and Lindsay focus their description more on the content and process of development of the book than its function.

Needless to say, the framework did not reveal all that goes into making therapy decisions. A view of those other important aspects of therapy rationales will have to wait for another book, or set of conference papers, or research projects in which the therapists are asked to reflect more philosophically on their own practices.

Other uses for the framework

In the above versions of the therapy framework, we, the editors, have taken the authors of the chapters' therapy descriptions and applied the framework to them. Our stance toward their writing is one of a naïve reader, who is not privy to the thoughts of the authors in this book. It is analysing what is going on from the outside.

It is our hope that the framework could also be of use to therapists who want to summarise and regularise their therapy descriptions for themselves or for others. This could help them illustrate the factors that have influenced their own thinking about their clients and their choice of therapies. It would work by analysing what is going on from the inside. (For an illustrative example of how this might work see Bunning's case examples explicating an earlier version of this framework: Bunning, 2004, pp. 93–104).

We would expect that, had the authors of these therapy chapters filled out their own framework forms, they would have come up with different factors and rationales from ours. This points to the fact that this sort of reflective thinking about therapies will differ depending upon the logical reasoning of the person doing the reflection. We do not see the aim of the framework as revealing a pristine, objective logic for therapies, but rather to uncover the sort of *personal logic* that goes into therapy decision making. We take this sensitivity to points of view as a positive characteristic of the framework, since its aim is to reveal the thinking that goes into decision making about therapy.

The framework entries will also differ depending upon when it is applied. In this study it was applied after the therapies were over. But it also has the potential for use when planning therapies. If it is filled out by the therapist prior to therapy, it could serve as a way to explain to clients how and why certain therapies were chosen. For example, the therapist could point to certain personal and situational factors that would call for certain therapies. It could also serve as a vehicle for therapists and their clients to talk about the various activity options available and to negotiate goals.

A less technical version of the framework could be filled out by the therapist and a client or group of clients together, prior to therapy. This would allow both parties to identify facilitators and barriers, and to create together a list of priorities and associated activities. Through these discussions, the rationales for different therapies could be formed. The framework could provide a way to assure that therapists' and clients' collaboration is seen as relevant and realistic.

Questions raised by the framework about how we write about people to whom we provide therapy

As is suggested in the last section, our hopes for the therapy description framework go beyond its use in this book. We would like it, or others like it, to be used to create reports of therapy that are more comparable and explicit, and that would lead to more opportunities for reflection. In this vein we call on you, our readers, to ask yourselves what the last therapy session that you engaged in would look like if examined in a framework such as ours, and what you might learn by reflecting on how you go about making therapy decisions. Here are a few questions that are raised by a framework such as the one we used to analyse this book's chapters.

When reporting on your therapies:

- Did you indicate factors that facilitate therapy? Do you need to?
- Did you describe barriers? When doing so, did you talk about barriers outside the person, such as ones that are due to context or

interlocutors? Should you have? Why?
- When describing your activities did you talk about how the activities were done and in what contexts?
- Which of the barriers and facilitators served as a rationale for designing your activities?
- Which facilitators and barriers did not apply to your decisions, and why?
- Did you describe how the person with aphasia was involved in determining the development of the therapy? Could you have done more to involve him or her? Would this have been a good idea?
- What outside influences affected your choices of factors to include in your description and your choices of therapy activities? For example, did you consider evidence-based research, ease of tracking data and evaluating progress, methods promoted by a mentor or your place of work?

But these questions do not uncover the full story. They only allow for reflections on therapies that have already been chosen. What still needs to be asked is where these therapies come from. What, for example are the values that led to their selection? (For more on the importance of values underpinning therapies see Byng, Cairns, & Duchan, 2002; Worrall, 2000.) What are the underlying philosophical frameworks and associated principles upon which the therapy is grounded (Byng & Duchan, 2005), and how can we make these explicit?

We feel that this book, like the one preceding it, is different from what is usually allowable in the literature on speech and language therapies. Many of the chapters, because they describe how therapists think, have more self-reflection than would be found in other therapy research reports. We invite people to continue along these lines, creating opportunities for discussing therapy collaboratively—examining not just what they did, but also why they did it. Such an examination would naturally lead to their uncovering what are perhaps the most important factors influencing their work as therapists—their underpinning values and philosophies.

REFERENCES

Bunning, K. (2004). *Speech and language therapy intervention: Frameworks and processes*. London: Whurr.

Byng, S., Cairns, D., & Duchan, J. (2002). Values in practice and practising values. *Journal of Communication Disorders, 35*, 89–106.

Byng, S., & Duchan, J. (2005). Social model philosophies and principles: Their applications to therapies for aphasia. *Aphasiology, 19*, 906–922.

Duchan, J. (2001). Impairment and social views of speech-language pathology: Clinical practices re-examined. *Advances in Speech-Language Pathology, 3*, 37–45.

Duchan, J. (2004). *Frame work in language and literacy: How theory informs practice*. New York: Guilford Press.

Petheram, B., & Parr, S. (1998). Diversity in aphasiology: Crisis or increasing competence? *Aphasiology, 12*, 468–473.

Weniger, D., & Taylor Sarno, M. (1990). The future of aphasia therapy: More than just new wine in old bottles? *Aphasiology, 4*, 301–306.

Worrall, L. (2000). The influence of professional values on the functional communication approach in aphasia. In L. Worrall & C. Frattali (Eds.), *Neurogenic communication disorders: A functional approach* (pp. 191–205). New York: Thieme.

Author Index

Subject Index